Evaluation of Health Promotion Health Education and Disease Prevention Programs

Second Edition

Evaluation of Health Promotion Health Education and Disease Prevention Programs

Second Edition

RICHARD WINDSOR
Birmingham, Alabama

TOM BARANOWSKI
Emory University
School of Public Health

NOREEN CLARK
University of Michigan
School of Public Health

GARY CUTTER
Pythagoras, Inc.

 Mayfield Publishing Company
Mountain View, California
London • Toronto

Library of Congress Cataloging-in-Publication Data
Evaluation of health promotion, health education, and
disease prevention programs / Richard A. Windsor . . .
[et al.]. — 2nd ed.
    p.   cm.
    Includes bibliographical references and index.
    ISBN 1-55934-243-9
    1. Health education—Evaluation.   2. Preventive
    health services—Evaluation.   3. Educational
    accountability.   I. Windsor, Richard A.
    RA440.5.E93   1994
    613—dc20   93-23540
                                                    CIP

Manufactured in the United States of America
10 9 8 7 6 5 4 3 2 1

Mayfield Publishing Company
1280 Villa Street
Mountain View, California 94041

Sponsoring editor, Erin Mulligan; *production management,*
Rogue Valley Publications; *manuscript editor,* Betty Duncan;
illustrators, John and Judy Waller; *cover designer,* Joan
Greenfield. This text was set in 10/12 Palatino by G&S
Typesetters and printed on 50# text white opaque by
Maple-Vail Book Manufacturing Group.

Contents

Chapter 6: Measurement Issues in Data Collection   197

Chapter 9: Cost Analyses   359

Appendix A: The Evaluation Report   391

Preface

This book presents a comprehensive discussion of the technical skills that staff of health promotion and education programs must have to evaluate their programs. It has been prepared for multiple audiences: (1) senior undergraduates and graduate students specializing in health education and health promotion and the social and behavioral sciences; (2) public health, nursing, and medical students enrolled in health promotion and education program evaluation courses; and (3) practitioners, health educators, nurses, epidemiologists, physicians, nutritionists, and allied health professionals who plan, implement, and evaluate health education, health promotion, and disease prevention programs.

Better documentation and assessment of program impact process and content will be needed as technology increases and budgets decrease, and as society and agencies expect reasonable returns for resources and effort invested. Public health programs will be expected to demonstrate effectiveness, and program planners will be held more and more accountable for their efforts, particularly in a period of finite and often diminishing resources. The expanding literature base for practitioners, policymakers, funders, and program planners of more rigorous evaluations of community health promotion/disease prevention programs provided the impetus for this text.

We used three documents as guiding sources for the content of this book: (1) *Promoting Health/Preventing Disease: Objectives for the*

Nation 1900–2000, by the U.S. Department of Health and Human Services; Public Health Service (1980 and 1990), which presents measurable objectives in twenty-two areas of particular salience to community health promotion programs for the year 2000; (2) "Guidelines for the Preparation and Practice of Professional Health Educators," developed by the Society for Public Health Education (1977); and (3) the role-specification section for evaluation of the *Initial Role Delineation for Health Education: Final Report,* prepared for the National Center for Health Education under contract with the U.S. Department of Health and Human Services (1980), reprinted as Appendix B of this book.

A dramatic improvement in the qualitative, quantitative, and analytic skills of practitioners in health promotion and education program evaluation occurred in the 1980s. Expectations of increased skill and sophistication in program evaluation is the norm in the 1990s. Those who lack technical competence will not reflect the state of the art in their practice and will not be as competitive in the marketplace. Through analysis of individual program experiences, evaluators will expand the knowledge base in the field; by sharing concepts, such as those discussed in this text, through the professional literature, they can improve the practice of health education and promotion. This may, in turn, improve an individual's or organization's ability to affect policies and resource allocations related to health promotion and disease prevention.

This book fills a clear gap in the literature on evaluation of health promotion, health education, and disease prevention programs. It is, however, primarily a synthesis and dissemination document for use in health promotion and education training programs and for application by public health practitioners. Health education specialists who develop the technical skills to plan, implement, and evaluate programs in multiple settings and to collaborate with other health professionals will achieve greater professional success, will enhance the profession, and will play a more significant role in achieving the health objectives of the United States in the years 2000–2010.

Chapter 1, "An Introduction to Evaluation," sets the stage by discussing the evaluation movement, particularly over the last two decades. The salience and examples of content of the Healthy People Objectives for the nation (1990 and 2000) and other important documents (e.g., *Clinical Preventive Services*) are presented. A common set of evaluation terms and a description of four interrelated levels of evaluation are introduced. The purposes and expectations of program evaluation are considered. Particular attention is given to encouraging program planners to set more realistic program objectives and to appreciate the role of politics in planning and evaluation. The philosophical and ideological orientations of program directors and planners and their impact on what an evaluator can accomplish are discussed. The realization that every program evaluation cannot and should not be conducted as a clinical trial (experimental study with randomized treatment and control groups) is stressed. Both qualitative and quantitative evaluation methods are important to improve the efficacy and effectiveness of health education and promotion programs.

Chapter 2, "Conducting Evaluations and Promoting Organizational Change," presents how to approach an evaluation as a staff member within an organization. Emphasis is given to identifying (1) the purposes of the evaluation, (2) the organizational structure and principal decision makers, (3) how major program decisions are made, (4) the role staff members see the evaluator playing, (5) what is necessary to encourage decision makers to promote and accept change in an organization, (6) who the evaluator's model audiences are, and (7) what behavior changes are possible within the organization and by the social group for whom the program is planned.

Chapter 3, "Program Planning and Planning for Evaluation," presents basic principles and steps of program planning as they relate to evaluation. Of concern here and in the real world is the question, Can the staff of this organization implement a program and evaluate it? The "staff" may consist of only one person, for example. The steps used to develop a work plan are identified, and methods, with examples, to create a plan are described.

Chapter 4, "Conducting Qualitative-Process Evaluations," identifies a number of procedures used to conduct a quality assurance review of a program. Periodic audits and expert panel reviews of the procedures used to implement a program must be performed. We examine in detail how to plan and conduct a formative assessment of program content, methods, materials, and media, using qualitative and quantitative approaches. Specific methods and case studies on how to conduct a process evaluation, readability assessment, and content analysis are presented.

Chapter 5, "Evaluating Program Effectiveness, " presents (1) the importance of selecting a strong evaluation design and (2) how to select an appropriate one. Getting the most out of what is available—which is usually more than program staff thinks is possible—is a theme of this chapter. Emphasis is placed on examining problems and constraints of the real world but also on the basic theoretical issue of causation. The concepts of internal and external validity, selection of a control or comparison group, and how to make a decision about sample size and statistical power are examined. Methods to adapt the scientific method to practice settings are explored. We suggest ways to organize a community program to control for common problems that may confound results. Complex concepts and procedures are distilled into basic and practical elements for use in meeting day-to-day program issues. Insight on dimensions and issues of design often unfamiliar to the practitioner but directly applicable to all practice settings is provided. Four case studies illustrate applications of all principles and methods presented.

Chapter 6 "Measurement Issues in Data Collection," deals with multiple, common problem areas faced in program planning and implementation: determining what data to collect and how to collect them. Special attention is given to how to select and develop an instrument or questionnaire and the importance of identifying existing instruments and data-collection methods from similar programs. Types of validity and reliability are discussed. Specifying what data are to be collected, collecting high-quality data, and employing sound methods of data collection are the core concepts emphasized in this chapter.

Chapter 7, "Data-Collection Methods," presents the various methods and identifies the strengths and weaknesses (biases) of each. Consideration is given to other issues in method selection. Several practical steps to develop an instrument and implementing a data-collection method are outlined. The various methods are considered in two broad categories: obtrusive and unobtrusive data collection.

Chapter 8, "Simple Methods to Analyze Program Data," presents commonly used statistical techniques to analyze data. The techniques and skills presented represent those within the capabilities of a graduate-trained person. Although individuals involved in large-scale evaluation research or clinical trial studies usually employ a variety of complex analytic techniques, most programs are faced with two or three basic questions requiring less statistical sophistication. The determination of program impact, however, requires a comprehension of statistical tests and the ability to apply analytic techniques to interpret data. The issue of program importance versus statistical significance is addressed in this chapter.

Chapter 9, "Cost Analyses," presents a basic primer on the different types of cost analyses. It identifies the steps that must be used to perform cost-effective and cost–benefit studies. Three case studies provide current examples of the application of the principles and steps presented in this chapter.

Appendix A, "The Evaluation Report," presents the basic purpose and elements of an evaluation report. Report writers need to determine in advance who should receive the report and learn the explicit expectations of key personnel (e.g., policymakers, administrators, and contract officers) before preparing interim and final reports. It is wise to reach agreement beforehand on the format, length, and depth of the report and its subsections.

Appendix B, "Specification of the Role of the Entry-Level Health Educator, U.S. Public Health Service," describes the minimum functions, skills, and knowledge (credentials) necessary to evaluate health education and promotion programs.

Acknowledgments

A special note of appreciation is extended to our colleagues, who served as reviewers for this edition, for their helpful suggestions and insights: Catherine Crooks, Middle Tennessee State University; Richard Petosa, The Ohio State University; and Yuzuru J. Takeshita, University of Michigan.

Richard Windsor
Tom Baranowski
Noreen Clark
Gary Cutter

Authors

Richard Windsor received his BS with honors (1969) in Health Education at Morgan State College and an MS (1970) and PhD (1972) in health education from the University of Illinois. He was an assistant professor, College of Education, at Ohio State University from 1972 to 1975. He received a post-doctoral fellowship and an MPH in maternal and child health, School of Hygiene and Public Health, Johns Hopkins University (1975–1976), and was an assistant professor, School of Hygiene and Public Health at Johns Hopkins (1976–1977). He was professor of Public Health and chair of the Department of Health Behavior, School of Public Health, University of Alabama at Birmingham (UAB) from 1977 to 1991. He was senior scientist (1978–1991) and associate director for the cancer prevention and control of the Comprehensive Cancer Center of Alabama at the UAB Medical Center (1987–1991). From 1991–1993, he was associate director for Prevention, Education, and Control of the National Heart, Lung and Blood Institute—NIH—U.S. Public Health Service. He has been the principal investigator or co-principal investigator of six randomized clinical trials funded by the National Institutes of Health (NIH) and NCHSR to test the efficacy and cost-effectiveness of public health education methods. He has been an advisor to the NICHD, NCI, NHLBI, IOM, CDC, Robert Wood Johnson Foundation, and to WHO, Ministries of Health of Canada, Ireland, Scotland, Singapore, and the People's Republic of China.

Tom Baranowski, PhD, is professor of health behavior and director of the Division of Behavioral Sciences and Health Education at Emory University School of Public Health in Atlanta. Tom received an AB in politics from Princeton University (1968) and an MA (1970) and PhD (1974) in social psychology from the University of Kansas. Tom's research has emphasized children's health-related behaviors within the context of the school and the family. He is currently principal investigator for two school nutrition education projects among elementary school children. He has consulted with several national health organizations and with the World Health Organization. He has over 80 publications, most concerning issues of measurement and evaluation.

Noreen Clark is professor and chair of health behavior and health education at the University of Michigan School of Public Health. Her research specialty is self-management of chronic disease, and she has conducted many large-scale evaluations of health education and promotion programs. Dr. Clark has served as president of the Society for Public Health Education and as chair of the Public Health Education Section of the American Public Health Association. She has been chair of the Behavioral Science Section of the American Thoracic Society, a member of the Pulmonary Diseases Advisory Committee for the National Heart, Lung and Blood Institute and a member of the institute's Advisory Committee on Prevention, Education, and Control. She is a member of the Coordinating Council of the National Asthma Education Program. Dr. Clark is a member of the board of directors of the American Lung Association (ALA) and chairs the ALA Technical Advisory Group on Asthma. She is the editor of the *Health Education Quarterly,* the preeminent scholarly journal in the field of health education. She is the recipient of the Distinguished Fellow Award, the highest honor bestowed by the Society for Public Health Education; the Derryberry Award for outstanding contribution to health education in behavioral science given by the American Public Health Association; the Health Education Research Award conferred by the National Asthma Education Program for leadership and research contributions in health education.

Dr. Clark's work in asthma self-management has made a significant contribution to the research literature and the field of practice by demonstrating that educational interventions can decrease hospitalizations and medical emergencies among low-income families. Her work with colleagues at Columbia University has resulted in model educational programs being distributed nationally by the National Institutes of Health and ALA. She is working with colleagues at the University of Michigan to develop and test model programs for self-management of the heart diseases by older individuals.

Gary Cutter received his Bachelor's degree in mathematics in 1970 from the University of Missouri, Columbia, his Master's degree in Biometry from the University of Texas School of Public Health in 1971 and his Ph.D. in Biometry from the University of Texas School of Public Health in 1974. He was Assistant Professor of Biometry from 1974–1978 at the University of Texas School of Public Health. He spent a year as a consultant to the National Cancer Institute's Division of Cancer Control in 1978–1979 and was Associate and full Professor at the University of Alabama School of Public Health in Birmingham, Alabama. From 1989–1991 he was Chairman of Biostatistics and Information Systems at St. Jude Children's Research Hospital. Currently, he is President of Pythagoras, Inc., a scientific research organization in Birmingham. Dr. Cutter has directed several coordinating centers for multicenter clinical trials and epidemiological studies. He has served on numerous NIH advisory committees including the Behavioral Medicine Study Section and the Clinical Trials Review Committee. He has been a reviewer for a variety of journals and served on the editorial board of Controlled Clinical Trials. His research interests include clinical trials and community studies, behavioral amd chronic disease epidemiology, and the logistics and design of research studies and large scale data bases.

1

An Introduction to Evaluation

"We know what health education programs to offer. The big question is, How do we evaluate them?"

"It was difficult to develop conclusions because the program kept changing as we were trying to evaluate it."

"The exciting part was to see our projections of effectiveness confirmed by the data, both statistically and in the comments of the people surveyed."

"It was rewarding to show our board that our program worked. Knowing about designs really helped."

This book explains the theories, principles, methods, and procedures to plan and evaluate health promotion and education programs. In this chapter, we present and examine the following:

The health objectives for the 1990s and year 2000 and the evaluation literature of the 1970s and 1980s.

Evaluation terminology—for example, *program evaluation*, a generic term used throughout the text, refers to the many different types and methods of evaluation used to conduct a comprehensive assessment of process, content, impact, and outcomes.

Four types of evaluation: process evaluation, formative evaluation, impact evaluation, and evaluation research; evaluation skills essential for a master's-trained public health professional.

Purposes of program evaluation, the role of evaluation in organizations, the importance of setting realistic objectives and developing feasible program plans, and the uses of program evaluation reports.

Professional competencies in evaluation of health education and health promotion programs.

Useful planning and evaluation references.

HEALTH OBJECTIVES FOR THE NATION: 1980–2000

In *Healthy People: The Surgeon General's Report of Health Promotion and Disease Prevention* (1979b), the surgeon general's goals (evaluation targets) were based on expert assessment of historical trends combined with an estimate of the extent to which interventions would accelerate potential gains. In 1976 the U.S. Department of Health, Education and Welfare established the Office of Disease Prevention and Health Promotion (ODP-HP) to coordinate health promotion/disease prevention initiatives in the Public Health Service. A multitude of health promotion and education programs in schools, communities, work sites, clinics, and other health care settings were implemented throughout the country to achieve these goals. This report, the first federal document to describe objectives in priority areas to improve the health of the nation, listed five national public health goals, classified by life stage, for 1990 (Table 1.1).

HEALTH OBJECTIVES FOR THE NATION: 1990

When the U.S. Department of Health and Human Services (DHHS) published *Promoting Health/Preventing Disease: Objectives for the Nation*

Table 1.1   Surgeon General's Goals for 1990

Life Stage	1990 Goal	Special Problems
Infants	35% fewer deaths* (less than 9/ 1000 births)	Low birth-weight infants Birth defects
Children (ages 1–14)	20% fewer deaths* (less than 34/ 100,000)	Growth and development Accidents and injuries
Adolescents and young adults (ages 15–24)	20% fewer deaths* (less than 93/ 100,000)	Fatal motor vehicle accidents Alcohol and drug misuse
Adults (ages 25–64)	25% fewer deaths* (less than 400/ 100,000)	Heart attacks and strokes Cancer
Older adults (ages 65+)	20% fewer days restricted* (less than 30/ year)	Influenza and pneumonia Ability to function independently

SOURCE: U.S. Department of Health, Education and Welfare (1979b).
*Relative to 1977

(1980c), 227 measurable objectives were specified in 15 health priority areas grouped into three major program areas—Preventive Health Services, Health Protection Services, and Health Promotion Services (Table 1.2). The objectives for each priority area represent, from an evaluation perspective, a macro (national) statement about the importance of establishing baseline data for each objective and monitoring data and trends over a 10-year period. With the establishment of an informational tracking system (ITS) in 1984, the ODP-HP was able to fulfill a key monitoring and evaluation responsibility. The ITS is an electronic data file that documents the status of measurable objectives. It provides annual information from all DHHS lead and collaborating federal agencies about individual national objectives.

Data related to achievement of health promotion/disease prevention objectives for each priority area are very useful for planning and evaluating health promotion programs. These data should be considered as one of several primary information sources in setting objectives in which several health outcomes are possible. These objectives include

Health status
Risk factors

Table 1.2   1990 Health Objectives for the Nation
Fifteen Priority Areas

Preventive Health Services
1. High blood pressure control
2. Family planning
3. Pregnancy and infant health
4. Immunization
5. Sexually transmitted diseases

Health Protection Services
6. Toxic agent control
7. Occupational safety and health
8. Accident prevention and injury control
9. Fluoridation and dental health
10. Surveillance and control of infectious diseases

Health Promotion Services
11. Smoking and health
12. Misuse of alcohol and drugs
13. Nutrition
14. Physical fitness and exercise
15. Control of stress and violent behavior

SOURCE: U.S. Department of Health and Human Services (1980).

Public and professional awareness

Utilization of appropriate clinical and/or screening services

Knowledge, beliefs, or skills

HEALTH OBJECTIVES FOR THE NATION:
1990—*A MID-COURSE REVIEW*

In 1986 the DHHS published *A Mid-Course Review*—data documenting the mid-decade status of the 1990 objectives and projections for
their accomplishment. It was anticipated in 1985 that 108 (48%) of the
objectives were likely to be met by 1990. It is worth noting that of the
226 objectives specified, 58 (26%) were written without baseline data.
Thus, the true number of measurable, achievable objectives was 168,
not 226.

HEALTH OBJECTIVES FOR THE NATION: *HEALTHY PEOPLE 2000*

Because of the success in achieving many of the 1990 objectives, a
new set of health promotion/disease prevention objectives was prepared. Between January and March, 1988 in Birmingham, Los Angeles, Houston, Seattle, Denver, Detroit, and New York, over 1000
people participated in 2-day regional hearings to provide input into
the revision of a draft "Year 2000 Health Objectives." This multiset-

Table 1.3   *Healthy People 2000:* Twenty-Two Priority Areas

Health Promotion
 1. Physical activity—injuries
 2. Nutrition
 3. Tobacco
 4. Alcohol and other drugs
 5. Family planning
 6. Mental health and mental disorders
 7. Violent and abusive behavior
 8. Educational and community-based programs

Health Protection
 9. Unintentional injuries
10. Occupational safety
11. Environmental
12. Food and drug safety
13. Oral health

Preventive Services
14. Maternal and infant health
15. Heart disease and stroke
16. Cancer
17. Diabetes and chronic disabling conditions
18. HIV infection
19. Sexually transmitted diseases
20. Immunization and infectious diseases
21. Clinical preventive services
22. Surveillance and data systems

SOURCE: U.S. Department of Health and Human Services (1990b).

ting was critical to ensure that the objectives specified have scientific validity and program feasibility. The U.S. Public Health Service (PHS) and the Institute of Medicine also convened the "Year 2000 Health Objectives Consortium" of more than 300 national professional voluntary organizations and state and territorial health departments to help guide the process. These organizations held special hearings and submitted written and oral testimony. A total of 800 people and organizations submitted testimony, with 318 testifying at the regional hearings. On September 6–7, 1990, the Secretary of Health and Human Services, Dr. Louis Sullivan, presented to the nation *Healthy People 2000: National Health Promotion and Disease Prevention Objectives* (1990b).

Table 1.3 provides a topical outline of the 22 priority areas identified in *Healthy People 2000,* and Table 1.4 lists some examples of the objectives for several age groups. As in *Promoting Health/Preventing Disease* and the *Mid-Course Review,* priority areas were grouped into three major categories: Health Promotion, Health Protection, and Preventive Services. A new category of special importance to program evaluation was established: surveillance and data systems. The existence of annual ongoing data-collection and reporting systems

Table 1.4   *Healthy People 2000:* Examples of Objectives

Type	Objective
Health Status	To reduce coronary heart disease deaths to no more than 100/100,000 people (age-adjusted baseline: 135/100,000 in 1987)
	To reduce deaths caused by alcohol-related motor vehicle crashes to no more than 8.5/100,000 (9.7/100,000 in 1987)
Risk Reduction	To reduce the initiation of cigarette smoking by children and youth so that no more than 15% of them become regular smokers by the age of 20 (30% of youth have become regular smokers by age 20–24 in 1987)
	To increase by at least 1 year the average age of first use of cigarettes, alcohol, and marijuana by adolescents, ages 12–17 (age 11.6 for cigarettes, age 13.1 for alcohol, and age 13.4 for marijuana in 1988)
Service and Protection	To establish tobacco-free environments and include tobacco-use prevention in the curriculum of all elementary, middle, and secondary schools as part of school health education (17% of school districts totally banned smoking in school premises in 1988); antismoking education was provided by 78% of the school districts at the high school level, 81% at middle, and 75% at elementary school
	To increase to 50 states that have enacted and enforced policies beyond those in existence in 1989 to reduce access to all alcoholic beverages by adolescents

SOURCE: U.S. Department of Health and Human Services (1990b).

through ODP-HP in the Office of the Assistant Secretary for Health is critical for monitoring national progress in achieving objectives. It and other similar systems can be developed at the state and country level.

THE EVALUATION MOVEMENT: THE 1960s AND 1970s

Evaluation of health promotion and education programs in the 1960s and 1970s paralleled a national interest in evaluation of public health, medical care, education, and social services programs. In the 1960s, Rosenstock (1960), Hochbaum (1962, 1965), Campbell and Stanley (1966), Suchman (1967), Deniston and Rosenstock (1968a, 1968b), and Campbell (1969) stressed the need to improve both the quality and the quantity of evaluation research. The close relationship between program planning and program evaluation and the salience of conducting educational assessment as part of the planning and evaluation process received consistent emphasis. The health promotion/disease prevention literature, however, reported almost no examples of rigorous, empirical evaluation studies. A concern often expressed was that the health education and health promotion professions relied on evaluations that measured effort and resource use—that is, structure and process evaluations. Evaluations of behavioral impact were seldom reported, and observed changes, attributable to program inputs, if documented, were often equivocal.

In the 1960s and 1970s, the gap between scientific theory and professional practice was another issue frequently expressed in social and behavioral science research and program evaluation literature. Rigorous quantitative methods, well described in evaluation research methods texts, were typically not employed.

Qualitative methods began to receive attention in the late 1970s. The problems of adapting the range of social and behavioral science methods to evaluations of public health programs and the influence of individual and organizational values on evaluation were as apparent in the past as they are today (Baric, 1980; Campbell, 1969; Mullen and Iverson, 1980; Windsor et al., 1980).

The *Report of the President's Committee on Health Education* (Larry, 1973) noted the paucity of evaluation literature in health education and health promotion and the need to document effectiveness and efficiency of programs in a variety of settings: schools, hospitals, community health clinics, and industries. The report from the Task Force on Consumer Health Education, *Promoting Health: Consumer Education and National Policy* (Somers, 1976), also stimulated national interest in evaluation. The need for greater precision in program evaluation was the basis for task force recommendation 6: "Provide federal support for research and development in consumer health education techniques, methodologies, and programs, and their evaluation" (Somers, 1976:40).

In a survey of 23 consumer health programs, Little (1976) indicated that the field showed an increase of evaluation studies. Program evaluation was identified as a required part of the health systems plan by the National Health Planning and Resources Act of 1975 (Public Law 93–641) and the National Consumer Health Information and Health Promotion Act of 1976 (Public Law 94–317). Presentations during the 1970s at national and international health education and health promotion meetings suggested that program evaluation methodology had moved beyond the basic stage and was improving in quality.

Several large-scale evaluation studies were conducted in the 1970s, representing successful first-generation models of large-scale community health education programs: the North Karelia Cardiovascular Risk Reduction Projects of 1972–1978 in Finland (Puska et al., 1979), the Stanford Heart Disease Prevention Study of 1973–1976 in California (Farquahar et al., 1977), and the National Multiple Risk Factor Intervention Trial (MRFIT) of 1974–1982 (Neaton et al., 1981). All studies point to the value and feasibility of planned designs and methods in evaluating health promotion programs and education efforts.

From 1960 to 1980, there was much discussion of the importance of evaluation. The literature, however, confirmed that application of evaluation principles, concepts, and methods in planning and evaluation of health education programs lagged behind the underlying disciplines of education, sociology, communication, psychology, and epidemiology. The 1970s was an early gestational period for program evaluation and evaluation research. Seminal work by Rossi and Williams (1972), Weiss (1972, 1973a, 1973b), Deniston and Rosenstock (1973), Green et al. (1975), Rosenstock (1975), Shortell and Richardson (1978), Cook and Campbell (1979), and Rossi et al. (1979) reflected increasing levels of sophistication.

THE EVALUATION MOVEMENT: THE 1980s AND 1990s

In the 1980s, the need to develop a literature base through the standardization of procedures, strengthening of designs, and replication of studies in a variety of settings was a strong, consistent theme. Zapka (1982) suggests the following strategies to expand the knowledge base:

1. Continued commitment to rigorously controlled experimental and quasi-experimental designs in evaluation research

2. Increased attention to and application of qualitative research strategies

3. Increased attention to integration of formative and summative approaches to evaluation design

4. Diversification of the settings and focus of evaluative research

5. Increased case studies by field practitioners, to demonstrate modest evaluation methods applied to well-planned programs

6. Evaluation studies placed in a larger, health education, quality assurance framework

7. Critical analysis of broader issues of research and evaluation

In the 1980s, there was a large expansion of the evaluation literature. Health program administrators were becoming more aware that formal evaluation, primarily a reflection of a broader national and federal interest, was one of the major methods to assess program accountability and to help in decision making (Michnich et al., 1981). The Evaluation Research Society in *New Directions for Program Evaluation* (1982) published standards for evaluation practice. At the onset of the decade, the World Health Organization (WHO) published *Health Program Evaluation: Guiding Principles for Application of the Managerial Process for National Health Development* (1980) and a companion book, *Development of Indicators for Monitoring Progress Toward Health for All by the Year 2000* (1981). These documents provided an international- and country-level focus on evaluation and reconfirmed the importance of using evaluations to improve public health programs and to guide planning and resource allocation.

The PHS prepared the *Report on the Standards and Criteria for the Development and Evaluation of a Comprehensive Employee Assistance Program* (1984). The essential elements of program standards and assessment criteria were developed to provide a framework for evaluating the effectiveness of federal and nonfederal programs. These standards, designed to be used as a management tool, helped federal managers when they addressed occupational and employee health issues in their agencies.

The Centers for Disease Control (CDC), in collaboration with state health departments, began in 1981 to conduct telephone health behavior surveys using CDC's standardized instruments, training, coordination, and data-collection methods to monitor the progress of health promotion programs at the state level. In 1993, 50 states and the District of Columbia conducted a Behavioral Risk Factor Surveillance Survey (BRFSS). This system represents another important evaluation development, providing useful data to document state progress toward the health objectives for the nation for the year 2000.

As part of its National Health Interview Survey (NHIS), the National Center for Health Statistics initiated the 1985 Health Promotion–Disease Prevention Study to monitor progress toward the DHHS's major initiatives. The NHIS is an ongoing cross-sectional national interview survey of more than 36,000 adults in eligible households (nonresponse rate = 7%). Multiple surveys have evolved from this 1985 NHIS, including the 1990 survey to track defined populations and for individual state programs or countrywide progress.

Concurrent with the national interest in evaluation of health promotion and education programs was the perceived need to evaluate outcomes of health care services used to prevent, diagnose, treat, and manage illness and disability. In 1989 the Agency for Health Care Policy Research (AHCPR), formerly the National Center for Health Services Research, was established to implement the Medical Treatment Effectiveness Programs (MEDTEP) within the DHHS. The principal objective of MEDTEP is to improve the appropriateness and efficacy of medical practice by developing and disseminating scientific information about the impact of use of health care services and procedures on patient survival, patient health status, functional capacity, and quality of life.

Multiple federal activities and initiatives and prevention, behavioral, demonstration, and education research programs of the National Institutes of Health—particularly the National Heart, Lung, and Blood Institute, the National Cancer Institute, and CDC—served as major sources of support for evaluation studies from 1980 to 1994 in specific risk-factor areas.

Numerous examples of evaluation reports reflecting variations in setting and populations became available in the 1980s. Iverson (1981) and Iverson and Kolbe (1983) provide a thorough discussion of the evaluation of health promotion strategies in schools. Kreuter (1985) presents a comprehensive discussion of the results of the School Health Education Evaluation, which was published in a special issue of the *Journal of School Health*. Stone et al. (1989) synthesize the behavioral research in cardiovascular youth health promotion programs. McElroy et al. (1984), in a Meta-Evaluation, provide new knowledge into the evaluation of stress reduction programs at the work site. Rimer et al. (1986) make an important contribution in their article, "Research and Evaluation Programs Related to Health Education for Older Persons." This report, covering approximately a 15-year period, presents a comprehensive review of the literature for this population and synthesizes the methodological and evaluation design issues and findings. Rocella and Ward (1984) report on the impact of the National High Blood Pressure Education Program. It provides documentation of the planning process used by a nationwide public health education program and the evaluation of its impact on rates of hypertension control, more appropriate use of physician visits, and the reduction of stroke-related mortality rates.

Two special issues of *Health Education Quarterly* are noteworthy in a discussion of progress in health promotion and education evaluation: "Integrating Qualitative and Quantitative Methods" (Steckler et al., 1992) and "Arthritis Health Education" (Daltroy and Goeppinger, eds. 1993). The first is one of the most recent, comprehensive presentations of the complementary nature of both methodological paradigms. It should put to rest the either/or debate and provide a foundation referent for future discussions. The second issue reflects the synthesis of 15 years of evaluation research. The work by Lorig and Holmen (1993) deserves special attention about how to use evaluation as a building block for knowledge.

Second-generation reports in the late 1980s and early 1990s became available from three large-scale community programs designed to improve health education of three populations in the United States: Minnesota, Rhode Island, and California. The Minnesota Heart Health Project (MHHP) (Blackburn and Leupker, 1980–1990) was designed to evaluate the reduction of cardiovascular disease using a comprehensive communitywide approach. The Pawtucket Heart Health Project (Carlton and Lassiter, 1980–1991) used a variety of community-based interventions including citizen participation at work sites, religious organizations, schools, grocery stores, and restaurants; screening education; and referral to mobilize community involvement in all aspects of heart health planning. The Stanford Five City Projects (Farquahar and Fortman, 1978–1992) principally used media interventions, both broadcast and print, and a wide variety of health education materials in their community-based programs. Each of these programs represents excellent models for community health education planning and evaluation.

Guyer (1989), in "Injury Prevention: Meeting the Challenge," a consensus statement of a conference held in 1985, provides a primary reference for planning and evaluation of injury-related health promotion and education programs. Two key themes were emphasized:

"Data are an essential element in effective program design; they can be used to pinpoint major injury problems to focus attention on the sources and to monitor and evaluate interventions."

"We must increase the use of interventions that have proven effective and make the evaluation of promising interventions a priority."

Green and Lewis added new insights to the evaluation literature in *Measurement and Evaluation in Health Education, and Health Promotion* (1986). Rossi and Freeman published their fifth-edition *Evaluation: A Systematic Approach* (1993). These books provide valuable information about how to conceptualize, design, and implement comprehensive evaluations for health promotion/disease prevention programs. Each provides full-ranging, complementary discussions about the technical complexity and political and programmatic issues related to planning, implementation, and evaluation. Finally, *Fourth Generation Evaluation* (Guba and Lincoln, 1989) and *Foundations of Program Evaluations* (Shadish et al., 1991) represent comprehensive discussions about the evolution of evaluation theory, methods, and practice. Both are essential references for the advanced student of evaluation.

The previous synopsis, designed to be eclectic rather than comprehensive, highlights the many new additions to the evaluation literature. A comprehensive description of the theoretical, methodological issues and practical problems to plan and conduct evaluations is available in almost all specialty areas. We know how to conduct rigorous evaluations in the 1990s for local, state, and national programs.

EVALUATION OF AIDS AND HIV EDUCATION PROGRAMS

The onset of the AIDS epidemic in the early 1980s and its prominence as an enduring public health problem deserve special attention. As Freudenberg notes, "Evaluation is the single most valuable way to learn what works and what does not work. It is the only way AIDS educators can develop a body of knowledge that can guide their practice" (1989:61). Unfortunately, as of 1994, the number of methodologically sound studies that document the validity and efficacy of AIDS education methods is limited. Public health education continues to be the primary and secondary prevention and control strategy to address this problem.

The report *How Effective Is AIDS Education?* (U.S. Congress, 1988), from the Office of Technology Assessment, represents one of the first documents to describe the state of the art and science. This document confirmed the importance of two principles:

> "No single intervention appears to have maximal effectiveness even within a single geographic area."
>
> "Effectiveness of interventions have been handicapped by program designs that do not lend themselves to evaluation."

Because it is beyond the scope of this book to discuss AIDS evaluation methods, the following references represent first choices in understanding the complexity of AIDS interventions and evaluation:

> *Evaluating AIDS Prevention Programs* (Coyle et al., 1991)
>
> *Preventing AIDS: A Guide to Effective Education for the Prevention of HIV Infection* (Freudenberg, 1989)
>
> *New Perspectives on HIV-Related Illnesses: Progress in Health Services Research* (Levee, 1989)
>
> *Health Services Research Methodology: A Focus on AIDS* (Sechrest et al., 1989)

The last two references are proceedings from conferences sponsored by the National Center for Health Services Research (now the Agency for Health Care Policy Research).

Coyle et al. (1991) provide the most comprehensive discussion in this area—*Evaluating AIDS Prevention Programs*. This book is a product of the Panel on the Evaluation of AIDS Interventions convened by the National Research Council Committee on AIDS Research and the Behavioral, Social, and Statistical Sciences. Six chapters cover the following topics: (1) design and implementation of evaluation research, (2) measurement of outcomes, (3) evaluating media campaigns, (4) evaluating health education and risk-reduction projects, (5) evaluating HIV-testing and -counseling projects, and (6) randomized and observational approaches to evaluating the effectiveness of AIDS prevention programs. Appendices provide extensive additional information on methodological issues in surveys, sampling, and other salient topics. The Freudenberg text, *Preventing AIDS* (1989), is an excellent companion reference on how to systematically plan, implement, and evaluate programs. Sepulveda et al. (1992) present a global picture in *AIDS Prevention Through Education: A World View.*

GUIDE TO CLINICAL PREVENTIVE SERVICES

In 1989 the U.S. Preventive Services Task Force published the *Guide to Clinical Preventive Services.* This guide, representing 4 years of review and analysis by 20 experts from medicine and related fields, is a primary resource for evaluators of prevention programs. It reviewed evidence for and against the effectiveness of screening tests, counseling procedures, and immunizations. Part II—Methodology is of special interest to the evaluator. Criteria to determine efficacy and effectiveness and the methodology to review the quality of evidence for intervention programs are presented. A major emphasis in the *Guide* was personal behavior and behavioral counseling. Of 169 interventions evaluated to prevent 60 different diseases, evidence from three categories were reviewed:

1. Screening: Forty-seven screening methods for nine disorders and diseases
2. Counseling: Eight areas—tobacco use, exercise, nutrition, prevention of motor vehicle accidents, prevention of household and environmental injuries, prevention of HIV infection, prevention of unintended pregnancy, and prevention of dental disease
3. Immunization and chemoprophylaxis: Five areas

A new guide is planned for 1994.

EVALUATION TERMINOLOGY

As in all technical fields, a set of common terms has developed in evaluation. Knowing the definition of each is essential to understand the evaluation literature. We use the following terms frequently in this text:

Intervention (program)   A planned and systematically implemented combination of standardized health promotion and education program content, procedures, and methods designed to produce change in cognitive, affective, skill, behavior, or health status objectives for a defined population at risk at a specified site and during a defined period of time.

Efficacy   An evaluation of the extent to which a *new* (untested) intervention produced an impact or outcome: Did the intervention produce change among a sample of the population at risk under *optimal* program conditions?

Effectiveness   An evaluation of the extent to which an *existing* (tested) intervention produced an impact or outcome: Did the intervention produce change among a large, representative sample of the population at risk under normal *practice* conditions?

Formative evaluation (pilot study)   An evaluation designed to produce data and information during the developmental phase of an intervention (program) to be used to improve it and to document the feasibility of program implementation, immediate (1 hour to 1 week) or short-term (e.g., 1 week to 6 months) cognitive, affective, psychomotor (skill), and/or behavioral impact of a program and the appropriateness of content, methods, materials, media, and instruments.

Process evaluation   An evaluation designed to document the degree to which program procedures were conducted according to a written program plan: How much of the intervention was provided, to whom, when, and by whom? A process evaluation, in clinical terms, can be called a quality assurance review (QAR).

Program impact evaluation (summative evaluation)   An evaluation designed to assess intervention efficacy or effectiveness in producing midterm (e.g., 12–24 months) cognitive, belief, skill, and/or behavioral impact for a defined population at risk.

Health outcome evaluation   An evaluation designed to assess intervention efficacy or effectiveness in producing long-term changes (e.g., 1–10 years) in the incidence or prevalence of morbidity rates, mortality rates, or other health status indicators for a clinically diagnosed medical condition among a defined population at risk.

Internal validity   The degree to which an observed change in an impact (behavior) or outcome (health status) rate (A) among individuals at risk (*B*) can be attributed to an intervention (*C*): Did *C* cause *A* to change among *B*?

External validity   The degree to which an observed change in an impact (behavior) or outcome (health status) rate attributable to an intervention can be generalized to a large, defined population at risk.

Evaluation research (ER)   An evaluation using an experimental or quasi-experimental design conducted to establish the efficacy or effectiveness—internal and/or external validity—and cost effectiveness or cost benefit of an intervention among a defined population at risk for a specific impact or outcome rate during a defined period of time.

Cost-effectiveness analysis (CEA)   An evaluation of the relationship between intervention–program costs (input) and impact (output): a ratio of cost per unit of impact.

Cost–benefit analysis (CBA)   An evaluation of the relationship between intervention–program costs (inputs) and program health outcomes, expressed in monetary benefits (outputs): a ratio of costs per unit of economic benefit and net economic benefit.

TYPES OF EVALUATIONS

You can use four interrelated types of evaluation to organize your approaches to evaluation of health promotion and education programs:

Type 1: Process evaluation

Type 2: Formative evaluation

Type 3: Program evaluation

Type 4: Evaluation research

Type 4 subsumes all characteristics of Types 1–3. Type 1 employs nonexperimental designs; Types 2–4 use quasi-experimental or experimental designs and Type 1 (process evaluation) methods. This book focuses mainly on Types 1–3: process, formative, and program evaluations. All types make demands for time, training, skill, and resources. The purposes, methods, and characteristics of each type are interrelated. General characteristics of Types 1, 2, 3, and 4 are presented in Table 1.5 and the next four sections of this chapter. A full discussion of the technical issues related to all types is provided in Chapters 4 and 5.

Table 1.5   General Characteristics by Type of Evaluation

Level	Selected General Characteristics
1. Process evaluation (feasibility)	Applies nonexperimental designs Monitors procedures-effort-activity Examines structure and process Conducts observational analyses Performs qualitative observations Monitors effort-activity Reviews: audits data and records
2. Formative evaluation (efficacy, short term)	Applies experimental or quasi-experimental designs Assesses immediate or short-term impact Field-tests measurement and intervention methods Emphasizes internal validity Employs qualitative evaluation methods
3. Impact evaluation (effectiveness, long term)	Applies quasi-experimental or experimental designs Assesses behavioral impact Emphasizes internal validity Uses simple analysis and comparisons Applies tested interventions Employs formative and summative evaluation methods
4. Evaluation research (efficacy, long term)	Applies quasi-experimental or experimental designs Tests hypothesis on behavior change Uses multivariate analyses Improves knowledge base Grounded in theory—tests new methods Emphasizes internal and external validity Assesses behavioral impact and health outcome

Type 1: Process Evaluation—Quality Assurance Review

Type 1 evaluation documents program feasibility: It assesses structure and process components to be delivered as part of a service. Part of a program quality assurance review (QAR) consists of observing and assessing the quality of procedures performed by program staff. This involves examining the situation, events, problems, people, and interactions during program development, implementation, and field testing. Evaluators assess components of the program for congruence between staff adherence to a written plan and participants' responses. This review should suggest ways from quantitative and qualitative data to improve the program design and operational plan.

Process evaluation activities include assessment of staff performance, periodic review of department functions, budget review, and evaluation of the performance of a new system for monitoring participants. In a process evaluation, criteria and standards for determining acceptable performance are derived from independent professional judgment, experience, or available guidelines from accrediting agencies, procedure manuals, consultants, and professional associations.

The review of interactions between program staff and clients should also be part of a QAR. It may be written participant appraisal or participant observation of staff performance in providing the educational service. Qualitative techniques should be used to define the content, methods, materials, and elements of a program (Cook and Reichardt, 1979; Mullen and Iverson, 1980; Patton, 1980).

QARs of selected elements should be planned, occur routinely (particularly in the early phases of project implementation), take a short period of time, expend modest resources, and be conducted as unobtrusively as possible. The QAR should be planned with full-staff input into its objectives, process, and scope. These sources will provide valuable insights about revising program structure and process. Chapter 4 provides an extensive discussion of standards and quality control procedures for conducting process evaluations.

Type 2: Formative Evaluation— Assessing Feasibility and Efficacy

Conducting a formative evaluation assumes that the methods and procedures to conduct a process evaluation have been completed and all intervention and data-collection methods are developed. A formative evaluation answers an immediate question: Can the program be implemented, and is it efficacious? Synonyms of a formative evaluation are a pilot test or field test: intervention and measurement methods for a health education and promotion program are tried in the field. Impacts most likely to be observed would be improvements in knowledge, skill, compliance behaviors, and immediate or short-term behavior change, for example, within 1 week or 1–3 months.

Data and information derived from this type of evaluation are used to revise intervention components and instruments and data-collection procedures. Types 3 and 4 evaluations must conduct a Type 1 and Type 2 evaluation before initiation. Failure to conduct a formative evaluation and a process evaluation are major reasons why programs fail.

Type 3: Impact Evaluation—Effectiveness Assessment

The objective of an impact evaluation is to determine if the intervention applied at a specific location to a defined population produced change. Because of time and resource limitations and because programs are (and should be) concerned about what works in their setting for their clients, greater emphasis is usually placed on internal validity than on external validity. An assumption usually apparent in an impact evaluation is that the *efficacy* of the intervention has been confirmed by evaluation research. A common problem that may contribute to a program failure is not looking at comparable, previously conducted programs in order to learn what level of skill or behavioral impact is possible to achieve.

Because randomization may not be feasible, quasi-experimental research methods are chosen and employed more frequently in a program evaluation. Another principal difference is that an evaluation of an existing program usually deals with a fluid situation and has to adapt to organizational and situational changes. Program evaluations also tend to be multifaceted. Evaluation research tends to be more rigid in its inputs and methods, attempting not to deviate from a protocol and research design. Capabilities are usually more limited among an ongoing program evaluation staff versus evaluation research staff. Although control for bias of program impact is an important issue, a control or comparison group may be more difficult to establish in conducting a program evaluation.

Evaluation of an existing program focuses primarily, although not exclusively, on internal validity of program results—*effectiveness*. Did the program work in this setting? Did it produce the observed change? In contrast, evaluation research is concerned with both internal and external validity: Did this program produce an observed change? Would the program produce a comparable impact at other sites with another comparably-defined population?

Impact evaluation attempts to determine the congruence between performance (i.e., what occurred) and objectives (i.e., what was supposed to occur) and to isolate the cause(s) of an outcome. Program evaluation and evaluation research can be similar in that both are generally designed to supplement real-world decision making and to add valid new knowledge to the health promotion and education literature.

Type 4: Evaluation Research—Efficacy and Effectiveness Assessment

The purposes and complexity of evaluation research (ER) demand extensive resources and staff capability usually beyond what a school, community, business, or hospital program has available. ER is almost always conducted by specialized centers of research as a collaborative effort of investigators with training in the psychosocial, quantitative, and health sciences: public health education, social and behavioral sciences, epidemiology, biostatistics, and medicine–nursing–nutrition specialists. Extensive skill training in measurement, evaluation design, statistical analyses, and research methods is essential for the principal investigator in ER.

The primary purpose of ER is to document the level of impact of a new intervention among a defined population at risk. ER is the primary method to test a theoretical model and to establish the feasibility, efficacy, and cost benefit of a health promotion and education intervention. The intervention may have single or multiple components and may apply individual, group, or mass methods of communication.

ER attempts to produce evidence to support or reject a research hypothesis and to demonstrate a cause–effect relationship between the intervention and the impact, or outcome. Because the researcher is concerned with both internal and external validity to answer questions with policy implications, ER must be designed to yield convincing, generalizable conclusions. Alternative explanations for an observed, significant impact must be ruled out by ER (Cook and Campbell, 1983). From practice perspective, ER represents the best method to empirically assess "age-old truths" and "new fads."

Another critical step to proposing and conducting ER is performing a thorough review and synthesis of primary source material and literature. A *meta-evaluation* or *meta-analysis* of a completed ER must be done (see Chapter 5). This gives the evaluator (principal investigator) and staff an understanding of the newest developments in a specialized area of health behavior change. Thus, an ER team develops interventions based on accumulated knowledge derived from a sound theoretical grounding. ER uses the following standard procedures:

1. Specification of research questions or hypotheses

2. Selection and definition of an appropriate population at risk to test the hypotheses

3. Selection of data sources and measurement of high validity and reliability

4. Selection of an evaluation design to maximize internal and external validity

5. Application of a data-monitoring system to produce early estimates of immediate and short-term program effects and estimates of long-range effects

6. Application of a standardized, replicable intervention

PURPOSES OF PROGRAM EVALUATION

Different people see program evaluation in different ways. To some, it is a means to ascertain the extent to which a program has succeeded or failed. To others, it is a management tool: a means to improve the planning and implementation process or to have an impact on policymaking. Many see it as collecting data from participants to determine their degree of satisfaction with or acceptance of the program's process and content. Still others believe it is a waste of time and money. Irrespective of the evaluator's viewpoint, pragmatically, most program evaluations have to be concerned with five broad questions (Rossi and Wright, 1979:20):

1. Is the intervention reaching the target population?
2. Is it being implemented in the ways specified?
3. Is it effective?
4. How much does it cost?
5. What are its costs relative to its effectiveness?

Most people expect a well-designed evaluation to confirm, with varying degrees of certainty, whether the program worked. Identifying reasons for nonsuccess may prove as fruitful for program development as a success, although obviously failures or partial successes are not as well received as successes. From the perspective of program efficacy, the sine qua non of evaluation is to determine the degree to which observed behavior changes can be attributed to the program. The ability of a program to demonstrate behavioral impact, however, is always related to the characteristics of the health problem, the setting, the population at risk, available resources (personnel and money), and time.

The following represent ten common purposes of evaluation:

1. To determine the degree of attainment of program objectives
2. To document strengths and weaknesses of program or components for making decisions and planning
3. To monitor standards of performance and establish quality assurance and control mechanisms
4. To meet the demand for public or fiscal accountability
5. To improve the professional staff's skill in the performance of program planning, implementation, and evaluation activities
6. To fulfill grant or contract requirements
7. To promote positive public relations and community awareness
8. To determine the generalizability of an overall program or program elements to other populations and settings

9. To contribute to the base of scientific knowledge about health education program design

10. To identify hypotheses about human behavior for future evaluations

Although it is not realistic to expect each evaluation to achieve all the listed purposes, an evaluator must consider the relevance of each purpose to each program. The creative and skilled practitioner can accomplish a number of purposes at once.

ROLE OF EVALUATION IN AN ORGANIZATION

In an organization, the interest in, expectations of, and funding for evaluations tend to have a tidal quality: ebbing and flowing. Some see evaluation as a necessary evil or meaningless exercise. Others believe it is a way to gain insight into what happened and why. In theory, an evaluation's objective is to provide evidence on the quality and impact of a program to be used in future decisions about resource allocation; however, in practice, scientific, economic, philosophical, and political orientations play an equal (perhaps greater) role in policymaking and resources allocation. Whatever the evaluator's position, he or she must deal with political realities. The evaluator who fails to recognize the political dimension of decision making and resource allocation is in for a rude awakening. Chapter 2 discusses this issue at greater length.

Program staff and evaluators need to recognize that the principal reasons for conducting a program evaluation differ from situation to situation and from site to site. Involvement of managers, service providers, and representatives of the target audience is an important step in clarifying the purposes of the evaluation. The expectations and demands of the various audiences for the evaluation will influence its purposes.

The purposes, organizational and programmatic, will help define the following issues:

1. The objectives to be evaluated

2. The type(s) of evaluation to be performed

3. The evaluation design to be used

4. The measures appropriate to program input, process, outcome, and impact

5. The types and amount of data collected

6. The analytic demands of the program

7. The time, staff, and resources needed to accomplish the evaluation

The evaluation process will be enhanced if program staff perceive an evaluation as an ideal opportunity for professional growth.

SETTING REALISTIC OBJECTIVES AND PROGRAM PLANS

One of the first steps in evaluation planning is to conduct a needs assessment and to prepare objectives. A comprehensive program evaluation may not be possible, given the time, resources, and circumstances of many ongoing programs. Program staff need to determine what a program can achieve and what it cannot achieve, and they also need to clarify reasonable expectations. In general, program staff should set more modest expectations for their programs than they do (Ogden, 1978, 1980). Trying to evaluate what cannot be evaluated given resources, time, and expertise; evaluating a program before it has had a chance to be established in a setting; or evaluating inappropriate outcomes—all represent common problems faced by program staff. One also needs to remember common sense. Every aspect of a program usually cannot and, in most cases, should not be evaluated.

You should recognize that there may not be a "perfect" evaluation design or definitive measurement method to apply to a program staff's situation. Designs and methods are better or worse, or more or less appropriate, for particular situations and behaviors. Data are of better or poorer quality or can be collected more or less easily or expensively in different situations for different risk factors. The best evaluation information, however, will be produced when methods and designs are matched to the program questions being asked.

Proof of efficacy derived from a sophisticated design—for example, a randomized clinical trial with experimental and control groups and with extensive resources—may also not provide a definitive answer to a specific research question. All programs and evaluation studies experience implementation problems. Another issue is that unequivocal proof of intervention effectiveness is difficult to document. The best an ongoing program evaluation may be able to do is rule out several less plausible reasons for an observed change and support one or two reasons why the program worked. The serendipity of positive and negative program outcomes also needs to be acknowledged.

Program managers and staff must agree on the criteria of success before conducting evaluations; compromise is often the product of this process. Plans must include both qualitative and quantitative criteria. Although criteria obviously will vary from organization to organization, most organizations and agencies in the 1990s will continue to be concerned about the effectiveness and efficiency of services rendered, often measured in economic terms.

Program evaluators need to approach the creation and revision of an evaluation plan with insights into how different parts, methods, and designs relate to one another conceptually and operationally. Adjustments in one component or method almost always affect another dimension. Attention to detail at the outset will, in general, improve the ability to revise and adapt the plan as it unfolds. Weiss (1973a:51) suggests that prior agreement on several issues is essential:

1. The goals of the program

2. The nature of program service and typical variations

3. The measures that indicate the effectiveness of the program in meeting its goal

4. The methods of selection of participants and controls

5. The allocation of responsibilities for participant selection, data collection, descriptions of program input, and so on

6. The procedures for resolving disagreements between program and evaluation personnel

7. The decisional purposes that evaluation is expected to serve

It is also important to remember that an evaluation plan (1) defines program objectives, outcomes, and impacts; (2) specifies tasks, methods, and procedures to be employed by whom, for whom, and over what period of time; and (3) describes what resources will be allocated to achieve the objectives. A good plan will assist the program and the evaluator in resetting objectives (if needed). Failure to specify and put into operation all major objectives is a common omission in a program plan. Writing one's objectives, discussing them, and then agreeing on the priority objectives will help staff set realistic targets.

When the evaluation plan is prepared, a number of decisions and assumptions are also made. Not all aspects of a program evaluation, however, are evident during the planning and early implementation stages. Opportunities to examine selected dimensions of a program may exist prior to or in the early stages of program implementation and may not exist at a later time. One purpose of this book is to improve an evaluator's ability to confidently participate in preparing or revising a program plan, realizing as fully as possible the alternatives and consequences of each alteration.

PROFESSIONAL COMPETENCE IN EVALUATION

The quality of an evaluation depends heavily on the competency and confidence of the evaluator. Training institutions and professional leaders in public health have consistently perceived evaluation competency as a major skill of graduate-trained health professionals. Evaluation has also long been identified as a critically important and integral component of school, public, and community health service programs by standard-setting organizations such as the World Health Organization (1954, 1969, 1980, 1981), American Public Health Association (1957), Association of Schools of Public Health (Boatman et al.,

Table 1.6 Guidelines for the Preparation and Practice of Professional Health Educators: Area Four—Research and Evaluation

Skill Area	Master's Level Function
1. Statistical methods	Collect and use quantitative data and perform standard statistical tests to understand and analyze the relationships between variables and draw inferences for work activities
2. Research design and research methods	Design and conduct studies on health-related behavior, health education methods, and behavior-change problems
3. Design methods of evaluative research	Design health education programs so that evaluative measures are incorporated, with provision for continuing process evaluation
4. Methods of data collection and analysis	Determine which data are needed to analyze a health problem and where they can be obtained Use standardized measurement instruments Analyze research findings relevant to health-related behavior change and draw implications for application Design action research and demonstration projects
5. Computer science; technologies for storage and retrieval of data	Understand appropriate applications of computer technology for planning, conducting, and evaluating educational activities
6. Knowledge and skills possessed by other professions and disciplines in research and evaluation, and how these resources can be utilized for health education	Use expert help as needed for design and conduct of research

SOURCE: Society for Public Health Education (1977b:75–89).

Table 1.7 Specification of the Role of the Entry-Level Health Educator

Area of Responsibility V: Evaluating Health Education

Function A. Participate in developing an evaluation design.
Skill   1. Specify indicators of program success.
          2. Establish the scope for program evaluation.
          3. Develop methods for evaluating programs.
          4. Specify instruments for data collection.
          5. Determine samples needed for evaluation.
          6. Select data useful for accountability analysis.

Function B. Assemble resources required to carry out evaluation.
Skill   1. Acquire facilities, materials, personnel, and equipment.
          2. Train personnel for evaluation as needed.
          3. Secure the cooperation of those affecting and affected by the program.

Function C. Help implement the evaluation design.
Skill   1. Collect data through appropriate techniques.
          2. Analyze collected data.
          3. Interpret results of program evaluation.

Function D. Communicate results of evaluation.
Skill   1. Report the processes and results of evaluation to those interested.
          2. Recommend strategies for implementing results.
          3. Incorporate results into planning and implementing results.
          4. Incorporate results into planning and implementation processes.

SOURCE: U.S. DHHS, Role Delineation: Final Report (1980:78–82).

1966), International Union on Health Education (Kaplun-le Meitour, 1973), American School Health Association (1976), Society for Public Health Education (1968, 1977a), and American Society of Health-care Education and Training (1990). The Society for Public Health Education (SOPHE) (1977a) described the research and evaluation skills needed by a health education specialist with a master's degree (Table 1.6).

The importance of having baccalaureate-trained educators assist in program evaluation has also been defined (SOPHE, 1977b; U.S. DHHS, 1980a). As noted in Table 1.7, the health education specialist is expected to perform a number of evaluation functions and be skilled in multiple technical areas.

CREDENTIALING AND PROFESSIONAL PREPARATION IN HEALTH EDUCATION

The President's Committee on Health Education, the U.S. Coalition of Health Education Organizations, and the leadership in the field of health education and health promotion throughout the 1970s called for improvements in training programs and competency of health educators. The leadership in school health education, public health education, patient health care education, and work-site health education agreed that major commonalities existed in the functions and skills of health education specialists. These deliberations produced a landmark meeting in April 1978, convened by the Bureau of Health Manpower, Department of Health Resources Administration: "Preparation and Practice of Community, Patients and School Health Educators." A National Task Force on Professional Preparation was established at this time.

Information presented in Table 1.8 reflects the critical events of the credentialing process. Two major initiatives of the National Commission for Credentialing are ongoing to promote improved competency: (1) professional certification of health education specialists (CHES) and (2) continued promotion and application of the "A Guide for the Development of Competency-Based Curricula for Entry-Level Health Educators" by more than 100 baccalaureate professional preparation programs and over 75 master's programs in the United States.

Table 1.8   Critical Events in the Health Education
Credentialing Process

Year	Critical Events
1978	Workshop: Commonalities and Differences in the Preparation of Health Educators, Bethesda, Maryland
	National Task Force on the Preparation and Practice of Health Educators, Inc., established
	Initial-role specification prepared
1980	Role verification and refinement document published
1981	National Conference for Institutions Preparing Health Educators
	Curriculum Development Project initiated
1983	"A Guide for the Development of Competency-Based Curricula for Entry-Level Health Educators" drafted and disseminated
1986	Workshop: Quality Assurance in the Delivery of Health Education Services: Credentialing the Health Education Specialist, Bethesda, Maryland
1987	Model for Continuing Professional Development of Health Educators developed
1988	National Commission for Health Education Credentialing, Inc., established
1990	Board of Commissioner appointed; CHES initiated

SUMMARY

Contemporary thinking dictates that the professional preparation and practice of health education and promotion be approached in the 1990s from both an experimental and qualitative perspective. Evaluation should serve as a mechanism not only to assess and improve programs but also to test new intervention innovations. It represents one of the most important channels for improvement of the health education profession and should become a major source of personal and professional growth.

Program evaluation and health education practice need to be perceived as the "spawning ground" for collaboration between trainers, trainees, and practitioners, regardless of setting. All types of evaluation, 1–4, have considerable potential to provide opportunities to bridge the existing gap between academically oriented and practice-oriented health promotion/disease prevention professionals. The work of professionals of both orientations improves or diminishes the technology and advancement. Although both groups experience frustration at the energy and sophistication needed to plan, implement, and evaluate a program with limited resources, individuals in practice and academic settings need to strive to do better with what they have so they can get more of what they need. This book is intended to provide structure and guidance for the process of resource development.

The development, implementation, and adaptation of an evaluation plan to unanticipated situations can be one of the most creative exercises in which a health professional participates. If health education and promotion are to continue to prosper as an integrated part of the public health, health care, work site, and educational systems of the United States, you need greater technical skill and improved sophistication. Responsibility for the extra effort it takes to master the technical skills to conduct health program evaluations rests with you. With improved skills and experience, you will be able to better perceive what is possible, probable, or impossible given available resources, time, and the existing political environment.

2

Conducting Evaluations and Promoting Organizational Change

"I worked for two years on that evaluation, and no one even read the report."

"We were the first to employ an elegant factorial design in evaluating this program, and the administration ignored our findings."

"The only reason the agency hired me is that the feds require an evaluator on staff. These people don't even know what an evaluator does."

"I really threaten our program people. They keep me at arm's length. I can't even get a meeting with them."

Professional Competencies Emphasized in This Chapter

• Analyzing political processes related to health and health education

• Identifying social, cultural, environmental, organizational, and growth and development factors that affect health behavior, needs, and interest

• Acquiring ideas and opinions from persons who may affect or be affected by the educational program

• Securing administrative support and the cooperation of those affecting and affected by the program

• Incorporating results into planning and implementation processes

• Contributing to cooperation and feedback among personnel related to the program

• Reconciling differences in approach, timing, and effort among individuals

Evaluation can be defined as the act of placing a value, positive or negative, on something. Negative value implies something is wrong, that is, improvement is needed. A less than fully positive value implies that the object of the evaluation can be improved through some change. Because program evaluations are almost always conducted by comparing a program's performance against a standard, most evaluations produce some negative value. The responsibility of the evaluator is to be an agent of change: working to improve a program in the many ways identified by evaluation results.

The comments at the beginning of this chapter point out the frustrations experienced by many evaluators in the real world in getting the results of their evaluations implemented. Program evaluators, usually working with other staff, spend many hours specifying evaluation objectives, considering alternative designs, laboring over instruments, analyzing multiple facets of data, and communicating results to multiple audiences. Despite this effort, their reports are frequently not used. Ineffective programs are rarely dropped. Obvious improvements are infrequently made. Effective programs may not be allocated additional money. Although evaluators might wish that an agency's operation were governed by a rational approach—evaluative data are applied and appropriate decisions derived—no such equation exists.

Table 2.1 Health Educator Evaluation Skills

Analyzing political processes related to health and health education

Identifying social, cultural, environmental, organizational, and growth and development factors that affect health behavior, needs, and interests

Acquiring ideas and opinions from persons who may affect or be affected by the educational program

Securing administrative support for the program and the cooperation of those affecting and affected by the program

Incorporating results into planning and implementation processes

Contributing to cooperation and feedback among personnel related to the program

Reconciling differences in approach, timing, and effort among individuals

SOURCE: Adapted from National Center for Health Education (1980: 1–31).

Thus, evaluators may become exasperated at the lack of immediate or long-term rewards for their technical expertise and extensive effort. These attendant conditions highlight the political nature of evaluation. Evaluations are conducted by people, for other people, about other people. All evaluations are conducted within a "social context" (Levine and Levine, 1977). The evaluator becomes a part of the struggles and movements in the agency and between agencies. To be effective, an evaluator needs a variety of skills related to the politics and interpersonal relationships of health promotion and its evaluation. Many of these skills were identified in the Report of the Role Delineation Project (National Center for Health Education, 1980) (Table 2.1).

The Joint Committee on Standards for Educational Evaluation proposes a standard for ensuring the political viability of evaluations:

The evaluation should be planned and conducted with anticipation of the different positions of various interest groups, so that their cooperation may be obtained, and so that possible attempts by any of these groups to curtail evaluation operations or to bias or misapply the results can be averted or counteracted. (1981:56)

We address these issues in this chapter. We present an overview of factors affecting the use of evaluation reports, delineate four kinds of program evaluations, and identify factors that promote utilization of evaluation findings. We provide a framework for understanding human service organizations and examine how evaluators might more effectively conduct single agency or multiagency evaluations.

FACTORS AFFECTING USE OF EVALUATION RESEARCH

A legitimate question commonly asked about an evaluation is, Is anyone going to pay attention to it? The literature on the use of federal education, social, or health program evaluations suggests that reported results have often exerted little or no influence on program and policy decisions. In the past, this situation was paralleled in the broad field of evaluation research (ER) and program evaluation. Discussing issues seldom examined in the health education/health promotion literature, Suchman (1967), Weiss (1972, 1973b), Patton et al. (1977), and Zweig and Marvin (1981) confirm the nonuse or underuse of ER by management and policymakers. Reasons for nonuse are varied. More than two decades ago, Wholey et al. (1970:23) described four basic reasons for underuse of ER reports by organizations:

1. Organizational inertia: Organizations tend to maintain the status quo and to resist change. Evaluation usually implies that changes are needed.

2. Methodological weakness: Poorly conducted studies produce poorly respected conclusions. Decision makers tend to trust their own instincts or experiences rather than the results of poorly done studies.

3. Design irrelevance: Critical program components and vital policy issues often are unrelated to the evaluation undertaken.

4. Lack of dissemination: Concerned policymakers and decision makers may not see or hear the conclusions of the evaluations. Sometimes the evaluation is deliberately buried to keep the information from being communicated to relevant individuals and organizations.

Lack of adequate definitions and explicit consensus on program impact may explain why decision makers ignore evaluation reports. Evaluators must assess more than impact or outcome variables. Both qualitative and quantitative assessments need to be performed to characterize a program's implementation success and effectiveness more fully—not just the presentation of a statistically significant increase at the .05 level. Although impact evaluation may help in the decision to continue or repeat a program, it is not (and should not be) the *sole* criteria of worth.

One primary purpose of evaluation reports is to help an organization make program and policy decisions related to resource allocation. Program staff who get too involved in their own objectives and activities may lose sight of or become insensitive to what they are doing, why they are doing it, and for whom. Appendix A, "The Evaluation Report," provides a description of how to improve the presentation quality. Increased use of ER and program evaluation results will come about, in part, by broadening the utility of response results to those who philosophically support and fund evaluation studies.

Another purpose of an evaluation report is the synthesis and translation of findings into recommendations. The report should, within the constraints of reality (data), attempt to persuade the reader or listener. Prudence suggests that an evaluation report should also identify program weaknesses and provide alternative recommendations for administrative and policy use.

Evaluators in both practice and research settings need to become more adept at communicating relevant information so that principal decision makers can answer their questions and respond to their agenda. In the 1990s, the profession must give much greater emphasis to improved translation. Increased concern about the effective dissemination of methods and results should increase the use of ER and program evaluations in health education and health promotion.

Boyer and Langbein (1991) reviewed the circumstances in which evaluation results would more likely be used. Similar to Wholey et al. (1970), they suggest the following characteristics of the report were associated with greater use:

There was high methodological quality to the research.

The report was clear in what it stated.

The results in the report were clearly relevant to the decisions being made.

They also suggest the following social circumstances were related to increased use of results:

The author had a good reputation as a researcher.

A strong advocate (within the agency) encouraged use of the evaluation findings.

Good communication (other than a written report) existed between the evaluators and the users.

There was conflict about the issue under consideration.

The report appeared at a timely point in the decision-making process.

Thus, although blaming methodological defects is easy when an evaluation's conclusions are not heeded, better methods are only part of the answer. Many factors affect a program, and evaluators of health promotion programs must fully understand them. Health promotion specialists must realize that improvements in the methodological quality and analytical sophistication of an evaluation by itself may not improve its acceptance, dissemination, or use. In fact, the methodological quality may receive little consideration among some people in an agency. Improved methods are important to ensure that we are making the right inferences, but they may not persuade a school superintendent, public health officer, or chief executive officer of a company to apply an evaluation's conclusions.

TYPES OF EVALUATION RESEARCH

Differentiating the types of evaluations and exploring the role of social and organizational factors in each type are helpful. In general, we can categorize most ER into four types, based on its purposes: (1) social science, (2) social policy, (3) agency decision making, and (4) consumer decision making. *Social science evaluation* includes studies conducted to contribute to social science knowledge on a problem or on the most effective methods to redress the problem. The interventions studied in this kind of evaluation are usually innovative, either designed by the investigator and based on some theoretical framework or designed by practitioners but taking a new approach (or considered as having done so). The research designs to evaluate these programs are usually experimental or quasi-experimental and focus on program outcomes, with process measurement as a check on the internal validity of the experimental program. This type of evaluation has generally been conducted by university-based social and behavioral scientists and published in relevant academic journals. Whether the evaluation is accepted depends on whether the research methods conform to prevailing scientific principles. Social scientists doing this kind of research need an organizational perspective to more effectively collect program evaluation data and to build better social science knowledge bases of how health and human services organizations function.

Social policy evaluation includes research conducted to enhance the formulation of policy at the state or national levels. *Agency decision-making evaluation* is research conducted to enhance a specific agency's ability to provide more effective services, either at the state or local level. *Consumer decision-making evaluation* is research usually conducted by consumer or client groups with the intent to help consumers better select from available services or to lobby for change in existing services. Table 2.2 lists the defining characteristics of these types of evaluation. This categorization helps to avoid the trap of ap-

Table 2.2 Differences in Four Types of Evaluation Research

	Social Science	Social Policy	Agency Decision Making	Consumer Decision Making
Purpose	To contribute to social science knowledge	To enhance formulation of social policy	To enhance an agency's ability to provide more effective services	To enable consumers to better select services or lobby for change
Type of intervention usually studied	Intervention designed by investigators: theory based; Innovative intervention based on practical or theoretical perspective	Establishing national need for a new program; Existing programs on a national scale	Establishing local need for a new program; Existing programs on a local scale	Programs serving a particular group at the national or local level
Usual research designs	Experimental or quasi-experimental outcome assessment; Process measurement check on internal validity	Reviews of existing program evaluations; Surveys of agency officials or clients	Process evaluation as primary focus; Single-group outcome assessment	Client surveys
Usual employer	University or private research agency	University, government, or private research agency	Agency staff or private research agency	Private research agency or consumer group staff
Usual publication outlets	Professional academic journals	Government reports or academic journals	Internal agency reports	Consumer publications (magazines or newsletters)
Tenets of acceptability of evaluation	Prevailing standards in social science	Prevailing standards in policy science	Meaningfulness to agency personnel	Meaningfulness to audience intended by group
Need for an organizational perspective	To improve quality of data collection; To improve knowledge of human service organizations	To enhance agency functioning at national level; To increase utilization of evaluation findings	To collect better data; To increase utilization of evaluation findings	To make agency more responsive to client needs

plying the same criteria to all evaluations and to better understand the phenomena at work in affecting social policy and agency functioning.

Because social scientists, social policymakers, local agency staff, and consumers all form different social groups, how they make decisions will likely vary. Different analyses have been conducted of decision making in the different groups.

Social Science Evaluation

Technical and social factors determine whether research contributes to the body of social science knowledge. The technical factors (methodological sophistication) are the topics of the rest of this text and many other social science research texts (Cook and Campbell, 1979; Sechrest et al., 1990). The study of how social factors affect the use of research findings has been called the *sociology of knowledge* (Crane, 1972) and is beyond the scope of this introductory text. Science, however, is not only a technical discipline. Social factors are important in all aspects of science and play a pivotal role in defining support (fiscal and policy) for the research spectrum—basic to applied sciences.

Social Policy Evaluation

Boyer and Langbein (1991) examined what aspects of evaluation affect decision making in Congress. Their results differed by factors affecting Congress's decisions versus congressional staff's decisions and the source of the study (the General Accounting Organization [GAO] or other). For all decisions and sources of data, the timing of the report (not appearing too early, nor too late) was important in whether a particular study was used or not. The report clarity was important for Congress, but not aides. The credibility of the methods was important for aides, but not for Congress. The social factors were important for reports coming from sources other than the GAO, indicating that the GAO, as an agency of Congress, already has extensive credibility among Congress and staff.

Agency Decision-Making Evaluation

Wholey et al. (1970) note that formal evaluation reports may not play a substantial role in organizational policymaking and programming for two reasons: they do not support the reasons for existence of the program or a bureaucracy, and they frequently communicate negative or equivocal results. A related and continuing problem is staff turnover in an organization, which impairs evaluation and program continuity. In addition, organizational goals, organizational constraints, and the role played by the health education practitioner in the planning and use of finite resources affect the valuing, conduct, and use of an evaluation.

Consumer Decision-Making Evaluation

Little information exists on the generation or use of evaluation findings by consumer groups, either to select better services or to work to improve the services available to them (Tripi, 1984). This is an area that deserves more attention.

Most students of health promotion/health education program evaluation will likely find themselves working in or with health agencies (as opposed to Congress). An analysis of social factors in your agency will help clarify how evaluations might be more effectively conducted and how the evaluation can contribute to agency growth or change.

DOMAIN AND INTEREST GROUPS

Agencies or organizations provide services. Agencies may have one service provider and a limited clientele (e.g., a private health education consultant and clients), or they may be large and complex with many clients (e.g., a state health department, Kaiser Permanente of California, or the American Heart Association). There are many models for agencies and many characteristics of interest to an evaluator.

The agency decides which services to provide; decisions and actions can be complex. To understand how professional human services organizations function, Kouzes and Mico (1979, 1980) found it useful to identify three domains of decision making and action: policy, management, and service. The *policy domain* usually consists of a board of directors; the *management domain* usually consists of agency administrators; and the *service domain* consists of agency staff members who render the services (Figure 2.1). For example, a state affiliate of the American Cancer Society (ACS) will have, at a minimum, a board of directors responsible for deciding statewide organizational activities (*policy*), a state vice-president responsible for raising funds and managing staff to achieve the board's objectives (*management*), and a statewide activity coordinator (staff) who motivates and organizes volunteers to conduct ACS activities (*service*).

Although a particular person in an organization may perform activities that fall within all these domains (e.g., the manager who makes some policy decisions, manages, and provides services), each domain has characteristic functions. The function of the policy do-

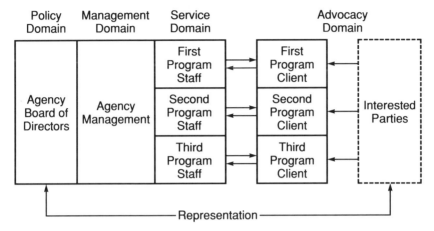

Figure 2.1 A Model of Agency Domains

main is to define the mission, set the direction, and prescribe operational guidelines for the agency. Questions addressed by the policy domain include: What services will this agency provide? With what other agencies should it collaborate? How and where should it seek funding?

The function of the management domain is to run the agency using guidelines set by policymakers. Questions considered by management include: Given the funds available, how many and what kinds of staff members will the agency hire? Where should the staff be located? How can the staff be organized to provide quality service?

The function of the service domain is to provide the specific services selected by policymakers and organized by management. Questions related to service include: What should each service include? How should various services available from this agency be best employed to meet the needs of a particular client? How does this agency define *quality* for the services provided?

An agency functions by providing service units to a clientele. The clients justify the agency. A dramatic example of the importance of this relationship occurred when the March of Dimes Foundation participated successfully in eliminating polio as a national scourge. The foundation had to find another target group to justify continuation of its extensive and powerful fund-raising organization. It did so by emphasizing birth defects and problems of pregnancy, delivery, and infancy. This new set of problems justified the effective fund-raising and service delivery activities of the March of Dimes.

The clientele has various interested parties, that is, groups interested in the welfare of the agency's clientele. For example, the Juvenile Diabetes Foundation is interested in young diabetics, the Citizens

Council for Hypertension Control is interested in hypertensive patients, and the National Welfare Rights Organization is interested in welfare clients.

In a sense, clients and their interested parties constitute a domain: the *advocacy domain*. If organized, clients can exert significant influence on agency activities (Tripi, 1984). To be *organized* means that a clientele has some political or self-help group that works for clients' interests. An unorganized client group may be able to exert substantial influence on an agency; lack of organization, however, tends to reduce the direct influence clients exert on the decisions and actions of the other domains. Questions related to advocacy include: What are the perceived needs of the client group? What new services are needed to meet the perceived needs of the clients? How might services be changed to better meet client-perceived needs?

Each domain addresses a different set of questions, and all questions are important to the agency's effectiveness. The concerns of one domain are no more important than those of another for the viable functioning of the agency.

Examples will give a clearer picture of how the domain ideas apply in specific situations. Three types of agencies are discussed: a health education staff in a local clinic, a division of a state health department engaged in a risk-reduction program, and a state affiliate of a voluntary health agency.

Example: Local Clinic

A locally run primary-care clinic will often have a board of directors, a central management unit, and a variety of service providers to meet local needs. The board of directors constitutes the policy domain. Boards are usually composed of individuals and representatives of groups interested in health issues and influential in the local community (e.g., representatives of local industry, labor unions, churches, potential health care consumers, and individual benefactors). Three reasons for inviting people to be on a board of directors are (1) they represent groups who can provide financial or professional resources, (2) they are sources of clients, or (3) they represent influential community opinions. Having these people on the board gives the agency more direct access to the resources represented and feedback on how the community perceives the agency.

Central management is usually composed of a director and other staff members, who manage the books, collect and pay bills, obtain funding and materials, maintain the buildings and facilities, hire personnel, and plan services and facilities to meet local community needs.

The service staff includes physicians, nurses, dietitians, health educators, technicians, and various other professionals who provide health services. These service providers are usually organized into divisions (e.g., pediatrics, radiology, and pharmacy). The directors of these divisions often experience role conflict because they operate in both the management and the service domains and experience the demands of both.

Clients in this system are patients who come for acute or chronic disease care and people who benefit from clinic outreach programs (e.g., weight-reduction programs and hypertension screening).

Example: State Health Department

Divisions that operate risk-reduction programs in state health departments present a more complex domain structure. The policy domain has several components with separate responsibilities. High-level policy for risk-reduction programs is formulated to one degree or another by Congress, the federal executive branch (the U.S. Department of Health and Human Services), the state legislature, and the governor's office. Policy guidelines from these sources tend to be broad enough so that local programs have latitude for action on specific needs. The state-level policy function is most often provided by the director of the state health department and a statewide risk-reduction advisory board. Advisory boards are usually composed of representatives of organizations that can contribute to a statewide risk-reduction program (e.g., voluntary health agencies, university departments, other divisions of the state health department, and individuals who have been particularly active in risk reduction).

Management is also complex. State health departments often have a variety of divisions concerned with management functions (e.g., finance and personnel). Like the service division director in a clinic, the risk-reduction program director has both management and service responsibilities.

Service staff in a statewide risk-reduction program includes the director of the risk-reduction program and all paid staff members promoting risk-reduction programs throughout the state. From the evaluator's point of view, the service domain also includes all people who volunteer their time to help achieve program objectives.

In a statewide risk-reduction program, all state residents are potential clients. Primary clients, however, are the groups targeted by specific risk-reduction projects (e.g., people with a high risk of stroke, smokers, or alcoholics).

Example: Voluntary Health Agency

In a state affiliate of a voluntary health agency, the policy domain includes groups that provide direction to the affiliate, most often the

Table 2.3 Operating Characteristics of the Domains in Human Services Organizations

Domain	Governing Principles	Success Measures	Organizational Structures	Work Modes
Policy	Consent of the governed	Equity	Representative Participative	Voting Bargaining Negotiating
Management	Hierarchical control Coordination	Cost efficiency Effectiveness	Bureaucratic	Use of linear process tools
Service	Autonomy Self-regulation	Quality of service Good standards of practice	Collegial	Client-specific problem solving
Advocacy	Client advocacy Agency oversight	Increased or improved services for clients	Varied, depending on history of development	Protest Conflict Participation

national (parent) organization, its representatives and staff, and the affiliate's own board of directors (e.g., local business people who volunteer their time and efforts) or board of professional members (e.g., physicians). These boards usually have committees to govern policy formation and implementation in many facets of the agency's activities.

The management domain consists of the director, staff, and volunteers assigned to management tasks (e.g., fund-raising and personnel). The service domain in a voluntary health agency is usually composed of a director and volunteers engaged in program activities. The clientele is all residents of the state with the particular afflictions targeted by the agency or residents at risk of developing the afflictions. A more specific client domain consists of afflicted or at-risk individuals for whom the agency has developed specific service programs.

In some cases, the board is also drawn from volunteers; the manager may also be a major service provider. In these cases, the same person may function in several domains. The rest of this chapter must be understood by considering one function at a time. Conditions in agencies vary so greatly that it would serve no purpose to detail the many possible functions and interrelationships. Domain is a useful concept for understanding the interests that intersect in agency operations and for dealing with them effectively.

OPERATING CHARACTERISTICS OF AGENCY DOMAINS

Why is it important to know about an agency's domains? Kouzes and Mico (1979) propose that agency domains differ in their operating characteristics: governing principles, success measures, organizational structure, and working modes. Table 2.3 summarizes the differences, which are overstated to clarify the ideal. Although no agency functions in exactly this manner, a clearer understanding of the ideal operating characteristics may help the evaluator work better with these domains in a particular agency.

Kouzes and Mico (1979) describe the policy domain as using the "consent of the governed" as their governing principle. This means that policymakers usually employ a parliamentary form of governing: All members are considered equal. In theory, the consumer representative is the equal of the physician in the policy domain. Policymakers often assess the success of their activities by whether some equitable (just) distribution of resources occurs among interests and concerns. Thus, members of the Heart Association board might be satisfied if the agency's resources were equitably distributed among hypertension, heart disease prevention, stroke, and heart disease rehabilitation programs. The structure for their meetings is representative (each member represents an interest) and participative (each member participates in policy deliberation). Setting policy is most often accomplished by persuasion, negotiation, and voting. Different interests may have different weights in setting policy due to personal, political, or economic influences. In some agencies, policy may be set by a malevolent or benevolent "dictator."

The management domain typically employs a hierarchical mode of organization: relationships among nonequals. People at the higher levels are considered to have more responsibility and skill. They coordinate the activities of people at lower levels. The clinic director may employ directors of finance, personnel, and purchasing, who employ staff, including support personnel. Management often uses a variety of analytic tools (e.g., budgeting systems and cost-effectiveness analysis), which have as their criterion of success some aspect of effectiveness or efficiency. This focus on efficiency and effectiveness naturally follows from the constraint that management provides services within the limits of resources. Thus, a risk-reduction program can work with only as many communities as its staff, printing, telephone, and travel budget will permit.

The service domain is most frequently composed of human services professionals, people who are as responsive to and interested in the values and activities of colleagues at other agencies as they are in the directives of their agency. These service providers belong to professional organizations at which standards are defined and discussed. The way professionals typically relate to one another is as colleagues: peers with similar skills and responsibilities providing complementary services with a common purpose. This is true *within* classes of professionals (e.g., physicians and nurses) but not necessarily *between* classes of professionals, a potential source of conflict. Service staff members tend to protect the professional autonomy of their own domain and class of colleagues. They prefer to control their practices through professional self-regulation. Peer review committees for professional self-regulation are common in a variety of disciplines. The work mode of professionals is characterized as client-specific problem solving; techniques for this are developed and defined by professional consensus.

Outlining the four organizational characteristics of the advocacy domain is more difficult. The measure of success is increased and improved services for agency clients. Hypertensive patients may want more and better hypertension-control services from the health department. The organizational structure, however, may be representative and participatory or autocratically ruled by a charismatic, bureaucratic, or even anarchistic leader, depending on the circumstances and leadership at the creation of the organization. The advocacy domain can provide a crucial impetus for improved agency performance, at least from the client's perspective (Dinkel et al., 1981). To implement the governing principles of client advocacy and agency oversight, clients may alternatively use conflict and participatory work modes, as appropriate. Conflict and protest were common work modes among client groups in the 1960s and early 1970s. In the mid-1970s, many agencies formulated rules (Windle and Paschall, 1981) and developed mechanisms (Zinober et al., 1980) to promote client and client group participation. There continues to be federal interest in methods for effectively involving clients in service programs (NIMH, 1991).

COOPERATION AND CONFLICT AMONG DOMAINS

A health promotion and education program can more easily be evaluated in agencies where each domain (1) cooperates with other domains to achieve agency ends, (2) has mutual respect for one another's operating characteristics, and (3) is open to the possibilities for growth and change. This state rarely exists, however, because conflict is more common than cooperation. The evaluator must understand the tensions within agencies to deal with them effectively.

The pattern of conflict and cooperation among domains is complex. For example, disagreement may exist about the long-term goals of an agency, but agreement and cooperative behaviors may exist on short-term goals. Domains may cooperate in some areas of activity, but conflict in others. Coalitions may form to cooperate on certain issues, but not others. Coalitions may be in conflict with other coalitions. A variety of factors lead to conflict or cooperation, including salary level, fringe benefits, and control over resources (power). Limited resources and funding are always in short supply; no agency has all the funds it would like. If one division or domain gets increased funding, that may mean less funding for the others. Colleagues do not shower prestige on everyone (or else it would not be considered prestige). Resources and incentives go to some people and not to others, to reward their effort and skill, to keep them working at a high level, and to demonstrate to others that increased skill and effort will be rewarded.

A certain amount of conflict in an agency is natural, a healthy outcome of competition for scarce resources. The desire for more salary, more benefits, more recognition from superiors and colleagues, or more resources is universal. At times, however, conflict can go beyond some poorly defined acceptable bound.

Conflict may also stem from structural differences among domains. People in one domain tend to relate to individuals in other domains by using operating principles that have worked in their domain. Imposing one domain's operating characteristics on another can have disastrous effects. For example, although it is possible to conceive of a clinic manager employing a completely representative, participatory management structure, there would be little specialization of activity under such a structure. Thus, secretaries may do accounting, accountants may do janitorial work, and janitors may make program management decisions. This is a violation of the "efficiency" measure of success, a strong component of management's operating characteristics. Similarly, it is difficult to conceive of physicians using voting as their work mode for deciding on the best therapy for a patient.

Different operating characteristics lead to conflict among domains. For example, improving the quality of health promotion or education programs often requires increased expenditures; increased expenditures may violate the cost-efficiency measure of success held by management. An extra expenditure of resources per unit of service may incur the wrath of managers who must take resources from other activities to meet the demands of the new activity. For example, health educators have been told by third-party payers that patient education programs can be implemented only if the costs of their programs reduce the cost of medical care by at least an equal amount (cost-effectiveness criterion) (Baranowski and Fuller, 1981).

THE EVALUATION DOMAIN

The domain concept is also useful in demonstrating the conflicts between health program evaluators and people in each of the domains, conflicts that lead to the types of comments at the beginning of this chapter. Although evaluation is usually located in the management or policy domain, the common conflict between evaluation and management (Connolly and Porter, 1980) indicates that evaluation has a unique set of operating characteristics, thereby justifying consideration as a separate domain. We will describe the operating characteristics of the evaluation domain in terms of dominant "ideal types"; few organizations manifest these characteristics precisely as characterized.

The evaluation domain can be structured in two ways. If the evaluator is based in a university, the organizational structure is often colleagial. If the evaluator works in a contract research organization or for the agency itself, the structure is likely to be bureaucratic, with some attempt to create a colleagial atmosphere. The governing principles are autonomy and self-regulation among university-based evaluators but hierarchical control and coordination among others. The primary work mode is the use of social and behavioral science methods within a client-specific problem-solving framework (rather than a hypothesis-testing framework). The evaluator attempts to address particular problems, case-by-case, using one or more social science tools. The measures of success often include direct use of the results in agency decision making, more effective agency performance (as a result of evaluative efforts), and production of a respectable report.

Conflicts with Other Domains

The identification of these evaluation operating characteristics points out differences from the other domains and highlights the conflicts that face an evaluator working within an agency. Conflicts have been recognized in the literature at the interface of the evaluation and management domains (Connolly and Porter, 1980). Cox (1977) reviewed the management literature and identified aspects of "managerial style" that sharply conflicted with evaluative style. He notes that managers must deal with vast amounts of information and make many different types of decisions in a short period of time. In contrast, evaluators intensively focus on a limited set of issues over a long period of time. The speedy managerial pace implies that the manager must deal with many issues in a brief and fragmented manner. The evaluator usually attempts to achieve some integrated conceptual whole. Managers are more interested in action, the evaluator in contemplation. Verbal communication fits more easily into the manager's style. To provide a comprehensive picture, written communications are more useful to evaluators. The manager prefers faster (less well-formulated) information to the slower, better formulated information preferred by the evaluator. Hawkins et al. (1978) empirically validate Cox's contention about the manager's preference for informal verbal information. Managerial style therefore comes into direct conflict with the more reflective, intensive, and written documented style of the evaluator.

Gurel (1975) identifies several conflicts encountered by evaluators. He notes that agencies are often caught in a dilemma: The organizational need for stability is in conflict with the need to understand and adapt to new problems. Managers and staff usually maintain stability. The evaluator is often working for organizational change. Gurel notes that, despite the popular perception of science (particularly the physical sciences but also the social sciences) as omniscient, the social sciences have not established a technology for promoting change. Agency people at all levels may thus have unrealistic expectations of how an evaluator can help them accomplish their goals. In addition, most people believe that effort expended in the service of a worthwhile end will produce positive results. Agency people find it difficult to accept predominantly negative evaluation findings. Such findings threaten the self-esteem of all agency domains and may threaten the financial security of particular projects. Gurel also notes that evaluations are frequently conducted on programs in serious trouble. Given the lack of effective technologies for change, evaluators and their methods can hardly assist such programs. From Gurel's perspective, the social setting in which evaluation is usually conducted generates tensions and conflicts before the evaluator has begun.

Weiss (1972) and Conner (1979) classify conflicts between the evaluative and management domains into major categories:

Personality differences

Differences in roles (management and commitment to the project as is vs. assessment and change of the project)

Lack of clear role definition (the activities and responsibilities of evaluators have never been clearly spelled out)

Conflicting goals, values, interests, and frames of reference

Institutional characteristics (primarily the conflict between the organizational structures and working modes of the two domains)

Aspects of evaluation methods and techniques (the obtrusiveness of questionnaires, random assignment, etc., into agency operations)

No one has reported on relationships between the evaluative and the policy, service, and advocacy domains. Undoubtedly, similar categories of conflict exist where these domains interface.

This brief overview of agency structure and interrelationships raises questions about evaluation. Is an objective evaluation always possible? Which domain's or faction's interests does a particular evaluation serve? What are the roles an evaluator can play in relation to other domains? How does an evaluator deal with all domains and factions in an agency?

Effects of Domain Conflicts on Evaluations

Clearly, evaluations employing objective techniques are not always possible. For example, a clinic manager may want to reduce the number of patient educators employed by the clinic. The manager may direct an evaluator to assess the demand for and effectiveness of educational services per unit of medical service. Money is not available for an observation study, however, so the evaluator must depend on specially designed forms completed by educators themselves. The manager and educators have a severe conflict of interest. The tension and conflict between these two domains may be so high that the educators may actively subvert the evaluation. They may provide responses to questions to improve their own performance image or devalue the manager's. Domains and factions tend to focus on a limited number of performance indicators to the detriment of overall performance (Campbell, 1975). The evaluator is thus always at the mercy of the people who complete the records to be used in an evaluative assessment. Unless a large evaluation budget and time are available, these record completers are always agency staff who are members of the various domains and factions with their vested interests.

Within a cauldron of conflicts and competitiveness, the perception of interest may be crucial. An evaluation introduced by one domain in conflict with another will be greeted with suspicion and defensiveness. In the preceding example, a full-blown evaluation focusing on patient educators' achievements may not be the best approach. Other evaluation options (reviewed in Chapter 1) are available that an evaluator may find useful.

Evaluations, program design, policy development, and the resource allocation are all value choices. Persons who direct or assist in program evaluation need to become adept at influencing an organization's written and unwritten agenda that determines what will actually get done. As Weiss notes,

> Only when the evaluator has insight into the interests and motivations of other actors in the system, into the roles that he himself is consciously or inadvertently playing, the obstacles and opportunities that impinge upon the evaluative effort, the limitations and possibilities for putting the results of evaluation to work—only with sensitivity to the politics of evaluation research—can the evaluator be as creative and strategically useful as he should be. (Weiss 1973a:50)

Possible Roles of the Evaluation Domain

Uzzel (1978) notes that the community agency researcher (this includes the program evaluator) can play four roles in relation to an agency and/or a research audience. Traditionally, the evaluator has played the role of "dispassionate outside observer or chronicler of social activity." An evaluator, however, might also play the roles of educator, broker of conflicts, or advocate of change. When each role is more appropriate will vary with circumstances. The evaluator may be in a position to remedy a knowledge deficit in the agency. When conflict exists between two domains, the evaluator may attempt to get each side to understand the other's position and may negotiate differences. Finally, an evaluator may be an advocate of his or her self-perceived need for change or may work with the advocacy domain to help its members achieve their perceived need for change.

This last role, advocate of change, identifies another sensitive evaluation situation. The common concept of the evaluator as an objective observer conflicts with the concept of an evaluator as change agent. This conflict reinforces the notion of evaluation as a separate domain. Evaluators, too, have vested interests in a variety of agency activities and actively pursue those interests. The interests include not only salary and fringe benefits but also influence in the agency, that is, utilization of evaluative reports in policy formulation, allocation of fiscal resources, agency management, and delivery of services. Maintaining the distinctiveness of the evaluation domain from the policy, management, service, and advocacy domains simultaneously may assist evaluation in being more "objective" in its findings and recommendations.

In the next section of this chapter, we discuss how an evaluator might conduct an evaluation to promote the changes identified in the final report, while negotiating the conflicting interests of the various domains and other vested interests in the agency.

UNDERSTANDING CHANGES THAT OCCUR NATURALLY

Change can be brought about in an agency despite conflict and the potential opposition of vested interests. Some change, after all, is a normal part of human experience. A change may be small and relatively insignificant (e.g., new typewriters, new time schedules for a service, or new record-keeping forms). Other changes, such as a new activity or procedure (e.g., contracting) introduced in connection with a prevention service (e.g., smoking cessation), have major impact. Some of these changes may occur naturally from changing circumstances, the decisions of leaders, or decisions made by other agencies. Other changes may be managed by individuals to achieve their own ends.

One approach to studying change that occurs naturally is associated with the theory of *diffusion of innovations*. This literature, reviewed by Greer (1977) in the area of health care organizations, has been primarily concerned with patterns in the introduction of a change to a set of organizations over time, rather than with the change process within a particular organization. Several authors have mapped the change rate in introducing a new practice, that is, the number of agencies adopting a new idea or practice over sequential units of time. This change rate has been labeled the *diffusion cycle*. Diffusion theorists have studied differences between those who adopt new ideas or practices early in a diffusion cycle (early innovators) and those who adopt them later. They have also studied differences in the characteristics of innovative ideas or practices that may result in quicker or slower change. Greer suggests that change occurs in three stages within each organization: (1) idea entry and consideration, (2) change decisions, and (3) change implementation. She describes these stages as follows:

> In the ideas stage, information and creativity are very important. This stage requires flexibility, circulation of ideas, a variety of perspectives, and freedom from threat of excessive discipline. At the adoption (decision) stage, other factors become important: motivation, resources, and the ability to reach a consensus. In the final implementing stage, such factors as perceived legitimacy, disruptiveness, displacement, and trust become important. (Greer, 1977:519)

Another approach to understanding change that occurs naturally derives from analysis of the conflict among domains and factions (vested interests). Greer reports on the principles of intraorganizational change propounded by Roos (1974), from a political analysis of organizational decision making. Changes occur "(1) when there are changes in the goals of powerful groups . . . ; (2) when the power of opposition groups is decreased . . . ; (3) when the power of proponent groups increases . . . ; (4) when the old structure becomes obsolete for achieving goals . . . ; (5) when performance gaps provide impetus for change" (Greer, 1977:525–526).

These general rules about relationships among domains or factions in promoting change apply to any agency. The health program evaluator should therefore know the goals of powerful groups in the agency, the relative power of these groups, how aspects of the organizational structure are used to achieve each group's ends, and differences between expected and actual performance for each group. The evaluator might be particularly valuable in designing alternative structures and might play an influential role by maintaining records of performance.

PROMOTING ORGANIZATION CHANGE

Porras and Silvers (1991) present a comprehensive model for promoting organization change. Three models for the management of agency change have been identified: the management consultant, the evaluator-managed, and the open-system problem-solving models.

Management Consultant Model

The management consultant model for promoting change through evaluation has been most clearly described by Ziegenfuss and Lasky (1975a, 1975b, 1980). The evaluator develops a relationship with the management domain and focuses primarily on management concerns in five areas: administration, agency services, fiscal management, legal matters, and service system. Ziegenfuss and Lasky's focus was not service outcomes but primarily organizational structure. Two examples of evaluative questions raised within this model are, Is there a statement of board roles and responsibilities? Are there procedures to protect the civil rights of clients, for example, protecting the privacy of people who attend health education programs?

Ziegenfuss and Lasky see this type of evaluation as useful early in the development of a program, to ensure that the program is developing along rational lines. For example, failure to protect privacy could result in the client's embarrassment or worse. Although all domains (except the clients') participate in self-assessment precipitated by evaluator questions, this method takes the easiest approach to evaluation: dealing primarily with one domain, management. The report is made primarily to the management. This can be an effective model early in an organization's development, when there is little conflict among domains and when the primary concerns of all domains are expressed in the report. There is no provision in this model for the resolution of domain conflict, but an evaluation of this type may result in clarification of potential problems.

Evaluator-Managed Model

Several authors (Schulberg and Jerrel, 1979) suggest that the evaluator align with management. This course is recommended because the manager is usually in the pivotal role, relating to all other domains and dispensing resources. Although attractive, this approach fails to recognize that management is not the sole domain to make decisions. Each domain makes decisions crucial to achieving agency goals: The board makes policy decisions; management makes management decisions; service renderers make service decisions; clients make advocacy decisions. A balanced evaluation should reflect the interests and perspectives of each domain. This will improve the evaluation, prevent one domain from foisting an evaluation on the others, and prevent one domain from subverting the evaluation.

Polivka and Steg (1978) provide examples of evaluator-managed change. They report on an overhaul of the organizational structure of the Florida Department of Health and Rehabilitative Services, placing the evaluation unit in a position to approve the continued funding and structure of all agency units and programs. An evaluation analysis and policy development process were established in which management and service domains of all programs periodically participate in evaluations to reach a consensus on recommendations for continuity and change. Many evaluators would find this an exciting model because they have "clout" in the agency's decision making. However, the authors report that, after 6 months, the evaluation unit was given more and more administrative responsibilities, becoming, in effect, part of the management domain. The danger of this approach is that evaluators may assume the conceptual styles, concerns, working modes, and the like of management and lose their perspective and objectivity on the needs and operating modes of other domains.

Open-System Problem-Solving Model

French and Becker (1975) see particular promise for an open-system problem-solving approach to managing change. In this model, the evaluator is no longer the "font of truth" but instead uses data collection and analyses, among other techniques, to clarify problems and to promote compromise, cooperation, and coordination among competing domains. Many authors have contributed to and commented on this approach (Argyris, 1970; Delbecq, 1978; Dickey and Hampton, 1981; Glaser and Taylor, 1973; Reppucci, 1973; Van de Ven and Koenig, 1976). We present Van de Ven's (1980a, 1980b) approach in greater detail because it encompasses the major ideas of the other authors and has been shown by experimental study to be superior to a method in which no systematic planning is conducted.

The basic problem-solving model was first presented by Van de Ven and Koenig (1976). They propose a seven-phase model for program planning and evaluation:

Phase 1, prerequisites to planning

Phase 2, problem exploration

Phase 3, knowledge exploration

Phase 4, program design

Phase 5, program activation

Phase 6, program operation and diffusion

Phase 7, program evaluation

Table 2.4 Characteristics of the Problem-Solving Approach to Program Evaluation

Phase	Task	Primary Participants	Strategy	Function
1. Prerequisites to planning	Establish a representative evaluation committee Identify the evaluation unit Agree to evaluation sequence	Leaders, all domains		Domain involvement
2. Problem exploration	Conduct an assessment of agency and program strengths and weaknesses	People, all domains	Inspiration	Problem appreciation
3. Knowledge exploration	Bring the best available expertise to bear	Experts	Judgment	Raising program staff's ideas
4. Evaluation design	Reach agreement on major issues Design an evaluation method	Leaders, all domains	Negotiation and compromise	Debate Negotiation
5. Evaluation implementation	Conduct the evaluation and produce a detailed report	Evaluators	Computation	
6. Evaluation dissemination	Work with all domains in reviewing evaluation findings	Leaders, all domains	Negotiation and compromise	Institutionalization of selected ideas

In later publications, phases 5–7 were condensed into a single phase (Van de Ven, 1980a, 1980b). Table 2.4 lists the primary characteristics of each phase in the problem-solving approach to program-evaluation.

Case Study 1: Smoking-Cessation for Coal Miners

At a rural primary-care clinic in a coal-mining area, the board of directors insisted that a smoking-cessation program be developed because of evidence that black lung disease (coal miner's pneumoconiosis) develops primarily among coal miners who smoke. The health educator on staff developed a program to be used by the nurses in the clinic with all coal miner patients (clients). Because implementation required considerable nursing time and other clinic resources, the board wanted to ensure that the benefits justified the effort.

In response, the health educator developed a program evaluation. As a first step (phase 1), the health educator arranged with the chairperson of the board and the clinic administrator to establish an evaluation committee. The committee included the board member who was most vocal in instigating the smoking-cessation program, the director of clinic finances (the person who raised the issue about the project's cost), the nurse who was most interested in implementing the program, a client with whom the program seemed to have been successful, and one with whom the program had failed.

The first meeting was spent primarily in having committee members get to know one another. At the second meeting (phase 2), the committee agreed that smoking cessation is a true need of coal miners. They also agreed that there were enough nurses to implement the program, but they were concerned that the nurses did not have adequate interest in and skills for the project. Several nurses had said they were overworked and didn't need additional responsibilities.

Two specialists from the local state university were invited to attend the third meeting (phase 3). The smoking-cessation specialist indicated that the methods employed in the program were standard and seemed to work well with volunteers who were smokers. The nursing educator specialist noted that nurses in high-volume, rural primary-care clinics were prone to "burnout" because of extensive responsibilities, seemingly endless demands on their time, and their perceived lack of control over specific tasks. The lack of control deprived them of the satisfaction of achievement.

The fourth meeting had to be canceled because the two coal miners on the committee had to attend a union meeting. At the fifth meeting (phase 4), the evaluation committee decided that three questions had to be answered in evaluating the project: (1) Was the program reaching miners? (2) Were miners stopping smoking at least as frequently as reported in the literature on smoking cessation in the general population? (3) How did staff nurses feel about the program?

Before the sixth meeting, the health educator designed a survey of nurses' attitudes toward the project and a survey of miners who had been in the clinic's care for the duration of the project. The miner survey aimed to determine if miners had been contacted by a nurse about smoking cessation and if they had given up smoking during this period. At the sixth meeting, the committee accepted the design of the evaluator's study and decided to expand the second survey to include a random sample of all adult clients (18 years or older) registered with the clinic. Data collection (phase 5) started following the sixth meeting.

At the seventh meeting, the evaluator reported on the progress of data collection. As a result, the nursing representative spoke to several nurses to speed their return of nursing questionnaires. The board and client representatives were asked to contact several noncooperating clinic patients to get them to agree to an interview.

At the eighth meeting, the committee learned that all nurses but two were antagonistic to the new smoking-cessation program, the program was reaching more nonminer clients (mostly women) than miners, and approximately 50% of all patients reached by the program had given up smoking for up to 2 months. The data indicated, however, that about 50% of people not reached by the program had also given up smoking in the last 6 months. In addition, 50% of the miners expressed interest in quitting smoking; of these, 75% preferred self-learning materials to an intensive clinic-based program.

Before the ninth meeting, the committee members discussed the evaluation results with members of their respective domains. The board member still felt that a smoking-cessation program was important for reaching miners and preventing black lung disease. The nurse educator was still excited about the program but was receiving very negative comments from her colleagues. The finance director was concerned about costs. Both patient representatives appreciated the attention given to all health care consumers at the clinic.

At the ninth and tenth meetings (phase 6), a compromise was reached. All but two nurses were relieved of responsibility for the program. These two, who had been most supportive, were assigned primarily to implementation of this project. The two nurses and the health educator were also asked to develop a smoking-cessation self-instruction package for miners. Once these materials were developed, the clinic clerical staff were to contact all miners in the clinic, find out which ones smoked, and discover who was interested in a self-instruction package for stopping smoking and who would participate in a smoking-cessation clinic. Miner clients were to be contacted over the next 2 years to avoid overburdening the staff. Other clinic clients were offered places in the intensive smoking-cessation group sessions, filling slots left empty by miners (thereby increasing efficiency).

The committee decided that some collaborative planning process should have been used in designing the original smoking-cessation program to avoid some of the problems that surfaced. The committee also agreed on an evaluation procedure that could be implemented with the start of the new smoking-cessation program (phase 7).

> This approach resulted in a smoking-cessation program for coal min-
> ers with greater chance for success, reflecting the interests and concerns
> of each domain. The committee was able to facilitate various stages of
> the evaluation process.

Why did French and Becker (1975) suggest that this open-system
model was such a valuable approach? Van de Ven (1980a) presents
data showing how it was used in 11 experimental and control-group
communities. The experimental communities performed better on
several outcome indicators. The open-system procedure effectively
dealt with social change by enabling conflicting interests to focus on
only a limited set of issues at one time and by negotiating and resolving the conflicts step-by-step (Van de Ven, 1980b). Dickey and Hampton (1981) argue that such a problem-solving evaluation model will
promote intraagency (interdomain) communication patterns that identify and solve problems more effectively.

Other studies support aspects of the open-system problem-
solving model. Weeks (1979) found, to his surprise, that the greater
the number of participants in an evaluation decision (especially early
in the evaluation-design process), the more likely it was that the
evaluation information would be used. Assessing five different models from a review of over 100 case studies of evaluation utilization,
Dunn found moderate-to-strong support for the following hypothesis: "The greater the overall influence of social scientists, policy makers and other *stake-holders* in each phase of the policy-making process,
the greater the knowledge utilization" (1980:530).

Windle and his colleagues (Windle and Cibulka, 1981; Windle
and Paschall, 1981) and others (Dindle et al., 1981; Zinober et al.,
1980) argue that clients and interested citizens have a right to participate in an agency's evaluation. They further hold that the evaluation
results will more likely be used if clients participate.

Under the open-system model, maintaining evaluation as a separate domain has important advantages. Evaluators will not be perceived as foisting one domain's set of operating characteristics or
interests on other domains. Working separately enables the evaluator
to facilitate resolution of the conflicts among other domains. What is
most important, evaluators can define and maintain the operating
characteristics appropriate to their own activities, which differ from
those of the other domains. In this way, the evaluation domain can
become a creative force within an agency, attempting to promote
change that makes the agency's program more responsive to internally and externally perceived needs.

Working as a separate domain also involves certain risks—isola-
tion of evaluators from other domains. Conner (1979) emphasizes the
importance of evaluators maintaining a cooperative and collegial

attitude to all evaluation participants and showing up at service-delivery sites to demonstrate a shared commitment to the project. Conner argues that these activities develop trust between evaluators and the other domains. This leads to their mutual respect and a minimum of conflict. Evaluators must appreciate the interdependence of all domains and work to promote trust, respect, and cooperation in the evaluative task. Guba and Lincoln (1989) in fourth generation evaluation provide a full discussion of how contemporary evaluations can address the issues raised by domains.

SUMMARY

In this chapter, we have emphasized one of the evaluator's many roles—agent of change. To promote change effectively, the evaluator must be aware of the domains and interest groups in an agency, their self-interests, and their operating modes. In working with domains and interest groups, the evaluator must promote a joint problem-definition and problem-solving orientation. This process requires the competing interests within an agency to collaborate in a phased sequence of steps in which problems are clearly defined, the greatest number of alternatives are clearly specified, and data are used to make selections from among alternatives. The project design must incorporate the most appropriate scientific approaches and data-collection methods for answering questions about the program under evaluation. The evaluator must be aware of the forces that tend to perpetuate the status quo and have the ability to control them. These propositions, if followed, are likely to result in evaluations that are on target, have the support of all concerned, and result in improvements to the benefit of all concerned.

3

Program Planning and Planning for Evaluation

"Why didn't we think of this before the program began?"

"Good grief, you mean we've been teaching breathing exercises to asthma patients, and these exercises have no relationship to improving lung function?"

"I thought this program would lead to fewer hospitalizations, but that outcome was never logically possible."

"I don't understand why the medical department won't cooperate in this program."

Professional Competencies Emphasized in This Chapter

• Describing the influence of the sponsoring organization on a health education program

• Describing the membership and usefulness of a health education planning network

• Defining needs assessment

• Analyzing a health problem and the logical connections between the problem, an educational program to address it, the impact of the program on learners, and related outcomes

• Defining the steps of health education program planning and a health education program plan

In Chapter 2, we focused on the role of the evaluator and the potential for evaluation to bring change within an organization and community. In this chapter, we discuss development of the educational program to be evaluated. In many, if not most, cases, the health educator oversees the planning, implementation, and evaluation of an educational program. The program plan is a road map—the blueprint to ensure that the program is logical, addresses learning needs, and can be evaluated. The plan consolidates staff thinking. Among the collaborators in planning, of course, are the population-at-risk. Frequently, involving probable participants directly in planning is possible. At a minimum, individuals who represent the population-at-risk's interests must be among the planners.

Besides ensuring that the program is well conceived, good planning also helps mobilize beforehand the information, people, and resources critical to program success. A plan is always necessary to secure funds. A plan provides guidelines for program instructors and enables programs to be replicated. The plan, then, is the comprehensive document to ensure that a program is sound and engenders the support needed for implementing it.

In this chapter, we focus on the steps to develop a program plan and emphasize program evaluation as part of the planning process. Initially, we discuss some important basic concepts for program developers: the organizational context for planning, the planning network, needs assessment, and the links from a program to new behavior and related outcomes. Later, we discuss a step-by-step process of developing the program plan.

THE ORGANIZATIONAL CONTEXT FOR
HEALTH PROMOTION AND EDUCATION

When researchers and academicians plan health education and promotion interventions, they try to manipulate the environment so theories can be applied and hypotheses tested. In the day-to-day operation of health education, however, practitioners must accept realities and try to build into their plan ways to manage existing situations. Often, staff have limited control over the conditions in which programs are developed and delivered. Nonetheless, a standard of practice is that programs need to be based on valid principles and theories. Successfully planning and evaluating a theory-based program can be difficult. For example, existing theory suggests that developing ongoing peer support groups with the same members meeting over time may enable chronically ill people to acquire the social support needed to manage their illness (Israel and Rounds, 1987). But, given the work schedules of patients, available meeting places, a limited budget, or other factors, it may be very difficult to apply this principle fully.

In practice, educators try to come as close as they can to theoretical conditions that enable positive change to occur. As discussed in Chapter 2, they continually try to bring about needed changes in employing organizations and communities, changes to enable them to come even closer to creating optimum conditions for behavior changes (Clark, 1978). Evaluation research, or Type 4 evaluation discussed in Chapter 1, manipulates the environment to test hypotheses. Program evaluations, or Type 3, contribute to the knowledge base of health promotion and education by assessing and describing the application of knowledge in similar settings and situations. Ultimately, the program evaluations you will conduct as part of your daily health work form the basis on which a theory becomes accepted as generally valid. The challenge for the field of health promotion and education is to develop programs and to conduct evaluations to bridge the theory-and-practice gap.

Philosophy of the Organization

Health promotion and education specialists are employed by health-related agencies and organizations to develop programs. Although this book has broad utility for a wide range of professionals, it is primarily to these professionals that this book is addressed. Working with an organization means that you must represent in programming not only your own view, objectives, and philosophy but also those of your employing organization. Sometimes there is conflict between what an individual believes and the goals of the organization. If you find yourself in such a quandary and no reconciliation of ideas can be achieved, you need to make a personal and professional decision about whether to work with organizational goals unlike your own. Deciding to proceed is likely to create a difficult situation and would probably preclude effective work. You may, instead, find another organization and setting where the philosophy and views are more in line with yours. Some educators volunteer their assistance to individuals and groups to develop programs that espouse particular political and philosophical views. Educators can then emphasize views they believe are particularly important, unencumbered by the need to represent an employer. In presenting the steps of program development in these pages, we assume that staff must pay attention to the mission and interests of an employing organization. We also assume that you will choose employment with an agency whose goals are consistent with your values.

Impetus for the Program

In the field of practice, there are three basic ways in which health promotion and education programs come into being. The educator sees the need to design a program: "We really need to develop a hypertension education program for the elderly. We've got to improve the quality and the cost effectiveness of our service. Shall I develop something for you and the budget people?" Or you are asked to design a program that, according to someone else, the agency's clients need: "Larry, given the data on hypertension in the elderly, the board of directors feels we should get a hypertension education program off the ground. Please develop something that we might get the budget to support." Or you are asked to design a program on the basis of what clients want: "Joan, what kind of health education do our elderly clients need and want? Find out and put together something. Then, let's see what kind of budget we'd need."

Orientation and Goals of the Organization

Regardless of who initiates the program, it is likely to be organized in one of two ways: (1) as part of ongoing activities providing related health services directly to clients and (2) as a project by groups that provide no direct medical or nursing service. For example, hypertension education may be part of the senior citizen program of a local health department. Health department physicians or nurses may be on staff and available to treat program participants diagnosed as hypertensive. Similarly, the program may be part of the services of a general medical clinic that has a large elderly population and where physicians routinely see hypertensive clients. In other words, health promotion and education is developed to be integrated into ongoing work of an organization with a wider set of health service activities.

On the other hand, the hypertension education program might be developed as an activity of a senior citizen center where the aim is to assist the elderly with many concerns, including health. In this case, participants will be referred elsewhere if they need medical or nursing services. Similarly, the community education program may be developed by a private voluntary agency, say Citizens for a Better Community, and directed to all the elderly in an area. Such a program might recruit physicians and nurses to participate, if they are needed, or might refer people to available services when necessary. The important aspect to note about these latter two examples is that health education is part of a broader community effort and not of medical or nursing services.

It is also likely that, in organizations where health promotion and education are part of a larger set of medical and nursing activities, health may be narrowly defined to mean primarily those conditions that document the absence or reduction of the diseases of organizational interest. Health related to hypertension, for example, may mean having normal blood pressure (120/80). In organizations where health promotion and education are not tied to medical and nursing services, health may have a much broader definition. Health for the senior citizens, for example, may include such things as practicing a range of good personal health habits (Simmons et al., 1989) or having social contact with other people (Shinn et al., 1984). In medical settings, health is frequently defined in light of medical or nursing objectives. In community settings, health is frequently defined more holistically.

The emphases of evaluations conducted by an organization will depend on how it defines health. Both the goals of health promotion and education and the goals of evaluations are greatly influenced by the orientation of the sponsoring organization. Organizations give priority to programs that further their primary goals. Health care organizations tend to be oriented primarily toward communities or individuals and toward disease treatment, management, or prevention.

If an organization serves individuals, it will tend to focus on what people can do to improve their health. Such an organization (e.g., a hospital) might develop patient education to assist diabetic patients to self-administer medications. The focus is on the individual and an individual solution to the health problem. If an organization has a community orientation, it tends to focus more on a broader kind of change; it looks for communitywide solutions.

As an example, assume a health problem exists in an area because health services are inadequate or because people cannot afford to eat nutritious food or buy necessary medications. A community-oriented organization might organize and educate people to work collectively to bring about changes in health care delivery or might develop cooperatives to cut costs of buying food or medications. In other words, health education favored by a community-oriented organization might focus on assisting groups of people to change conditions in the physical, social, or political environments that have a negative impact on their health.

For the program planner, a cardinal rule is to know the organizational context well before starting a program. You must understand organizational goals and orientation as they relate to the problem in question.

As you consider your program in light of the variety of organizations that sponsor it, you may ask a question frequently posed: Is the objective of education always behavior change? We would answer yes in the sense that behavior change is sought within the context of social change. Rarely is an individual's behavior under that person's total control. Public health education almost always tries to stimulate organizational and community changes to enable people to acquire the resources and services necessary for healthful living (Clark and Wolderufael, 1977). This is particularly apparent when education has a community-action orientation; but it is also the case, as discussed in Chapter 2, when the program is oriented toward individual change.

All programs operate on the assumption that people will be different as a result of their participation. This assumption is easy to understand when a program focuses on individuals and disease management. Hypertension education for an elderly woman, for example, should enable her to reduce her sodium intake—to behave in a new way. It is more difficult to see behavior change as the goal if the program focuses on communities and prevention. Assume, for the sake of discussion, that your program wants to help people improve inadequate housing in a community. A goal may be to organize groups to demand service from the city housing authority or to bring suit against recalcitrant landlords. Although housing may improve because the housing department or landlords send workers to make repairs, participant behavior has presumably led to this outcome. Even when the goal is to change the conditions that obstruct good health, it is people who bring about the change by behaving in a different way. These behaviors may include such things as being more assertive, being more vocal, exercising more community leadership, and participating more in cooperative activities (Clark and Gakuru, 1982;

Clark and Pinkett-Heller, 1977). An important part of planning a program evaluation is to anticipate what changes in behavior may occur and what other related changes might occur and to determine if and how such changes might be measured. We will discuss this further in a later section.

THE HEALTH PROMOTION PLANNING NETWORK

Regardless of the type of sponsoring organization, planning is very rarely a unilateral activity. The design, implementation, and evaluation of a program always involves a network of people: representatives of the target group, you (the program planner), others in your organization, and representatives of outside organizations who provide needed services and resources. Another cardinal rule of program development is that to be effective they should always be planned with the participation of major interest groups.

If a program fails to account for the learner's perspective, it cannot possibly appeal to potential learners' motives or enable them to see the relevance of the learning to their situation. Without the participation of potential participants, it is entirely possible to plan a program that misses the vital ingredient that will enable participants to behave in a new way or will change conditions that inhibit healthful behavior (Bruner, 1973). Without the views of those who provide needed related services, it is very difficult to mobilize the resources and cooperation to carry out a comprehensive program.

Good health seems to be everyone's goal, but views on what it is and how to get it differ enormously. Therefore, part of program planning is to reach some agreements with those who will collaborate with you in the program. Figure 3.1 illustrates the network of contacts you need to establish when planning a program. You will want to involve representatives from some or all areas when making decisions about learning needs, program objectives, learning activities, and evaluation procedures.

NEEDS ASSESSMENT

The program planner seeks to match the needs and wants of the target audience, the sponsoring organization, and the community. Therefore, needs assessment comprises a large part of your first steps of program planning. *Needs assessment* is generally defined as the process by which the program planner identifies and measures gaps between what is and what ought to be. Some educators refer to service needs and service demands or wants (Brehony et al., 1984; Kurtz and

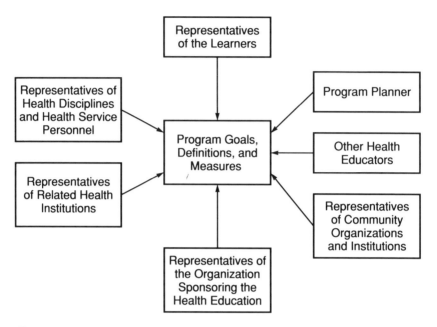

Figure 3.1 The Program Planning Network

Boone, 1981). Generally, *service needs* are those things health professionals believe a given population must have or be able to do in order to resolve a health problem. *Service demands* are those things people say they must have or be able to do in order to resolve their health problem. Service demands also include things a patient wants in order to be more satisfied with health services.

Real needs and perceived, or felt, needs also must be assessed. Real needs, like service needs, are determined by using clinical and epidemiological data, health service utilization statistics, or other empirical data. Perceived, or felt, needs, like service demands, refer to problems as viewed or understood by the people who experience them. Neither category of needs is infallible or inherently correct. Programs must account for both. Consider, for example, an asthma education program designed to teach parents how to manage their young children's disease. Physicians are likely to describe the real, or service, needs as knowing how to correctly use asthma medications and how to set up an appropriate schedule of medical visits. Parents are likely to feel that they need to know how to decide which physical activities a child with asthma can undertake. Both "real" and "felt" needs are critical to successful asthma management (Clark et al., 1980).

During the process of needs assessment, you must look ahead to what ought to be, collecting and analyzing data to set your objectives. Conversely, in a program evaluation, the evaluator looks back on what was, collecting and analyzing data on what occurred in a program, given what was expected. There can be no effective program or program evaluation without a good needs assessment.

A needs assessment is carried out on two levels. The first level is to document what is and to compare it to what ought to be. As noted in Figure 3.1, several groups must be involved. The second level is finding a fit between the needs and what the sponsoring organization can do. As you develop a program, keep in mind that it must provide some benefit to your organization, or the organization will have no reason to continue sponsorship. A program that benefits the organization at the expense of the patient, however, rarely will succeed.

Needs assessment can provide data on how collaborators in the program will benefit, if goals are met. To illustrate, consider the conclusions drawn by planners of two actual programs, after they analyzed their needs assessment data. First, in a project sponsored by a large metropolitan hospital to help families with a child who has asthma to learn to manage the illness better, planners asked, What do families need and want in regard to this problem? What does the hospital need and want? Existing and newly collected data provided the following picture: Asthma is the leading chronic illness of childhood in terms of the number of children it strikes and the days of absenteeism from school that it causes (Hill et al., 1989). Fear associated with asthma is the source of much disruption and stress within a family. Having asthma can lead to excessive emergency room visits. Asthma has been said to detract from a child's positive view of himself or herself (Freudenberg et al., 1980). From this picture, the planners could postulate the following benefits: If a family were assisted to develop confidence and expand its range of asthma management skills, the family might experience lower stress and increased normalization of activities of daily living, that is, an improvement in the quality of life. The hospital might benefit by reducing the number of inappropriate and expensive emergency room visits. The community might benefit by lowering school-system costs because of chronic absenteeism. Medical and nursing personnel might benefit because patients are more involved in their own care and "do better" in their treatment plans.

The second example is an employee diet-and-exercise program for cardiovascular risk reduction. Again, the planners in a large insurance company asked, What do employees want and need? How would the company benefit from such a program? Employees, they determined, might benefit more by simply feeling and looking better than from the knowledge that they theoretically would reduce their chances of heart attacks (Morris, 1980). Families might benefit by having a happier, healthier member. Employers might benefit because employee satisfaction with work might increase and worker illness and absenteeism might be reduced (Klesges et al., 1989).

In short, it is reasonable to believe that participation will produce rewards and that a program will answer needs, real and perceived. It is also reasonable to believe that evaluators will be able to measure the extent to which a program met the needs that it was expected to meet.

THE CONNECTION BETWEEN PROGRAM, IMPACT, AND RELATED HEALTH OUTCOMES

The purpose of needs assessment is to look forward, to determine what ought to be, and to set program objectives. The primary purpose of evaluation is to measure the impact of the program. Impact is the extent to which behavior is changed as a result of program participation. You also want to know if new behavior is associated with improved physiological and psychological health. In addition, you want to know if changes in behavior led to health status outcomes. In an asthma education program, these may include reduced number of hospitalizations, fewer emergencies, and lower medical costs. If the education is for community action to improve housing and nutrition, outcomes may include an increased number of repairs to correct housing violations, increased membership in a food-buying cooperative, and a permanent positive change in the services of local health facilities. Presumably, your program will change behavior, and the new behavior will stimulate other changes. As illustrated in Figure 3.2, a logical sequence exists that underlies program development.

As an example of how the logical connections can be made, consider again the case of asthma education. Following a needs assessment, planners may decide that intended new behaviors should include using breathing exercises and productive cough before and after an asthma attack. Improved health status will be defined as improved pulmonary functioning and fewer severe wheezing episodes. Parents who learn to use breathing exercises and productive cough with their children, and who learn to distinguish minor from serious symptoms may be less fearful during a child's wheezing episode and may be better able to calm the child. As a result of less fear and improved ability to distinguish symptoms, families may seek emergency services less often. Consequently, the hospital may save money or spend less on emergency services for children with asthma. In other

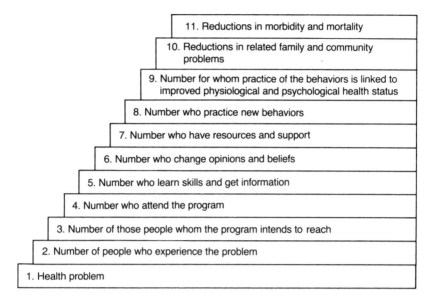

Figure 3.2 Logical Relationship of a Health Problem, a Program, and Anticipated Outcomes

words, the program and program evaluations must be planned in a logical sequence making links from the problem to learning activities to new behavior to improved health status and related outcomes.

You can see immediately from this example that, when programs are planned to introduce people to new behavior and to realize related outcomes, the educator must depend to a greater or lesser degree on the knowledge and actions of professionals in different fields. You must determine what encourages or hinders a family in adopting new behavior. You must know, for example, what conditions, factors, information, and skills will enable the family with asthma to practice breathing exercises. Similarly, you must know how to organize and deliver a program to help a family increase its information, develop skills, change conditions, and behave differently. You will often count on colleagues in other fields—you must turn to medical colleagues for knowledge of the factors linked to improved pulmonary functioning and the symptoms of severe wheezing. Suppose basic epidemiological research and clinical trials do *not* confirm that breathing exercises improve pulmonary-functioning level or that the association is equivocal. Thus, the pulmonary health status of children in the program may not improve even if the children regularly practice breathing exercises.

The measure of the success or failure of the asthma health education program is the occurrence and extent of new behavior among the children. The positive effect of the behavior on the physiological status of the child is a measure of medical success. If the connection between behavior and health status does not exist, you should not include the behavior in a program aimed to change health status. If the connection is questionable (basic research has shown both a connection and no connection), you must usually depend on the consensus of colleagues with expertise about the efficacy of a new behavior (attributable risk). In the case of asthma, for example, breathing exercises have not been shown to have a definitive connection with pulmonary functioning. There is general consensus, however, among patient educators and physicians that other psychological benefits result from the exercises. These benefits include increasing a person's ability to relax, providing a sense of control over the illness, and feeling that he or she is taking an action (not being passive) in the face of the illness (Clark et al., 1986).

When you evaluate the occurrence and extent of outcomes related to changes in behavior and health status, you also have to depend on the judgment and decisions of others. If, for example, needed health services are not available, are too costly, or are inappropriately organized, it will take much more than an asthma education program to realize desired outcomes. Assume that the optimum management of asthma (management that is least disruptive and time-consuming for families) entails periodic preventive visits to a clinic. Assume also that health services in the community are financed in such a way that it is cheaper for a family to visit the hospital emergency room in a time of crisis than it is to visit the clinic on a regular basis. An asthma education program may provide valid information that preventive visits are best. However, the structure of services at the hospital may not make such behavior beneficial to families. If this is the case, emergency room visits and related costs to the hospital will likely not decrease as a result of the program. Planners might then decide that the program must be preceded by changes in the hospitals' financial arrangements or that a more appropriate health education program would inform and organize families to push for changes in the structure and financing of community health services.

The efficacy and effectiveness of a health education program, then, is affected by the knowledge and actions of people in other disciplines. By involving professionals from relevant disciplines in the planning process, you obtain the expertise needed to forge clear links between the program, new behavior, and related outcomes. In planning the program evaluation, the knowledge of professionals in relevant fields is critical to help you determine which changes can and should be measured. Because new behavior is the objective of all interventions, it has priority for program evaluation. Once you have planned how to document the occurrence and extent of new behavior, you can decide which related outcomes can and should be evaluated.

THE BASIC PROGRAM PLANNING QUESTIONS

To design a program to meet the needs of a group of learners, a sponsoring organization, and a community, you must find answers to several questions, posed below. In securing answers to questions 1–6, you are doing a needs assessment. In answering questions 7 and 8, you are planning the program evaluation. Answers to questions 9 and 10 will give you a good idea of what educational methods and materials will be effective. Questions 11 and 12 deal with administrative aspects of a program. Their answers will help you plan training, logistics, and finances.

1. What are the condition-specific and people-specific dimensions of the health problem?

    a. Condition-specific: How does the health problem in which you are interested (e.g., cardiovascular disease) occur in the group-at-risk (e.g., middle-class senior citizens)? What is the incidence and prevalence rate? What aspects of the problem are unique to the group? How might the rates change if the health problem were addressed through education? How would people's behavior have to change to reduce the health problem?

    b. People-specific: What is the health problem of greatest priority for the group-at-risk? What is the rate of the health problem in that group? What would you expect the situation to be if the problem were addressed through education? How would people behave? What would their lives be like regarding the problem? How would conditions be different?

2. What specific behaviors must be acquired or strengthened to reduce the effect of the problem?

3. What information and skills must a person have to be able to behave in the new way?

4. What resources, personal and material, must a person have to behave in the new way (e.g., children will not learn to brush their teeth well and regularly without encouragement and a toothbrush)? Are these resources available, or can they be obtained at a low cost?

5. What kind of health or community services or other circum-

stances are needed to enable people to change to the desired behaviors? Are they available, or can they be arranged?

6. Which behaviors can be addressed by an education program? What learning objectives would be consistent with your organization's capabilities, orientation, and goals?

7. Which behavior changes can and should you try to measure? What specific measures will you use? When will measurements be taken?

8. What wider changes in conditions and situations would you expect to see if the group-at-risk adopts the new behavior? What changes would you see in individuals, families, and communities? How can these outcomes be measured? Which will you try to measure? When will you take measurements?

9. What theories of behavior and learning are most relevant for the population, problem, and behaviors to be learned? What learning principles are the bases for your program?

10. What educational techniques based on the learning principles will best present information, develop skills, provide support, and create an appropriate learning environment, given your particular audience and the desired behaviors? How can you monitor the quality and efficacy of the educational activities?

11. What organizational and logistical support arrangements are needed? What kind of orientation or training is needed for personnel?

12. What budget do you need? Can you provide the program with the existing budget? What cost is your organization willing to bear?

THE STEPS OF PROGRAM PLANNING

Following a set of program-planning steps will help you find the answers to these 12 questions.

Step 1: Analyzing the Health Problem Among the Population-at-Risk

In evaluation research, which is designed to develop a profession's knowledge base, there is a high degree of freedom to select problems and specify hypotheses to be tested. In the usual practice of health education, however, the educator generally selects or is given problems based on the missions, interests, and immediate objectives of the employing organization. These problems tend to be people-specific or condition-specific. The more narrowly defined the problem is and the more narrow the focus on a specific group-at-risk, the higher the chance of successfully documenting change. Although some health educators continue to mount general information programs for a general audience, the relative value of these efforts in achieving behavior change is difficult to ascertain. The relationship between general information programs and broader community change is almost impossible to document.

A goal of the first step of program planning is to define the health problem in specific enough terms to know how education may help resolve it. Similarly, you must know enough about the population-at-risk to be sure you see the problem the way they see it. The intervention must be relevant.

Assume, for example, that the health problem of interest to your organization is sedentary lifestyle—lack of activity. Obviously, this problem and a program to address it are quite different for senior citizens than for schoolchildren. They would be different for residents of a middle-class suburban community than for those of a poor, urban one. The information, skills, resources, and support needed to change behavior vary from group to group. This is not to say that there are no differences within groups; there are. The first step, however, is to describe the group of people with whom you will work, in terms of some pervasive similarities and common experiences with the problem: demographic, geographical, cultural, psychological, physiological, or historical. Similarities may also relate to the way people use health services, what they expect about health, or similar factors that give rise to common experience.

As discussed earlier, you may decide to begin with condition-specific planning. In that case, start with the health condition, lack of adequate exercise, and determine, from the range of clients you serve, for which group is the condition a priority problem. Alternatively, you may decide on people-specific planning and select a condition only after you analyze a particular group and determine what is the highest priority for them. You might find, as a result of step 1, that exercise is not an important concern to your particular group, but diet, increasing social contacts, safety, or some other issue is important.

Through the needs assessment process (steps 1–5), you will come to see a problem comprehensively. You will learn, for example, that controlling asthma is not just a matter of having a patient take medicines as prescribed by medical personnel; rather, there is a complex interplay of factors and conditions, not within the domain of physicians and nurses, that the family must control. You will begin to understand that controlling asthma is largely a matter of self-management, which is influenced by a person's beliefs and values and by certain skills. You will develop an idea of what self-management entails and of how difficult or easy it is for a particular group, for example, low-income families.

Through initial analysis of the problem and the population-at-risk, you are doing your homework, becoming versed in theoretical and empirical explanations of the problem and the kind of behavior change that may best address it. At the end of step 1, you should be able to describe the following:

1. The health problem in detail
2. The behavior associated with resolving it
3. The learners you are interested in
4. The relative importance of the problem to the learners and their perspective of it
5. The kind of program learners will be motivated to take part in to address the problem
6. The social, behavioral, and/or medical science base of the problem
7. Collaborator in related fields who might help address the problem
8. How collaborator see the problem
9. The willingness they have to work with you
10. The benefits of a health education program to the learners, your colleagues, and your own organization

You should be able to describe in detail the logical chain connecting a problem to a health education program to expected change in behavior to expected related health outcomes.

Data Collection. Whether you begin with a particular group of people or a particular health condition, there are basically two kinds of data to use: secondary data, available from other sources, and primary data that you collect.

Secondary Data. Program planners frequently use epidemiological data to determine the importance of particular health conditions, the kinds of problems arising in given segments of the population, the factors associated with health conditions, and characteristics of people who experience them. Government agencies, research institutes, or academic centers often make these statistics available. Currently, for example, the diseases causing the greatest number of deaths among U.S. citizens are heart disease, cancer, and stroke (National Center for Health Statistics, 1990). These are accepted as major national health problems precisely because many people experience them. The toll taken by heart disease is particularly high among middle-aged men, and, as a result, you may decide to provide public health education on heart disease for that group. Frequently, the government provides funding only for programs on problems that have a wide impact.

Epidemiological data, however, need not be national in scope to signal a problem for particular groups. Spiegel and Lindaman (1977) reviewed New York City Health Department records and documented falls by children from windows as an important source of morbidity and death. Rosenberg in 1977 reviewed hospital medical records and noted a high incidence of morbidity caused by lead paint poisoning among low-income children seen in the emergency room (personal communication, 1979). Each finding led to the development, implementation, and evaluation of successful health education programs.

Other secondary data from surveys, systematic observations, and experimental studies are available to define problems. Research results appear in professional journals and are presented at conferences. With increasing frequency, they are also reported on television and in print media. What do the experts and the literature say about the problem? Such data are widely available and call attention to the existence of health problems, the groups of people at higher risk, and potential solutions.

Primary Data. Despite the range of secondary data, you often must collect data yourself to fully understand a problem. You may know, from secondary data, which problems are widespread and which group of people is most affected by a particular health problem. However, you may not know how the problem is viewed by those people, how they specifically behave in relation to the problem, or what specific factors enable or inhibit desired behaviors. Sometimes you will be interested in problems for which few data exist. Even if much information is available, you may want to collect additional data from a subgroup to ensure that they see the problem as important. You might want to begin with a recognized problem and show the association of another one, for example, one found to be important in the epidemiological data. Motivation to learn is obviously much higher when the subject interests the learners.

The range of methods available for collecting needs assessment data is not different from that available for evaluation. Quantitative and qualitative methods can be used for both. Qualitative approaches are discussed at length in Chapter 4 and quantitative in Chapter 5. They are mentioned here briefly and in light of their usefulness for program planning.

Discussion Groups. If your aim is to discover how problems are perceived or which problem is most important to a group, you can form a *discussion group.* Representatives of the learners in which you are interested should comprise the group. Group members are volunteers who agree to discuss the issues they find most pressing or aspects of a health problem that concern them most. Members might be people who hold a position with community health groups or other organizations, or they may simply be interested individuals who experience the problem and are likely to know the viewpoint of their peers. Such a discussion group has the advantage of allowing people to discuss and even vote on something of immediate interest.

When conducting group discussions for needs assessment, make clear what actions your sponsoring organization is prepared to take in light of the perceptions and concerns of the group. If your organization can provide little or no assistance for the problems directly uncovered by discussion, sometimes you can help group members locate appropriate assistance. Indeed, the whole domain of community organization and action within the field of health education is based on this role and function. McKnight (1978) has used a very effective approach combining discussion groups, analysis of secondary data, and action. He assists members of community organizations to translate statistics from their local hospital, health department, or some other source into a picture of the actual problems experienced in the neighborhood. By examining available data, community representatives explore how the particular problem occurs in their area and then can select one aspect of the problem to address in action.

Sometimes health educators convene meetings specifically to discover the priorities of individuals or community groups. In such a meeting, group members, led by the educator, determine which problem or aspects of the problem are most important. In situations where varying points of view must be reconciled, health educators frequently use the Nominal Group Process, Delphi Technique (Delbecq, 1974), or a similar approach. These techniques enable group members to select problems and reach consensus on aspects of problems without letting individual views dominate.

A disadvantage of discussions by volunteers is that you never know exactly whose views the group members represent. Some representatives of organizations may have clear-cut constituencies, and statements by them may accurately present the case for their constituents; but this is not always the case. Similarly, concerns expressed by unaffiliated individuals may be uniquely felt. The views and attitudes of one suburban mother of young children do not necessarily reflect those of similar women. In other words, it is difficult to know how far to generalize the opinions and experiences of these volunteers. If a disparity eventually emerges between the views of the representatives and the learners you aim to reach, fundamental problems can plague your program. Nonetheless, discussion groups can generally shed much light on the problems potential learners confront, can help establish priorities among these problems, and can provide rich insights on dimensions of the problems.

Focus Groups. A *focus group* is a discussion among people similar to the target populations you wish to reach about specific aspects of a problem or program. The term is borrowed from marketing where groups of consumers are convened and paid to tell manufacturers or advertisers the characteristics of products they prefer or the elements of advertisements that capture their attention. Focus group techniques have been adapted in health education program planning (Basch, 1987). The primary difference between a focus and discussion group is the specificity of issues the members of the group are asked to consider. The focus group leader guides the attention of the discussants toward particular issues or questions concerning the program planners. The intention is to discover useful information about which product (program) is likely to be most attractive to the learners. No consensus is required. Ideas generated are used to tailor the program to learners' expectations. As in discussion groups, focus group members may not represent the opinions of other learners.

Surveys. The purpose of a *survey*, whether a mailed or telephoned questionnaire or a face-to-face interview, is to elicit specific information from a specific group of people. Like information collected from discussion and focus groups, survey data are used to delineate the problem and describe the population of learners. If the survey is of the exact people who will eventually be in the program, the answers can also be used as baseline data for measuring change.

In conducting a survey, the health educator generally samples a population. Sampling has been defined as the selection of a few observations that will serve as the basis for general conclusions (Kish, 1987). Sampling is used to overcome the problem of representativeness (remember the disadvantage of discussion and focus groups). By selecting people (e.g., women who come to the organization for counseling) at random or using a systematic procedure (e.g., every third woman who visits), you have a basis for expecting the data to be representative. The sample women's views are likely to be similar to those of people not surveyed, whereas volunteers might be different in some respect from the larger population you hope to reach. Sampling and techniques for conducting different types of surveys are also discussed in Chapters 4, 5, 6, and 7.

Fieldwork and Observation. Other ways to assess needs from primary data include *fieldwork* and *observation*. These methods have the advantage of not interrupting the normal events surrounding the target audience and the problem you are interested in understanding. Doing fieldwork means becoming part of the natural events where the problem occurs. Fieldwork, however, can be costly (time and staff) and can only reach small numbers of a potential population-at-risk. Nonetheless, fieldwork can generate rich planning data. For example, you might decide to observe an asthma clinic or participate in the activities of a family where a child has asthma. Using checklists, protocols, or a log, you might systematically record your observations and experiences. Being systematic and thorough in the way you collect and analyze data are crucial. Often, if the people observed are the same ones who will take part in the education, data from checklists and observation schedules can be used as baseline measurements.

Analyzing Secondary and Primary Data. Through analysis of the data collected in step 1, you should begin to see whether there are linkages between certain information, skills, and conditions on the part of particular groups to certain behaviors and whether specific behaviors are linked to specific health outcomes. During this initial step, you also identify the theories that describe why people with a particular problem behave as they do. You must locate and analyze the theories that predict your target behavior. Available theories may explain how people change their behavior. Every health promotion and education program should be based on sound, empirically tested, theoretical assumptions about behavior change.

Steps 2 and 3: Delineating Behaviors to Resolve the Health Problem and Delineating Needed Information and Skills

In these steps of a needs assessment, you must zero in on specific behaviors to help the group-at-risk manage or resolve the health problem and the information and skills learners will need.

The following set of circumstances illustrates how needed behaviors, knowledge, and skills are delineated. Assume that you have been hired to develop an employee health promotion and education program. Data show that middle-class men, 45–60 years of age, employed in sedentary office jobs, who smoke, are overweight, have high blood pressure, and do not get adequate exercise, are at high risk for cardiovascular disease. Your employer, a large, urban insurance firm, wants to develop a cardiovascular risk-reduction program for its male employees. You expect that the target population will benefit from such a program by looking and feeling better and being more active. The company is expected to benefit by increasing employee satisfaction and health. In the long run, the company also expects some benefit from reduced costs of cardiovascular-related illness among its employees.

The physicians and nurses of the employee health service are cooperative. Employees express interest in such a program. Most who do not engage in "good health practices" admit that they don't and feel as if they should. You have carried out step 1. You have read the risk-reduction literature, including critical factors predicting behavior and describing the kind of learning shown to bring about change. You have convened a representative discussion group of middle-aged, men from each department of the company to discuss risk-reduction issues. You selected a random sample of employees and surveyed 200 of the 2000 men who fit the description "middle-aged, with a sedentary job." To reflect employee concerns, you used a questionnaire partially developed from data collected from the employee representatives in the group discussion. The questionnaire also included questions addressing concerns of the medical professionals in the employee health service. You led the group discussions and constructed the questionnaire using principles discussed in Chapter 6 and 7 and based on factors discussed earlier in this chapter. The return rate from the survey was 84%. You calculate that about 40% of the male employee population is at moderate-to-high risk—engages in one or more negative health practices.

You begin to sift the primary and secondary data for the specific factors associated with changing behavior. You have four separate but interrelated risk-reduction behaviors you will consider: smoking, lack of exercise/daily activity, and high blood pressure. To illustrate how to find the behavior dimensions to include in a program, we will select being overweight as the health risk.

Assume that 20% of the population you surveyed are at least 20 pounds overweight for their age and height. No man in the group has associated physiological problems to account for the weight. You set an objective: Within 12 months, at least 10% of the overweight employees will lose and keep off at least 10 pounds for a 12-month period. What do all your data reveal about losing weight? Assume the data show the following:

1. The group's knowledge level about low-fat foods is low.
2. Most of the men eat breakfast and dinner at home and eat whatever is prepared for them.
3. Most have many business lunches in restaurants and must travel.
4. Most believe that the phrase "healthy food" refers to vegetarianism.
5. Many claim to have little time or inclination to exercise during weekdays and are too tired on weekends.
6. About 65% express an interest in exercise but say it is difficult to fit into a busy schedule, and some claim not to be the exercise "type."
7. Most believe that middle-aged men are susceptible to cardiovascular problems but believe they are not at much risk.
8. They report that the most important things to them are their families and advancement in the company.
9. About 95% say they believe that being healthy benefits their families and improves their work.
10. About 80% do not consider being overweight a deterrent to "getting ahead."

By carefully synthesizing your data, you should get a behavioral picture of the target group, of how they behave, and of how they perceive the seriousness of the problem. The accuracy of this picture depends on the relevance and completeness of your initial data.

Assume you know, from the literature and from discussions with your colleagues in nutrition, that the desired health status (lower weight) is, except for those with psychological or physiological problems, a function of eating the right combination of foods, eating the right amount of food, and getting adequate exercise (Glanz et al., 1990). What new behaviors, given your population and the context in which it functions, do these men need to acquire? You can diagram the problem as shown in Table 3.1. Begin with current behavior and behavior to be changed that is instrumental to ideal behavior. What are the behaviors to be learned by the overweight men? You know that nutrition knowledge is associated with receiving clear, accurate information. The men must learn which foods to eat and how much food to eat. They must be able to (1) select from a restaurant menu

Table 3.1   Three Types of Behavior Included in Program Planning

Current Behavior	Instrumental Behavior (Behavior to Be Learned)	Ideal Behavior (Outcome Behavior)
Eating "wrong" foods	Selecting correct foods, combinations, amounts	Eating "right" foods
Getting little exercise	Finding and practicing exercise that fits one's temperament and schedule	Getting adequate exercise

foods beneficial to their diet, (2) recognize "fat" foods from "skinny" foods, (3) distinguish too big a portion from an adequate portion and choose the latter, and (4) substitute foods they like or at least favor for foods they prefer but are too fattening. The men must rethink their behavioral patterns regarding exercise. For example, they must (5) be able to find time and fit exercise into their busy schedules, (6) choose, and even rehearse, a type of exercise suitable to their temperament and personality, and (7) determine an appropriate routine for its regular use.

Your initial data have also made clear that the men hold strong values and beliefs about health and nutrition. Most of these men, for example, reported that they highly value family and job. There are some theoretical connections between maintaining weight, maintaining health, and perceived benefits to a man's family and work. Men who accept the connections would also likely value losing weight. The employees who will take part in the program may come to accept the connection or reject it. In either case, the program should provide the opportunity for them to analyze the relationships and understand their own views. Many of the employees in the group do not consider themselves susceptible to cardiovascular accidents. You know, from your literature review, that people who believe themselves susceptible are predisposed to new health actions (Janz and Becker, 1984). The program, then, should enable the men to recognize overweight as a risk factor and recognize that overweight coupled with additional negative practices places a man at high risk.

In these examples of planning steps 2 and 3, we have used only a fragmented behavioral picture. When reviewing all the data collected in step 1 in the way recommended, you are likely to find an even wider range of information and skills that the potential learners need. This is especially so in a risk-reduction program that also addresses other problems (e.g., smoking and blood pressure control).

In step 2, you must try to be comprehensive about the problem and its associated behaviors. Carrying out this process enables you to see the people, the problems, and the needed information and skills in a larger context. When the time comes to select a smaller number of behaviors as the target of the program, you will understand more clearly how one behavior or set of behaviors relates to another.

Steps 4 and 5: Identifying Needed Resources and Related Services

If your program is to help people change behavior, you need to recognize the kind and extent of resources, both personal and material, available to the learners. For example, again consider the weight-loss component of the employee risk-reduction program. The literature review shows that a primary influence on the way a married man eats is the nutrition behavior of his spouse (Brownell et al., 1978; Rosenthal et al., 1980). Further, the potential participants, almost all of whom are married, have reported that at home they eat mainly what their wives prepare. Clearly, the educational program will have to find a way to reach these spouses. The literature review also shows that peer support is important to people who change behavior (Gottlieb, 1987). Because eating is significantly associated with business, the employees will have a more difficult time if their colleagues and bosses do not acknowledge the value of their efforts to lose weight. The employees also might not stick to their diets if they continue to equate eating healthful foods with "vegetarians or health nuts." Behavior is always influenced by others in the work setting who might give or withhold support. Your program must appreciate this fact.

Potential participants are likely have access to healthful food. Assume that they earn enough money to afford balanced meals and they live in an area where fresh fruits and vegetables and a range of other foods are readily available. These employees probably have other needed material resources. Most have a bathroom scale to monitor their weight. Most reside in communities where recreation facilities and parks exist, where they can exercise. These material resources could not be assumed in a poorer population, however, and their lack would need to be a factor in planning.

Assume, as well, that needed health and community resources are available to the group. For example, the physicians on your planning committee are likely to recommend a physical exam for each man before beginning a weight-loss program. Assume your group can be examined by the employee health service at no extra cost. Should physical problems be detected, they will be referred for service. The costs will likely be covered by their employee health plan. Assume that your group has the services available and financed in a way appropriate to their needs. Often a program to help people learn to behave differently entails an initial phase of securing needed related services, and, especially with low-income populations, this can be the most inhibiting factor of all.

In steps 4 and 5, you review each ideal and instrumental behavior, while asking, What personal and material resources must potential learners have in order to change? What services must they have? This process helps you see outside factors that will enable or inhibit the change. A goal at this stage is to identify ways to obtain needed social support, resources, and services. In the hypothesized case, it is evident that most resources are plentiful, but somehow your program will need to engender support from the spouses and colleagues of the men to foster change.

From steps 1–5 of the planning process, you will have amassed considerable information:

A comprehensive picture of the people and the problem

A comprehensive list of outcome behaviors—the "ideal behavior" to resolve or manage the problem

A corresponding list of instrumental behaviors—what people must learn to do to behave in a new way

A compilation of the information and skills that are entailed— the content of what must be learned

A compilation of the factors outside the individual that will most inhibit or enable learning—personal and material resources and needed health or community services

Step 6: Enumerating Expected Changes and How to Measure Them

In step 6, you further lay the foundation for evaluation. This is the time to identify which changes might occur and how they might be measured. Continuing with the weight-loss example, previous steps identified the kind of behavior that resolves or reduces the problem of being overweight. Next, the measurable outcomes related to new behavior must be identified.

The first change to be evaluated is the impact of the intervention. The impact of education on the patient (remember our earlier discussion) is what they do differently. Did participants change their eating and exercise patterns? You will also want to know if they lost weight and kept it off. Related changes in psychological health status might also be observed—for example, did the employees feel better, think they look better, think better of themselves—increase their self-esteem (Sonstroem, 1984)? Physiological and psychological changes are likely.

Now envision a number of these newly thin, happy, healthy employees. What related changes might be expected? The men may reduce their risk of cardiovascular-related illnesses, that is, they might get lower scores on risk-assessment tests. Over time, there may also be a reduced number of cardiovascular illnesses in the group, but that outcome is measurable only over a 10- to 15-year period. Some men may feel a higher degree of job satisfaction, due in part to their increased self-esteem and in part to receiving health education as an employee benefit (Holzbach et al., 1990). There may be less absenteeism due to illness (Yen et al., 1992). In other words, this phase of planning involves outlining the anticipated results of successful education of the men to eat "right," get exercise, and consequently lose weight.

At this point, you must think carefully about how each of these changes might be measured. Although many changes might occur theoretically, only some can be easily measured empirically. The following are examples:

Measure whether eating patterns change; ask participants to keep dietary diaries or recall their typical meals for a period of time, for example, 1 month preceding and following the program.

Telephone spouses on a few random occasions before and after the program and ask for a description of the meal the participant ate the night before.

Measure the outcome of weight loss by having the men weigh in and weigh out before and after the program.

Measure cardiovascular risk reduction by conducting an assessment before and after the program.

Measure job satisfaction or self-esteem before and after by developing an index or using a standardized one.

Measuring actual reductions in cardiovascular disease, in almost all cases, is not possible in the short term.

The focus, depth, and extent of evaluation of related outcomes are a function of how much time and what resources are available. Following step 6, however, you will have a very good idea of which outcomes seem most likely, which can be measured empirically, and how difficult and expensive evaluation will be.

Step 7: Selecting Behaviors to Change and Outcomes to Measure

Step 7 in the planning process might be called a "reality test." This is the time when you and your colleagues in planning must agree (get out the consensus exercises) on the specific goals that your program can indeed achieve. Although it is desirable during the initial steps to touch on all aspects of behavior related to the problem and although those planning steps may have revealed the complexity of the problem, paradoxically, now is the time to narrow the problem and to arrive at a feasible, manageable, affordable set of behaviors and outcomes to address and measure in the program.

The importance of taking a detached look at the emerging program cannot be overstressed. You must ascertain the appropriate scope for your program, given all you know about the problem and what is needed to resolve or reduce it. You must reassess whether the direction in which you are moving is appropriate for your organization.

Assume, for example, you are sure by this stage that one set of instrumental behaviors to bring change has to do with a wider kind of action, that is, something more than just personal health behavior of the learners. In the asthma example used earlier, suppose analyses have made you conclude that several equally important factors are involved in better management of childhood asthma: Taking medicine in correct doses at correct times, practicing relaxation exercises, using prearranged and rehearsed strategies in the face of an attack, and maintaining a favorable living environment. These practices, in large part, involve personal instrumental behaviors; however, analysis may reveal that maintaining a suitable environment is exceedingly difficult for the particular targeted learners because they are poor, urban residents of substandard housing. They cannot afford to rebuild their living quarters to eliminate falling plaster. They cannot afford to move to other apartments to get away from the broken-down elevators, dampness, and lack of heat that contribute to the onset of infections and wheezing.

Based on analysis of the data, you may feel that reaching desired outcomes depends on the ability of families to change these conditions. This, however, takes much more than one parent's effort; it takes collective action. The tenants might, for example, collectively sue the landlords who are failing to keep buildings in good repair. They might contribute time and materials and help one another repair their apartments. They might organize into a tenants' association and demand services from the city housing department. In other words, people might learn about and be assisted to take legal, cooperative, and political actions that would bring about a favorable living environment for their children. This need for wider action must be somehow addressed if significant change is to occur.

There are several options for accommodating this kind of need. Your organization may see the health promotion and education program for community action as part of its regular health education responsibility, and you can develop the appropriate activities as an integral part of the program. Your organization may not engage in community action and outreach of this type, but one of your collaborating organizations may; you might develop an action component with them. If no collaborating organization is willing, you may be able to refer learners to groups in the area who handle legal and political action. On the other hand, the objectives of your organization might be more in line with fostering collective action than with developing the personal, individual behaviors that are needed. In such a case, at this point, you would need to explore the possibility for addressing the latter dimensions. In some way or another, however, the major needs must be addressed, and you must form your expectations of change according to how well they are addressed.

Several criteria determine which behaviors to include and measure in the program. They have to do with what is relevant, appropriate, and feasible for the learners, for you as the educator, and for your organization. A behavior is a priority if the answer to most of the following questions is yes:

1. Is the behavior free from outside factors that would inhibit its development, or can you accommodate the important outside factors in your program? (For example, if you include eating correct foods at home as a behavior in a cardiovascular risk-reduction program, can you involve the person who controls at-home meals?)

2. Is the behavior critical to achieve the desired effect?

3. Is the behavior important, or could it come to be recognized as important by the population-at-risk?

4. Do the collaborators (members of the planning network) agree that the behavior is important?

5. Is the lack of this behavior pervasive? (If only one or two people are not already doing the behavior, individualized learning may be more effective than making the behavior a focus of the program.)

6. Is educational, medical, or other expertise available to design the needed educational activities?

7. Are needed related services available to support the change?

8. Is the cost of implementing education to change the behavior reasonable? How about the cost to measure the impact on the learners (the change in behavior that might occur)? What is the cost to measure related health outcomes?

By completing this step in the process, you have not only narrowed the list of behaviors to address, using criteria of feasibility, appropriateness, and relevance, but also specified which changes to assess. At this point, you also begin to explore the appropriate evaluation design. (Designs are discussed in detail in Chapter 5.)

Step 8: Designing Educational and Behavioral Interventions

Successful health education and promotion programs are based on an understanding of why people behave as they do relative to their health and what causes or enables them to change. A variety of theories of health behavior and learning exists to provide the theoretical underpinning for a program. Some theories predict behavior—posit that if certain conditions obtain, a person will behave in a certain way. The health belief model is an example of such a theory (Rosenstock et al., 1988). It assumes, for sake of illustration, that overweight men are more likely to lose pounds if they believe that they are *susceptible* to a health problem because of their weight, deem the health problem to be a *serious* one, and can see more *benefits* than *costs* in carrying out the recommendations your program will make.

Some theories explain what causes behavior to change. Social cognitive theory is an example (Bandura, 1986). In this theory, the factors influencing adoption of new behavior include the following:

Feelings of self-efficacy—that is, confidence that one can perform the recommended behavior

Vicarious learning from models in the social environment—other people who demonstrate the positive consequences of the behavior (perhaps the men in your proposed weight-loss program might be influenced by other men in the workplace who have successfully lost weight and feel better)

Mastery—successfully achieving a behavioral goal (e.g., your program might have a graduated weight-loss plan where individuals get much support and encouragement for losing the first few pounds; this mastery is likely to increase feelings of self-efficacy and motivate the men to continue with the plan)

Ability to self-regulate—being able to observe one's own behavior in relation to a problem, judging what new behavior would resolve the problem, and reacting with confidence after initially attempting the new behavior

Verbal persuasion—compelling information and encouragement from a credible role model

The program planner must be familiar with prevailing theories of learning and behavior change such as these so that he or she can select the theoretical principles most relevant to the people, problem, and program goals in question. The available theories considered in light of the data you have collected, the behaviors that have been selected as the objectives for the program, and the nature of your target population will dictate the type of learning techniques and materials most likely to be effective.

For example, the data from the potential participants in the cardiovascular risk-reduction program revealed that they discounted the importance of certain healthful foods. Assume one instrumental behavior you want to address is selecting healthful foods from a typical restaurant menu, and you plan to include learning activities to develop this skill as part of the program. You also know that participants will be unlikely to select foods they view as "health nut foods" or "wimp foods." They associate healthful food with social role models they do not admire. Your program may need to provide different role models—successful executives who follow prudent diets.

You also know that the support of spouses who prepare at-home meals will be needed for behavior change. You can organize discussion groups, information sessions, demonstrations of food selection and preparation, or other activities that include the spouses and that introduce new ways to improve family eating patterns. You can establish a mass information campaign at work, focused on colleagues and supervisors in the participants' social environment, to enlist their support of the men's efforts to change. In other words, for each behavior that you want to help the men develop, select the learning principle and approach best suited to its development and maintenance.

You need to satisfy two levels of concern when designing interventions: the content of the material (in the above example, health promotion, diet, and exercise) and the processes by which people learn to behave differently (mastery, vicarious learning from role models, self-regulation, verbal persuasion, etc.). Process and content are interrelated. A group discussion to provide social support among participants, if led by a trained facilitator, may also be the best means to present one or two nutrition messages and even to rehearse skills such as selecting low-fat foods from a list.

When evaluating programs, evaluation researchers think that it is "cleaner" to assess different interventions separately (Green, 1991)—that is, to discern whether rehearsal of skills is a more effective intervention than problem-solving groups or individualized counseling. In the daily practice of health education, this separation of approaches makes sense only if previous studies and your own experience say it is the most effective way to proceed. Answering the effectiveness question is currently an important area for evaluation research. Theoretically, combined approaches should be better. In designing learning events, however, the behavior to be learned dictates the approach and determines the resources and materials needed to support the approach.

Materials in health education (slides, films, tapes, written documents) in and of themselves are *not* learning methods. Learning is a process supported by materials. Materials can provide information, stimulate discussion, and reinforce information provided. You can choose the kinds of materials needed only after you have decided on the learning objectives and theoretical approach.

For each learning event, you must determine how participants will demonstrate that they have learned the behavior. Often, this is simple. Participants in the diet-and-exercise program might, for example, complete a checklist of low-fat foods at the end of their session on menu selection. Sometimes, monitoring learning activities is more difficult. For example, some participants may be unwilling to express how they feel about some aspect of nutrition at the end of a group discussion. For each learning event for which there is a specific objective, however, you must decide how to determine if the objective has been achieved to a satisfactory degree. Monitoring provides important benchmarks of mastery for both learners and program personnel (Bandura, 1986). There must be signs that the program has momentum and is moving the participants along.

The duration and frequency of learning sessions and of the program itself are of great concern to program developers in terms of both learning and cost. Some studies have shown that important behavior change has occurred in a single learning session (Green, 1977; Weingarten et al., 1976). At least one study has found that attending more sessions was associated with change in one setting (Clark et al., 1981) and fewer sessions were associated with similar change in a different setting (Evans et al., 1987). Green (1974) postulates that extended health education reaches a point of diminishing returns. Wang et al. (1975) found this to be the case with nutrition counseling and education delivered at home. Current data suggest that programs of more than one session that are not overly long may yield the greatest degree of change. Highly focused, standardized 10- to 15-minute counseling sessions and the provision of self-help materials can also be very effective (Windsor et al., 1985, 1993). Unless specific data are available from evaluation research to suggest a particular time frame for the type of education you are planning, this determination should be based on the following criteria:

1. What is best for the participants in their view?
2. What have previous studies and programs of a similar type shown to be effective?
3. What is manageable, given the context in which the program must operate?
4. What in your previous experience has been effective?
5. How much material must be covered?
6. What is the location of the program in relation to the participants?

The location of interventions is an important consideration. If the intervention site is not the place where people spend the bulk of their time (i.e., school, home, and work), then you must consider a practical question: How often and for how long can people be expected to travel to and from a site? If education is part of other health services, then the location and frequency of sessions may be geared to them—for example, the sessions will coincide with monthly clinic visits. If school, work, or home will coincide with the site monthly, more frequent educational sessions for shorter durations may be the best. You need to base decisions on available data and what makes most sense for participants. It is standard practice, during step 1 of program planning, to ask potential participants what time and what location are best for them.

Similarly, the number of participants to include in a program is based on three criteria: the number best suited to the educational approaches selected, the number of the population to be reached, and the practicalities of cost and manageability.

Assume that you have decided on group discussion as a format for the employee program on diet and exercise. From the review of the literature in step 1, you know that 6 to 8 members in a group is optimum to ensure full participation in discussion. However, there are almost 1000 men to be reached eventually. Therefore, you may decide to hold information sessions for medium or large groups (30 to 50) with numerous visual aids, self-tests, and a lecturer. These will alternate with discussion and support groups of small numbers (5 to 20) of men. In this way, you hope both to reach a big audience with information and to meet the necessary conditions of the more intensive learning approaches within a reasonable cost.

One of the most enjoyable steps in program development is designing the learning events. There is a rich and growing literature on both learning and health behavior. Your knowledge of theories and studies, coupled with creativity, can produce excellent learning activities and effective deployment of materials.

Table 3.2 presents a sample summary of goals, objectives, and anticipated outcomes for the asthma education program used as an example in this chapter. The table illustrates planning steps 1–8, the logical progression from a problem to a program to outcomes. From analysis of the problem, the people, and their behavior, the health educator identifies the kind of learning needed to help learners behave in a new way.

Step 9: Developing Organizational Arrangements, Logistics, and Personnel Training

If you have involved members of the program-planning network in the planning process, by step 9 the resources and support needed to mount the program should be evident and available. If, early on, the employee health service has agreed to give medical checkups to employees enrolling in the weight-loss program, now is the time to work out the details of referral, record keeping, and so on. If you have developed a program alone, without external input, expect trouble at this point in trying to secure assistance.

This is when you determine administrative and logistical details, from recruiting participants through evaluation of the program. What departments, people, and resources are needed and available? Which people must give their approval before the program proceeds? Which facilities are needed for learning events? Have all the parties needed to implement the program committed themselves and, where necessary, put the extent of their participation in writing? Have all organizational and legal constraints been considered?

Consider, again, the asthma education example. Assume you have decided to evaluate reduced school absences as a related outcome of better management. Will the local school let you use its records? Will parents sign needed releases? Assume you have decided to invite tenant organizers to the clinic to talk with parents about improvements in housing. Will the organizers need passes to visit the clinic? Must these visits be noted as referrals in clinic records? Each step of the program you have designed must be reviewed while you ask, Have we accounted for the administrative, legal, and logistical aspects of this element? You should undertake step 9 with the confidence that, because the planning network has been used, major aspects were considered and adequately addressed in earlier steps.

Table 3.2 Synthesis of Planning Steps: A Program for Managing Childhood Asthma Among Low-Income Families

Problem	Determinants of Family Behavior	Learning Objectives (Instrumental Behavior)
Disruption, stress, and high cost to families and communities resulting from childhood asthma *Goal* Increased ability of parents and children to manage asthma and reduce its negative effects on family life	Knowledge of potential management behaviors Level of skill in managing Belief in one's ability to control the illness Belief in one's ability to make judgments Perception of effective management measures Availability of personal support to self-manage Availability of material resources	*Learners will be able to* Demonstrate relaxation exercises Identify signs and symptoms of asthma Describe signs of a severe attack Describe strategies for managing a severe attack Identify basic ways to prevent infection Use guidelines for negotiating with the child to set limits Demonstrate ways to question the physician Complete an information sheet for the school Express confidence in their own ability to manage Express belief in their own judgments Describe criteria for seeking medical assistance Identify allergens Seek assistance from relevant community services

Program	Impact on Learners (Ideal Behavior)	Related Outcomes
Content Taking medicine Setting realistic guidelines for the child Getting information from the physician Keeping the child healthy Helping the child to do well in school Managing an attack *Process* Group problem solving Peer discussion Presentation of accurate information Rehearsal and practice of skills Peer support Counseling Parent and child discussion Parent and child practice of skills together	*Increased self-management—learners will* Practice relaxation exercises Accurately assess wheezing severity Take actions appropriate to wheezing severity Use criteria for seeking medical assistance Take actions to promote health and prevent infections Seek information and assistance Remove allergens Set realistic limits for the child Communicate with the physician Establish relations with the school	Reduced stress and fear in the child and the parents Reduced school absences Increased adjustment of the child in school Reduced emergency visits Reduced hospitalizations

At this juncture, you must also determine what kind of training of personnel is necessary to implement the program. Each member of your staff who will have an influence on the participants must be oriented. Many may need special training to implement education, to collect data, to keep records, and so on. Those who will facilitate discussion groups must be trained. Every program and group of participants is different. The educators must be prepared to work with the particular group of people in the specific context.

The design of personnel training, like the education program, operates on two levels: those who must be briefed and oriented regarding the content or health condition and those who must be trained in the learning process. Physicians who play a role as counselors in an asthma education program may be very well versed in clinical aspects of asthma but need training in counseling. Health educators may be highly skilled in facilitating discussion groups but need a background in the clinical dimensions of asthma.

A rule of thumb is not to assume that health personnel possess the requisite information and skills to educate patients. In most situations, personnel have uneven levels of skills and information. Orientation and training should fill this deficit. If different groups of personnel will undertake different tasks, train them separately. It is almost always necessary to bring all program personnel together for combined sessions or orientation. If tasks will cut across types of personnel (e.g., physicians, nurses, schoolteachers, and health educators, who must all provide the same basic messages when counseling), it is reasonable to train them all together. The extent of training is determined by the tasks to be performed, the information to be provided, and the existing skill level of the personnel.

Step 10: Developing a Budget and Administrative Plan

When a program is developed, certain costs and administrative needs result simply because the program is new. Costs of planning and development of methods, materials, and evaluation tools are, in large part, one-time expenses. The configuration of personnel needed to carry out initial planning and development may be different from the pattern needed when the program becomes institutionalized or part of an organization's routine.

The elaborateness of your program is likely to be proportional to the resources made available. Failure to allocate sufficient money has been cited as a major reason for the limited success of some health education programs (Green, 1991). A budget should provide justification for each person or tasks to be undertaken during program development and delivery. The budget justification should convince the sponsoring organization or funder that initial allocations are warranted and that the program will be affordable over time.

The first concern in step 10, then, is to think through carefully what staff will be needed to develop the program and to carry it out initially. Next, job descriptions must be written and personnel costs estimated. The following kinds of personnel may be needed: a program director to assume overall responsibility, program coordinators to manage logistics, consultants in particular areas (content specialists, educational methods specialists, materials specialists, data-collection and analysis specialists, etc.), educators to carry out the learning program, and secretarial and clerical staff.

Many of these people may be available in the organization or members of the planning network. Individuals from other organizations may participate, and their services will show on the budget as contributions. To determine the cost of personnel, the simplest method is to estimate the number of hours per week, month, or year a person will need (percentage of effort) to devote to program activities and to compute the amount that person will be paid per week, month, or year.

A budget must show not only the direct cost of personnel, the money they will receive to spend, but also the cost of fringe benefits provided by the sponsoring organization. All organizations have established rates for figuring these costs. There are also other unseen costs in a program. What is the cost of housing the program? What about services provided by other divisions or departments of the organization, such as the financial office and the personnel office, to support program personnel? The indirect cost of these services must be computed; again, the organization is likely to have an established rate for doing this. One person (e.g., you) will also likely have several program responsibilities. A health educator might serve as both program coordinator and instructor. If so, this fact must be spelled out in the budget rationale.

Items other than personnel services will be needed to develop the program. Some will be ongoing expenses, but others will be required only during program development. Expenses likely to be incurred initially include space, if program housing is not available; equipment—typewriters, desks, and so on; supplies—paper, pencils, and other office needs; telephone service and postage; photocopying; acquisition of studies, articles, and books (i.e., secondary data); printing costs for primary data–collection and evaluation materials; printing costs for educational materials; computer costs for data analysis (if a computer is available); travel costs to and from learning sites; and training costs.

Once you have determined who and what are needed to carry

Table 3.3 Budget for Program Development and Implementation: Year 1 (1994)

Personnel	Hours/ Week	Percent of Effort	Salary/ Annum	Fringe Benefits[a]	Total		Amount
Program director Susan Greenbaum	40	100	$50,000	$10,000	$60,000	—	—
Program coordinator/educator (To be named)	40	100	36,000	7,200	43,200	—	—
Program evaluator James Sinclair	4	20	6,000	1,200	7,200	—	—
Secretary Robert Murphy	40	100	20,000	4,000	24,000	—	—
Consultants Carlos Velez (educational materials)	2	5	—	—	—	Contributed by Heart Association	—
Rachel Polanowski (data analysis)	2	5	—	—	—	Contributed by university	—
Total personnel costs							$134,400
Costs other than personal services							
Books, materials, and acquisition of background data							1,000
Printing of questionnaires and evaluation materials							2,000
Telephone, postage							2,400
							$139,800
Indirect costs[b]: [Total direct costs (× .30)]							$ 41,940
Total year 1 request							$181,740
Total year 2 request (.04)							$189,010
Total year 3 request (.04)							$196,759

[a] Computed as 20% of salary.
[b] Computed as 30% of total direct costs.

Personal Services

Program Director Susan Greenbaum will devote 100% time during year 1 of program development. She will assume overall responsibility for the program, maintain links with all cooperating agencies, and oversee day-to-day program activities. The yearly department budget provides for the cost of the program director. In years 2 and 3, it is estimated that Greenbaum will spend approximately 10% time supervising ongoing program implementation.

Program Coordinator-Educator A person will be hired at 100% time to coordinate all day-to-day aspects of program development and to carry out the actual teaching in the program. The cost of the coordinator-educator is requested at 100% for all years of the program. After the first year of program development and evaluation, the program coordinator-educator will devote 100% time to the ongoing program and to its expansion to four sites by year 3 of program implementation.

Program Evaluator James Sinclair will spend 10% time in all years of the program and will coordinate all evaluation tasks.

Secretary Robert Murphy will spend 100% time handling correspondence and record-keeping tasks. The department budget provides for the cost of this position.

Consultants Each cosponsor of the program, the local Heart Association and the local university, will contribute the equivalent of 5% consultation time by Carlos Velez and Rachel Polanowski for development of educational materials and for analysis of initial survey data, respectively. In years 2 and 3, consultation will be provided regarding program expansion and evaluation.

Other Than Personal Services

Books, Materials, and Background Data Although many resources are available in our own resource center and in the library of the nearby university, we will need to acquire some specialized materials from outside sources. This collection of materials will need to be updated yearly.

Printing of Questionnaires and Evaluation Materials Most of the materials that will be needed for the program are available through existing sources, such as the Heart Association and other cooperating agencies. However, some costs will be incurred in the printing of specialized questionnaires to be used for needs assessment and for evaluation; these costs are likely to be incurred yearly.

Years 2 and 3

To compute costs for years 2 and 3, the year 1 budget has been increased each year by 4% to cover inflation and salary increases.

Figure 3.3 Budget Rationale

out the program, the budget must be developed. Table 3.3 illustrates how you might show program costs for the first development year and the following 2 years. Figure 3.3 presents the rationale that might accompany the budget to explain why the amounts are requested.

Table 3.3 shows that the formula the sponsoring organization

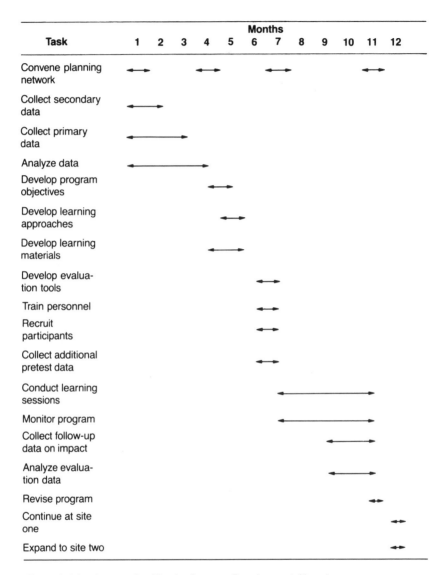

Task	Months 1	2	3	4	5	6	7	8	9	10	11	12
Convene planning network												
Collect secondary data												
Collect primary data												
Analyze data												
Develop program objectives												
Develop learning approaches												
Develop learning materials												
Develop evaluation tools												
Train personnel												
Recruit participants												
Collect additional pretest data												
Conduct learning sessions												
Monitor program												
Collect follow-up data on impact												
Analyze evaluation data												
Revise program												
Continue at site one												
Expand to site two												

Figure 3.4 Implementation Plan for Program Development, Year 1

uses to compute fringe benefits is 20% of a person's salary. In this example, indirect costs are determined to be 30% of total direct costs. Outside contributions are included in the budget with an indication that no funds are requested from the department for the services listed. Showing contributed time in the budget more accurately reflects the percentage of effort that will be expended. The bottom of the budget notes that requests will be made in years 2 and 3.

The budget rationale explains that, after the first year, the program director will spend 100% time administering program activities. This is likely to be considered a reasonable ongoing program expense. The rationale also states that, in the next 2 years, the program will be expanded to four sites with no addition of staff. Each year the budget has been increased by 4% to cover changes in salaries and prices of materials.

Once you have developed the budget and budget rationale, you need to outline the time frame for carrying out major tasks. Figure 3.4 gives an example of how the first year of tasks might be presented. Note that representatives of organizations and groups from the planning network will meet regularly over the first year of development. The program will also be monitored continuously during the 3 months it is operating and will only be expanded to the second site after evaluation and revision.

With a program description, including the evaluation plan, an outline of personnel and their responsibilities, a time frame, a budget, and a budget rationale, you are ready to seek funding, or, if money is in hand, to implement the work plan. In addition, on completion of the evaluation, you should be able to conduct cost analyses (see Chapter 9) of your program.

By undertaking planning steps 1–10, you prepare to carry out a program that is headed for success and to conduct an evaluation of sufficient rigor to document the extent of success. Through careful planning, evaluation becomes a fundamental, integrated element of the program, not something added at the end. If, for some reason, you find you must assess a program after it is in operation, you will need to engage in the planning steps (ex post facto) by reviewing the processes that led to the program. Only then will you be able to determine how the program might be evaluated. To make that determination, you must discern the logical chain—the links from program to new behavior to related outcomes. These links must be forged and assessed if health education is to be worthy of the learners it purports to assist.

SUMMARY

In this chapter, we have discussed the influence of the sponsoring organization on the health promotion and education program. We have emphasized the need to establish and use a program-planning network. We have defined needs assessment and suggested some approaches to assessing needs. This chapter has also underscored the importance of using the program plan to forge a logical link from a health problem to the education to expected outcomes. Finally, we have described and discussed ten steps the planner must undertake to ensure that the program addresses important needs, can be evaluated, and is feasible for the sponsoring organization to undertake. A detailed discussion of cost, cost effectiveness, and cost–benefit analysis is included in Chapter 9.

4

Conducting Qualitative-
Process Evaluations

"My hospital is looking for a new coordinator for our community health promotion center. What kind of skills should this person have?"

"If we use behavioral impact as the only indicator of success, I think our program is in trouble. Aren't there methods we can use to look at our program?"

"Our administrator was really pleased with our qualitative evaluation. She wants us to put more emphasis on satisfied consumers."

"I don't have the foggiest idea of how to conduct a process evaluation. How do you do it? What methods do you use?"

Professional Competencies Emphasized in This Chapter

• Defining quality, quality control, and performance standards

• Differentiating between efficacy and effectiveness

• Specifying standards of practice

• Selecting and applying quality control methods

• Describing key program procedures for program quality review

• Describing key components and methods for conducting a process evaluation

• Describing pretesting methods

• Applying readability and content analysis methods

The need to examine program procedures and skill and training levels of personnel who plan and deliver health-related programs has been confirmed by Donabedian (1966) and Greene (1976) on quality of medical care; Inui (1978) on quality assurance issues in patient education, physician training, and medical care; and Green and Brooks-Bertram (1978) on quality assurance and health education. A judgment based on existing performance standards is required to evaluate the content and quality of the delivery process. The need to know what a program has done to and for a patient, employee, student, or consumer and how well it was done is the primary objective of a process evaluation. The health education/health promotion literature emphasizes the need to conduct a process evaluation but provides limited guidance on what or how to conduct one.

As Table 1.5 shows, process evaluation (Type 1) (1) applies nonexperimental designs, (2) defines structure, process, and content, (3) documents delivery of procedures, (4) conducts observational analyses of program sessions, (5) performs qualitative observations, (6) monitors program effort or activity, and (7) reviews or audits data systems and records for participants. The primary dimensions to define in conducting a process evaluation are the strengths and weaknesses of a program and the procedures to which participants are exposed. This type of evaluation assesses how an outcome is produced rather than a statement of cognitive, skill, or behavioral impact. It answers questions about why a program succeeded or failed, (efficacy or effectiveness) and suggests what part(s) need to be revised. It also describes what actually happened as a new program was started, implemented, and completed. It uses existing standards of acceptability for each procedure defined in the literature and/or derived by professional consensus through internal or external review. A process evaluation is by definition descriptive and ongoing: a method used to explain the dynamics of a new or continuing program.

In this chapter, we identify normative criteria and procedures that you should regularly consider when planning and implementing your health education/health promotion programs. At the end of several sections, we provide practice standards to help you assess the quality of program (intervention) and process evaluation components.

QUALITY ASSURANCE

In a discussion of process evaluation in health promotion and education, several terms need to be defined: quality, quality control, and performance standards. *Quality* is the appropriateness of a set of professional procedures for a problem and objectives to be achieved. *Quality control* is the methods used to produce documentation of the quality of program procedures. A *performance standard* is the minimum acceptable level of performance set by experts in a specialty area to judge the quality of an individual's or program's professional practice (Green and Brooks-Bertram, 1978).

A quality assurance review (QAR) of a program should be viewed as a multidimensional process. At a minimum, it demands (1) documentation of the technical competence of the service provider and (2) the preparation of policy and application of methods to improve critical dimensions of health education practice determined to be inadequate. Two concepts are also frequently mentioned in discussions of program quality: efficacy and effectiveness. *Efficacy* is the maximum power of a program, applied under *optimum* conditions, to favorably alter the history of a risk factor (behavior) for a defined population-at-risk. *Effectiveness* is the normal power of a program, applied under *typical practice* conditions, to favorably alter the history of a behavioral risk factor for a defined population-at-risk.

An example of the contrast between efficacy and effectiveness is a comparison of the behavioral impact of the Multiple Risk Factor Intervention Trial (MRFIT) to the behavioral impact of a typical, community-based smoking-cessation program offered by a voluntary health organization at a work site or a health care institution. One major purpose of the MRFIT was to determine the efficacy of its smoking-cessation component. The intervention consisted of two parts: (1) ten sessions of 90–120 minutes, with 6 to 12 men attending each, and (2) a continuous, individual nonsmoking maintenance program for a 4-year period. A behaviorist (master's- or doctorate-trained staff), a nutritionist (in many cases, with a master's degree), and a physician formed the intervention team. This project reported a smoking-cessation rate of 46% after 4 years among approximately 6000 men (Hughes et al., 1981): one of the most successful, biochemically confirmed long-term smoking-cessation rates. MRFIT demonstrated the efficacy of a maximum resource intervention in altering the smoking behavior history among a sample of men aged 35 to 57. A typical community-based group process program focusing on smoking cessation would be expected to demonstrate an effectiveness level of approximately 20% cessation among men at a 6-month follow-up (US Department of Health, Education and Welfare, 1980b).

Distinguishing between efficacy and effectiveness is important. Statements of the quality of a program reflect value judgments. Therefore, statements of impact expectations should be made with a degree of realism, within the context of time, resources, and empirical evidence. If one program reports a 10% rate of smoking cessation after 6 months for junior high school students and another program for a similar population reports a 25% cessation rate, this strongly suggests a real difference in program effectiveness and quality. It confirms a need to determine why the rates were different. Assuming comparable samples, data, and intervention methods, the observed difference strongly suggests a difference in program quality and/or provider competence. These two additional, interrelated dimensions of quality assurance—provider program adequacy and competence—need to be carefully considered when an organization makes a decision to create a program.

QUALITATIVE EVALUATION METHODS

For well over two decades, qualitative evaluation methods have been discussed in evaluation literature. Cook and Reichardt (1979), Windsor et al. (1984), Mullen et al. (1986), Steckler (1989), and Patton (1990) have all made important contributions. In this section, we provide a synopsis of qualitative methods and their utility. Both quantitative design and qualitative methods should be used to comprehensively evaluate health promotion, health education, and disease prevention programs. A special issue of *Health Education Quarterly* provides an excellent set of eight papers on "Integrating Qualitative and Quantitative Methods" (Steckler et al., 1992).

The quality control methods, discussed in this chapter, include (1) expert panel review, (2) internal audits, (3) program utilization and record review, (4) community surveys, (5) participants surveys, (6) programmer or session observations, (7) focus group interviews, (8) component pretesting, (9) readability testing, and (10) content analysis. Each method provides important information about the sequence of events and the interaction and linkage between participants and a program. They provide empirical data reflecting the qualitative aspects of the program, including acceptance and participation rates by target groups for a specific setting. Data from these qualitative methods place the program manager in a more knowledgeable position to discuss "how well the program is doing and how well the program worked."

Dispelling the misconception that the use of the word *qualitative* implies a lack of quantification or lack of empiricism is important. In the planning phases, skilled health promotion and education specialists should be able to put into operation and measure all important dimensions of a program. They, in collaboration with staff, should be able to describe what qualitative information to collect, how it is going to be collected, who is going to collect it, when it's going to be collected, and what instruments and observational methods will be used. These steps will produce a richer insight about what happened with the program. Qualitative evaluation allows you to go beyond the simple statements of a 10% difference between an experimental group and control group.

TYPE III ERROR

A major qualitative concern in all programs is implementation success—program feasibility or failure. Basch et al. (1985) describe the failure to implement a health education intervention as a "Type III error." Steckler (1989), in an insightful discussion of Type III error, used the qualitative case-study approach to monitor data to complement an impact evaluation. The subject of this report was the implementation success of a cancer control program at industrial plants of the United Rubber, Cork, Linoleum and Plastic Workers of America.

The application of qualitative-process evaluation methods and the examination of the degree to which Type III error had occurred is discussed. Steckler collected two types of qualitative evaluation data. The first was data from in-depth case studies from one intervention plant; the second was the monitoring of training activities and educational events that occurred at all experimental (E) and comparison (C) industrial sites. Other methods, well described in the literature (e.g., Patton, 1990), were used, including (1) site visits, (2) participant observations, (3) interview with key decision makers, and (4) record reviews of reports and documents related to program planning and implementation. Four additional types of monitoring data were also collected at all industrial study sites: (1) running records, (2) consultation logs, (3) phone logs, and (4) correspondence. A general plan of how the project was intended to work was examined. This case study found that the cancer control programs were not used to any great extent by employees at the ($\underline{C}$) group plant nor by employees at most of the (E) group plants. Significant change did not occur among intervention plant workers because of inadequate implementation of the planned health education program. It was concluded that a Type III error had occurred.

The following conclusion should *not* be made about this cancer control program: Its content and structure were inappropriate for this industrial site and for this type of worker. A more appropriate inference to draw is that, for this situation and at this time, other critical organizational barriers that prevented the introduction of this type of program existed among and between management and workers. Without this kind of qualitative insight, evaluators cannot know why a program did or did not produce an impact. With such insight, however, evaluators are in a stronger position to attribute observed change (if any) to the health education intervention. In cases where implementation is not successful, the qualitative information collected must provide the insight about why and why not.

PROVIDER TECHNICAL AND CULTURAL COMPETENCE

There is a long-standing, historical concern about the need to improve the quality of professional preparation and practice in health education and health promotion. In commenting on this concern from a legal perspective, Easton et al. (1977) refer to the lack of professional competence as educational malpractice. They argue that this can be as serious in consequences and costs as medical malpractice.

Understanding the unique characteristics of groups, communities, and individuals-at-risk is an established principle of planning and evaluation. The evaluator's methodological and technical skills must be balanced and influenced by an appreciation for the richness and diversity of the ethnic groups served by our health promotion and education programs. Many resources are available on this topic, but the following two represent current and accessible choices: (1) "Cultural Competence for Evaluators" (U.S. Department of Health and Human Services, 1992a, ed. Orlandi) and (2) "Health Behavior Research in Minority Populations" (U.S. Department of Health and Human Services, 1992b).

Provider competence can be assessed through internal or external peer review mechanisms, examining the program provider's academic and professional training, program experience, professional products, and current activities in the development, implementation, administration, and evaluation of health education and promotion programs. A brief synopsis of this topic and the credentialing process was discussed in Chapter 1. Codification of the skills for good health education practice continues to evolve. Widely disseminated documents, however, confirm that the professional competencies are well defined. Using the report of the initial Role Delineation Project (National Center for Health Education, 1980) on professional preparation in health education as a referent, two dimensions of provider competence can be examined: (1) up-to-date knowledge and (2) technical skill.

Knowledge of the State of the Art

Although knowledge development is always in flux, the literature in health promotion and education and related disciplines offer a body of knowledge about human behavior in sickness or health for most major diseases and behavioral risk factors for many large populations-at-risk. Accordingly, directors (senior staff) of health promotion and education programs need to know what has been done, what can be done, and how it should be done. Functioning as a good practitioner without a knowledge of the most up-to-date literature germane to your program(s) is impossible. Commonly cited reasons for program failure include program staff lack of knowledge of what level of impact is possible or probable and lack of academic coursework or field experience in applying program skills: ignorance of published work and insufficient theoretical grounding about behavior change. These deficiencies exist, in part, because of the diverse backgrounds of staff engaged in planning and providing health promotion and education programs, the unique characteristics of a setting, target audience and health problems, and lack of organizational clarity or direction in offering such programs. Employers also don't hold common views about appropriate academic and professional credentials in the recruitment and appointment of program personnel.

Technical Skill

As noted in Chapter 1 in the report on "Guidelines for the Preparation and Practice of Professional Health Educators" and the report of the initial Role Delineation Project, health education/health promotion staff should be able to demonstrate competence in a number of areas. Competent planners, directors, and program coordinators should be able to provide evidence that programs under their direction reflect high standards of practice and, within the context of available resources, reflect the latest knowledge.

PRACTICE STANDARD: Staff responsible for planning, managing, and evaluating health promotion and education programs should provide documentation of appropriate baccalaureate and master degree training and skill in being able to:

1. Define and interpret data on the extent and distribution of a selected health problem or risk factor for a defined geographical area, location, setting, and population, using available and/or derived sources of data (needs assessment).
2. Derive and describe, from available or collected evidence and expert opinion, the behavioral and nonbehavioral risk factors associated with a specified health problem (priority setting).
3. Describe, from the related literature, the current knowledge about health education and promotion interventions for the specified risk factor or health problem and defined population at risk and the degree to which a behavior or risk factor(s) is amenable to change (definition of objectives).
4. Define and describe, from the scientific evidence in the literature and from an educational–behavioral assessment, the contributing factors found to be causally associated with the health behavior or risk factors, including

   a. Target group characteristics: predisposing factors such as attitudes, beliefs, values, and channels of communication.
   b. Situational or setting characteristics: enabling factors such as availability and accessibility and cost of health education services.
   c. Program or service provider characteristics: reinforcing factors such as staff attitudes, behaviors, and skill in health education (behavioral diagnoses).

5. Synthesize, interpret, and translate the information, data, and evidence collected from steps 1–4 into a program plan (specification of intervention and implementation plan).
6. Design, implement, administer, and evaluate appropriate communication, community organization, and organizational development-training and educational–behavioral methods to produce change in the contributing factors and the behaviors identified in steps 3–5, in collaboration with other health professionals, organizational personnel, and consumers (specification of evaluation plan).
7. Prepare project reports of a publishable quality based on appropriate analytical methods (preparation of program reports).
8. Conduct professional activities in an ethical manner, reflecting appreciation for human rights, quality control methods, and standards of peer reviews established by organizations that set professional performance standards and guidelines (implementation using ethical practices).

The level and type of academic training that should produce a person with these competencies is the master's degree in public health–

community health education–behavioral science: MPH, MSPH, MS, or MA.

PROGRAM ADEQUACY

Methods for examining the adequacy of a health care program were first set forth by Donabedian (1966, 1968), modified by Starfield (1974), and described by Greene (1976). Their application to health education and promotion was discussed in detail in Windsor et al. (1984). The focus of this body of literature is how to apply quality assessment procedures to program structure, content, process, and impact-outcome. In this chapter, we focus on the first three components of a program. In Chapter 5, we focus on the impact-outcome.

In a structural assessment of a program, an evaluator examines the resources, facilities, and equipment for the delivery of services and asks, Are they adequate to deliver the service? Is the staff delivering the health promotion program qualified? In a process assessment, the ultimate questions are, What procedures were used to develop and implement the program? Are they consistent with normative criteria: criteria developed by a consensus of experienced peers in health education with established professional credentials? A process assessment using normative criteria is indirectly an examination of provider competence. It provides an examination of the professional activities of the provider from the perspective of peer group judgment. As in the practice of nursing and medicine, the key issue is, What constitutes good practice (care) for a specific health problem and population? How should a professional intervene?

In 1987 the American Public Health Association in collaboration with the Centers for Disease Control published "Criteria for the Development of Health Promotion Programs." This document presents a set of criteria intended to serve as guidelines for establishing the feasibility and/or appropriateness of programs prior to a decision to implement in a variety of settings: industries, hospitals, work sites, voluntary and official health agencies, and so on. These criteria noted in Table 4.1 are not intended as prescriptions to ensure success of a health promotion program. They suggest the kinds of issues to be considered in the decision-making process leading to resource allocation or the setting of program priorities.

QUALITY CONTROL METHODS

Practitioners need to conduct qualitative evaluations of health promotion programs in a systematic and technically acceptable fashion. The project staff can use a number of techniques to gain insight into

Table 4.1 Criteria for Development of Health Promotion Programs

Description

1. A health promotion program should address one or more risk factors that are carefully defined, measurable, modifiable, and prevalent among the members of a chosen target group, factors that constitute a threat to the health status and the quality of life of target group members.
2. A health promotion program should reflect a consideration of the special characteristics, needs, and preferences of its target group(s).
3. A health promotion program should include interventions that will clearly and effectively reduce a targeted risk factor and are appropriate for a particular setting.
4. A health promotion program should identify and implement interventions that make optimum use of available resources.
5. From the outset, a health promotion program should be organized, planned, and implemented in such a way that its operation and effects can be evaluated.

SOURCE: Adapted from American Public Health Association, "Criteria for the Development of Health Promotion" (1987): 89–92.

how well the program is being implemented, how well it is being accepted by a target group, and what adjustments in methods and procedures might be made. One quality control technique is not necessarily superior to another. Each is useful in program planning and implementing. Each serves a specific purpose and provides unique information about the structure, content, and process of an ongoing program. All require allocations of resources: staff and time. Because of this, selecting the most appropriate and feasible methods for a specific program is important. To conduct a thorough review of program quality during implementation, a combination of methods is recommended: (1) expert panel review, (2) internal audit of resource allocations, (3) program utilization and record review, (4) community and participant surveys, (5) program or session observation, (6) process evaluation, (7) focus group interview, (8) component pretesting, (9) readability testing, and (10) content analysis.

Expert Panel Reviews

The importance of reviewing an evaluation plan during the early stages of preparation cannot be overstressed. An expert panel review (EPR) is an efficient way to assess program elements. It assumes that a written program plan exists: Program objectives, methods, activities, procedures, and tasks are described in detail. It delineates program staff, time, place, and target group. Table 4.2 presents examples of standards to be used in an EPR.

Table 4.2 Key Program Categories for an EPR

Standard	Rating[a]
1. Documentation of the use of published studies pertinent to the health problem and the population in planning the program	1 2 3 4 5
2. Consultation with state or local agencies or experts where specific data, literature, resources, or staff experience is lacking	1 2 3 4 5
3. Use of target group representatives and affiliated local program agencies in planning	1 2 3 4 5
4. Program planning and adaptation reflects staff input	1 2 3 4 5
5. Planning based on empirical needs assessment concerning the knowledge, attitudes, and practices of target groups	1 2 3 4 5
6. Written support statement of program objectives and behavioral–educational intervention content and methods	1 2 3 4 5
7. Staff tasks clearly delineated and performed according to the program implementation plan	1 2 3 4 5
8. Documentation of the target group by number, characteristics, and proportion reached	1 2 3 4 5
9. Documentation outreach plans to recruit specific target groups according to priorities dictated by the objectives	1 2 3 4 5
10. Description of the data collection plan prior to implementation	1 2 3 4 5
11. Recordkeeping system and forms pretested prior to the initiation of program services	1 2 3 4 5
12. Monitoring system in place and used to assess completeness of pre- and postprogram data	1 2 3 4 5
13. Instruments and observation methods pretested and their validity and reliability assessed	1 2 3 4 5
14. Communication media and educational materials pretested and evaluated when implemented	1 2 3 4 5
15. Allocation of resources according to the implementation plan; identification of costs per participant	1 2 3 4 5
16. Description of evaluation designs	1 2 3 4 5

[a] 1 = poor; 5 = excellent.

An EPR can only be conducted when staff members have followed a systematic process to plan a program. The EPR examines major components, activities, materials, and procedures during program implementation, comparing documentation with a set of standards, using professional ratings. The total program and individual components are reviewed—for example, the implementation plan, evaluation design, data-collection procedures, mass-media components, instruments, or methods and content of the intervention.

An EPR is particularly useful during planning and early stages of implementation (Rossi et al., 1979; Simmons, 1975; Windsor et al., 1984). A review by one or two experienced consultants, once in the first 6 months and again each year for a project, should provide sufficient, independent insight into program progress. Practically speaking, it is important to have a small review panel. One or two experts from the local area or state can be asked, in many cases on a voluntary basis, to examine a program. Although EPR panel members must have experience with the health problem or risk factors the program is addressing, they need not be national leaders.

Common standards used by program staff and expert panels are listed in Table 4.2. The panel reviews materials and discusses and rates each salient program component of a written implementation plan. Key questions are, Were each of these activities performed? Were they performed in a timely manner? Evidence from written documents and discussions can be gathered by panel members individually and as a group from the staff. In addition to ratings, the panel can provide comments on the degree of adequacy observed and suggest program revisions. This information gives the program staff an overall qualitative judgment of the structure and process of the ongoing program. The EPR should be a collaborative activity with staff and external reviewers. It should provide practical suggestions for immediate program improvement.

> PRACTICE STANDARD: Health education/health promotion programs should document an EPR during the first 6 months of operation and at least once a year thereafter.

Internal Audit

An administrator must have some idea of what proportion of time staff members have spent on implementing a program and what nonpersonnel resources are being used. The issue is accountability. Although the actual time a person spends on a program may vary from month to month, all organizations require assessment and documentation of the level of staff effort. Business, industry, and education staff members routinely document monthly estimates of percentages (hours) of their time spent in categories of activities.

A program audit determines the consistency between the implementation plan and reality. Table 4.3 presents an example of an implementation plan for a high blood pressure program. The number of programs developed, sessions offered, participants recruited, and participants completing the program should be routinely reported. Documentation of a staff member's performance or the program's performance might consist of data on whether the objectives of a specific instructional program were accomplished. For example, did the pa-

Table 4.3   Implementation Plan Worksheet

Activity: Develop a county detection and treatment center

Implementation Strategy

Who Does What	When
1. Director of ambulatory services develops proposal for detection/treatment center	1/1
2. County board of health funds proposal	3/1
3. County renovates facilities	6/1
4. Director hires staff, including administrator and medical director	6/15
5. Administrator and medical director develop protocols and procedures, including special effort to motivate residents to participate and to follow up	8/15
6. Administrator acquires equipment and supplies	8/15
7. Data specialist develops patient record forms	9/15
8. Health educator develops education materials	9/15
9. Staff and volunteers are trained by medical director, health educator, and head nurse	10/1
10. Administrator tests methods and materials with county residents	10/15
11. Staff begins detection and treatment services to county residents	11/15
12. Administrator evaluates detection and treatment service	11/15

SOURCE: U.S. Department of Health, Education and Welfare (1977:37).

tients become more skilled in urine testing, or did pregnant adolescents in a school-based prenatal care program hear of or see the antismoking campaign for pregnant women? To document this, program planners must provide for assessments of immediate cognitive or performance objectives of the participants. Are there opportunities to receive feedback on participant interest and motivation and on staff performance? Because many health promotion programs are carried out in service-oriented settings, the major program objectives may be knowledge, information, or improved skill. If materials distribution is the component of a program being examined, how much of what material was distributed to whom should be documented. Procedures need to be developed so that planners can examine how well an element of a program is being applied, being accepted, and working (Deeds et al., 1979; Simmons 1975).

PRACTICE STANDARD: Health promotion programs should provide monthly, quarterly, and annual documentation of the type and amount of resources allocated, including staff time, media, and educational materials.

Program Utilization and Record Review

Health education programs often have too much or too little information collected on participants. The information collected is often not used. Despite the difficulty that may be encountered, a record-keeping system is an essential component of program implementation. The system should not overtax participants and program staff, particularly if the staff is small, for example, one person—you. All program-monitoring and data-collection systems should be compatible with ongoing data systems.

Program utilization and record reviews encompass four topics: (1) monitoring program participation or session exposure, (2) improving record completeness, (3) documenting program or session exposure, and (4) monitoring the use of information services.

Monitoring Program Participation. Inherent to setting up a monitoring system is the need to define who the program is attempting to serve and an estimated number of eligible participants for the target area or location. All target populations must be enumerated. This allows you to answer the questions, How many of those eligible were served? Were the people who participated those for whom the program was designed?

Improving Record Completeness. For some programs, standard record forms may be mandated. Programs almost always need minimum demographic and psychosocial characteristics and data concerning participants. Although this responsibility may seem to present major difficulties, if staff members agree about the types of information needed on each participant and pay particular attention to efficiency in information collection, they should be able to gather complete documentation on service use (Broskowski, 1979; Windsor, Roseman, et al., 1981).

Table 4.4 illustrates the amount of information that can be lost by a poor instrument and record-keeping system. A retrospective 12-month review of medical records of patients at a 40-bed hospital was computed to determine the quality of patient educational assessment data of admitted diabetics (Windsor, Roseman, et al., 1981). Although it was hospital policy to assess each patient on admission, only 394 of 996 patients (39%) had a baseline assessment on file. These 394 forms were reviewed to determine the quality of the assessments performed. A major problem identified, beyond nonperformance of the assessment, was data incompleteness. From the standpoint of assessing educational needs, preparing an educational prescription, or evaluating program effectiveness, data abstracted from the forms for this

Table 4.4 Completed Items in Records of Diabetic Patients, in Rank Order

Item	Decile of Forms with Item Completed
Diabetes instructor	90–100%
Age	
Put on _____ calorie-ADA diet	80—89%
Diabetes mellitus diagnosed—year	
Demonstrated drawing up and injection of insulin	70–79%
Has been taught to use _____ urine test	
Personal hygiene and foot care items taught	
Educated in diabetic control	
After learning to use a urine test, knows how and when to test urine for sugar	60–69%
Knows how and when to test for acetone	
Knows how to use dextrostix	
Understands causes and symptoms of reactions, acidosis	
Understands need to call doctor if acidosis develops	
Attitude on admission	50–59%
Understands insulin adjustment for reactions etc.	
Attitude on discharge	40–49%
Can test urine for sugar accurately	
Knows how to use booklet to follow diet	
Patient or member of family has been taught to use glucagon	
Pretest score	30–39%
Class attendance—insulin	
Class attendance—personal hygiene and foot care	
Class attendance—reactions and acidosis	
Class attendance—diabetes	20–29%
Class attendance—urine checks	
Diet restrictions	
Knows representative foods and amount of each exchange group	
Class attendance—diet	
Patient's physical or learning handicaps	10–19%
Post-test score	0–10%
Incapable of drawing up own insulin or testing urine	

SOURCE: Windsor, Roseman, et al. (1981:468–475).

period were of no use. Serious questions about the quality, validity, and reliability of the data collected were apparent. Findings of this record review are not uncommon in health care and public health settings (Deeds et al., 1975).

Health promotion programs will improve their recording systems by developing a monitoring mechanism that meets both staff and evaluation needs. It should be compatible with data processing or allow data to be aggregated by hand for quick periodic assessment, for example, monthly or per session. A record-keeping system is the only mechanism by which program evaluators can confirm how many of which demographic groups of clients were served. It is an essential process evaluation element to examine.

Documenting Program or Session Exposure. Another dimension to consider in examining program records is participant exposure to program sessions. A baseline and follow-up assessment of all participants or a sample should be conducted. Without exception, a health promotion program must document who received how much of what and when.

The observation form in Figure 4.1 was used to confirm patient

Rm.	Patient						
	Mon.	Tues.	Wed.	Thurs.	Fri.	Sat.	Sun.
a.m.							
p.m.							

Rm.	Patient						
	Mon.	Tues.	Wed.	Thurs.	Fri.	Sat.	Sun.
a.m.							
p.m.							

Rm.	Patient						
	Mon.	Tues.	Wed.	Thurs.	Fri.	Sat.	Sun.
a.m.							
p.m.							

Rm.	Patient						
	Mon.	Tues.	Wed.	Thurs.	Fri.	Sat.	Sun.
a.m.							
p.m.							

Rm.	Patient						
	Mon.	Tues.	Wed.	Thurs.	Fri.	Sat.	Sun.
a.m.							
p.m.							

Figure 4.1 Observation Form for Closed-Circuit Television Programming in the Diabetes Hospital

Table 4.5 Patient Exposure to Closed-Circuit Television Programs

Day	Program	Patients Exposed	Potential Patients	Percentage Exposed
Monday	1	19	29	34
	2	3	31	10
Tuesday	1	5	31	16
	4	3	29	10
	5	6	27	22
Wednesday	11	6	28	21
	7	6	30	20
Thursday	8	4	30	13
	9	7	31	23
Friday	10	4	30	13
	11	10	31	32
Saturday	4	6	31	19
Sunday	13	8	31	26
	14	7	30	23
Total	14	85	419	20

exposure to a closed-circuit educational television (ETV) program for diabetic patients in a 40-bed hospital. For a 1-week period, patients' rooms were observed to determine whether the patients were viewing the ETV programs presented twice daily. Using this method, the staff confirmed the proportion of patients exposed to each program and the proportion of programs to which each patient was exposed during the 1-week observation period.

As Table 4.5 indicates, on average, only 20% of approximately 30 eligible patients per day watched the closed-circuit programs, documenting a very low level of patient exposure to this channel of communication. These data confirmed a need to examine why so few patients used this program method.

PRACTICE STANDARD: Health promotion programs should document levels of participant or target audience exposure to each intervention component.

Monitoring the Use of Information Services. Some health promotion programs provide health information or counseling services. For data to be routinely collected for each contact, a record-keeping system for monitoring use must be set up with concern for accuracy, quality, and consistency. The Caller Data Form (Figure 4.2) is an example of a simple, two-sided instrument used throughout the 1980s by the Alabama Cancer Information Service (CIS). It was established to gather and process by computer complete and essential data on the more

BIRMINGHAM COMPREHENSIVE CANCER CENTER

CIS CALLER DATA FORM

CASE I.D. [1][ ][ ][5][ ]   DATE [6][ ][ ][ ][11]

1. START (MILITARY TIME) [12][ ][ ][ ][15]   2. DAY OF WEEK: [16][ ]   3. SEX (M-1, F-2) [17][ ]

4. CALLS FROM:

☐ CaPat-1   ☐ Gen Pub-4   ☐ OtherHPro-7
☐ RelCaPat-2   ☐ MD-5   ☐ StudHPro-8
☐ FrCaPat-3   ☐ RN-6   ☐ OtherStud-9
                                  ☐ Other (Specify)-10   18 19 [ ][ ]

DESCRIPTION OF CALL:

5. TYPE OF INQUIRY:

		20 21 [ ][ ]
☐ SiteSpecInfo-01	☐ Treat-Rad-07	
☐ BCCC-Info-02	☐ Referral-08	22 23 [ ][ ]
☐ CIS-Info-03	☐ Symptoms-09	
☐ RiskFactor-04	☐ GenCaInfo-10	24 25 [ ][ ]
☐ Agency-Serv-05	☐ Ed-Info-Mat-11	
☐ Treat-Chemo-06	☐ Other (Specify)	

6. PRIMARY SITE(S) DISCUSSED:

			26 27 [ ][ ]
☐ Breast-01	☐ Skin-07	☐ Hodg-12	
☐ Lung-02	☐ Melan-08	☐ Brain-13	28 29 [ ][ ]
☐ Col-Rec-03	☐ Pros-09	☐ Lym-NHodg-14	
☐ Leuk-04	☐ Bone-10	☐ Pancr-15	
☐ Uterus-05	☐ Kidney-11	☐ Blad-16	
☐ Cervix-06	☐ Other (Specify)		
Not applicable			

7. PRIMARY TYPE OF SERVICE(S) PROVIDED:

		30 ☐
☐ Info-1	☐ Referral-3	
☐ Counseling-2	☐ MatNeeded-4	31 ☐
☐ Other (Specify)		
☐ Caller emotionally upset:	☐ yes-1 ☐ no-2	32 ☐

8. PRIMARY (FIRST) SOURCE OF INFORMATION ABOUT CIS

					33 34 [ ][ ]
☐ TV-01	☐ ACS-05	☐ RN-09	☐ HlthDept-13	☐ PrevUser-16	
☐ Radio-02	☐ Rel-06	☐ ProjHELP-10	☐ LeukSoc-14	☐ BCCC-17	
☐ Newsp-03	☐ Friend-07	☐ PhoneBk-11	☐ NCI-15	☐ UAB-18	
☐ PrintMat-04	☐ MD-08	☐ CoopExt-12	☐ Other		

Side 1

Figure 4.2 Alabama Comprehensive Cancer Center CIS Caller Data Form—1980

than 7000 individuals who initially used this information service from 1980 to 1982 (Windsor et al., 1983).

In establishing a form to monitor use of a health information service, program staff should first conduct a thorough review of existing instruments and record-keeping systems. Planners should adapt existing instruments and record-keeping systems for their purposes.

9. PREVIOUS USE OF SERVICE ☐ No-0   ☐ Yes-No. of times in past year

In order for us to know whether we are serving
all people in Alabama, we need to know your: Age: _____

Race: 1-B, 2-W, 3-0 _____

35 ☐
36 37 ☐☐
38 ☐

---

10. FOLLOW-UP SURVEY (MONTHLY)
It is very important that we evaluate our Cancer Information Service. Would you
be willing to fill out a short 1-page Questionnaire to be sent to you in the
next month to evaluate our service and the information you have just received?

39 ☐

☐ No-2   ☐ Yes-1   IF NO—TRY AGAIN

If no, why not: _____

ASK FOLLOWING INFORMATION:

Print
Name _____   Address: _____

_____

Phone: ☐☐☐ ☐☐☐☐ (40, 46)   County: ☐☐ (47 48)   Zip: ☐☐☐☐☐ (49, 53)

TIME ENDED CALL: _|_|_|_

CLOSED OUT (XA: ☐

TOTAL MIN. _____

OPERATOR NO. _____

54 55 ☐☐
56 57 ☐☐

---

11. FOLLOW-UP:

Mail follow-up needed?   ☐ Yes-1   ☐ No-2

Phone follow-up needed?   ☐ Yes-1   ☐ No-2

List follow-up action(s). Describe and note date completed. Include Xeroxed
materials sent.

_____

_____

_____

58 ☐
59 ☐
60 61 ☐☐

---

12. CLOSE OUT:

REFERRALS: _____

COMMENTS: _____

OPERATOR NO. _____

MILITARY TIME-CLOSEOUT _____

TOTAL TIME SPENT SERVICING REQUEST AFTER CALL: MINUTES _____

DATE: ☐☐☐☐☐

62 63 ☐☐
64 65 ☐☐
66   69 ☐☐☐☐
70 71 72 ☐☐☐
73   78

Side 2

Staff members need to remember that any form they develop may be
compared to a national standard of quality for similar programs. A
form must be acceptable to the program staff and participants who
must fill it out or file it. A major problem in many health education
and promotion programs is the apparent neglect to details such as
ease of use by staff and time in setting up a system. Existing CIS

monitoring systems were examined in the development of their data form. CIS staff input was continuous and extensive during the development process. In the final record system, the director of evaluation (Windsor) set a quality control standard of 95% as the acceptable level of data completeness for each item.

Programs that are not provided the resources, that ignore the importance of the procedures described, or that plan or implement an impractical or inappropriate system either reduce or eliminate the possibility of evaluating program process and effectiveness. From the standpoint of structure, the key question is, Does an information-gathering system exist? In terms of process evaluation, the question is, How good is it? Poor record keeping indicates a poor-quality program. If no resources have been provided to collect the needed information, program staff will not be able to document who was served, how well they were served, or what changes—cognitive, belief, skill, or behavioral—occurred from exposure to the program. The documentation and evaluation expectations of program staff and directors must then be modified accordingly. Poor data-collection and record-keeping procedures are major compromisers of program and process evaluations.

PRACTICE STANDARD: Health promotion programs should provide documentation of a 95% level of data completeness for all program participants and for each data record item.

Community and Participant Surveys

Program evaluators often need to survey target groups in a community or samples of participants in an organization. Although the purposes of a community survey will vary, it attempts to find out whether a program has (1) reached a target audience, (2) increased the target audience's awareness of the program, (3) increased the level of community interest, (4) increased the number who use the program or service, and (5) provided a satisfactory service (Rossi and Freeman, 1993; Windsor et al., 1984).

Representativeness of your sample and accuracy of data are important issues to address in conducting a community survey. The program staff must carefully consider the limitations and disadvantages of using nonrandom sampling methods. Selecting a representative sample of respondents is always preferable, but you can use a number of practical, less rigorous approaches to obtain qualitative data on audience needs and perceptions of a program prior to or during the early stages of implementation.

A community assessment may involve the use of a range of methods, from a random sample of households to a convenience sample. Of the possible techniques by which an evaluator may systematically gather qualitative information about a program's progress, four are feasible: (1) opinion leader survey, (2) community forum survey, (3) network (pyramid) survey, and (4) central location survey. Each can be conducted in a short period of time at little cost; each has advantages and disadvantages. They do not provide a representative statement of the opinions of a defined population. We will present more detailed discussions on sampling procedures and other technical details of data collection in Chapters 6 and 7, but in the sections that follow we describe each community survey method and its limitation.

Opinion Leader Survey. Key lay or professional community informants, persons who should be familiar with the program, are selected as participants in an opinion leader survey. This type of survey is relatively easy and inexpensive to conduct. It is particularly useful in the discussion, planning, and early implementation stages of a program when support and interest from community leaders are crucial for program success. It may also generate familiarity with awareness of and interest in the program among these leaders. Generally, data from this survey are generated from person-to-person interviews. Using a nominal group process is also effective (Delbecq et al., 1975; Ross and Mico, 1980).

Written questions should be prepared to elicit key information from the leaders about their impressions of a proposed or ongoing program. An opinion leader survey usually solicits a broad range of information. Results from it reflect the degree of consensus about the program from knowledgeable community people. This method plays an important role in assessing the political support for a program. It may be invaluable to an innovative program in identifying program barriers, acceptability, and initial enrollee satisfaction. Using this method, program planner should be able to document community and organizational input to and support for the program.

Community Forum Survey. In the community forum approach, several locations are selected for public meetings with a specific target audience. Community forums are inexpensive and usually easy to arrange. They usually take 1–2 hours. The meetings may be open or by invitation. This method can be used to educate the current participants and to gather their impressions of the diffusion, acceptance, and levels of participation in the program. A list of key questions must be prepared as a basis for eliciting audience input (Ross and Mico, 1980:257–272).

The forum method is most efficient when the meetings are small or when the audience is divided into smaller groups with a staff member or trained layperson acting as facilitator and recorder to ensure maximum participation. The forum encourages a wide range of community expressions about the problem. Its major disadvantages are (1) one group or individual may control the discussions or use the forum exclusively for expression of a grievance or opposition to the program and (2) attendance may be limited and information covered very biased.

Network Survey. In a network (pyramid) survey, key individuals—for example, those identified as "hard-to-reach," having characteristics representative of a special target group (e.g., black, female, under age 18)—are selected from existing records or they are program participants. A program may start off with a list of five to ten persons on file. As part of the survey, these subjects are asked to identify two friends with the target group characteristics who have not used the program. Each individual is surveyed and also asked to identify one or two people with backgrounds similar to theirs, until a given quota (e.g., 30 to 50) is met. This method elicits an increasingly broader selection of people who tend to be demographically homogeneous but not easily accessible to the program staff.

The surveys can be conducted in a short period of time (month) to collect data about target audience beliefs about the health promotion topic or program or the community's perception of the problem. Use of this method may also provide an estimate of community awareness of the program among those with whom little contact has been made. It should help uncover reasons why individuals with characteristics similar to program participants have not participated (Windsor, 1973; Windsor, et al., 1980).

Central Location Survey. The central location survey is another technique commonly employed to gather information quickly and efficiently from a large number of people (100 to 200) in a community. Typically, multiple sites (two to ten) are selected that are frequented by a large number of people who possess the characteristics of the target audience for the health promotion program: a shopping center, movie theater, beach, or other pedestrian high-traffic areas in a metropolitan city or rural county. Interviewers identify a specific group (e.g., women of a certain racial or age group) and conduct short interviews (2–5 minutes) of the people on the spot. Questions may concern the person's familiarity with a health problem, knowledge of the availability of the program and its purpose, or interest in a special program. Views are elicited from a specific number of people (U.S. Department of Health, Education and Welfare, 1978b).

PRACTICE STANDARD: Health promotion programs should provide documentation of having conducted surveys of community, consumer, and participant awareness of and satisfaction with the program.

Program or Session Observations

The purpose of observational data is to document the activities that took place at a specific time and place. These data also describe the people who participated and examine what happened between participants and staff during a session. A highly accurate appraisal of the interaction can be derived from observational techniques. The interpersonal skills of staff members are, in part, reflected in their interactions with an audience. The audience may be consumers of a health education program, the providers of a health care service, a group of administrators, or community leaders who play a principal role in setting organizational policy or providing community support. One quality control issue is the adequacy of verbal and nonverbal communication and group process skills demonstrated by staff members.

There are a number of ways to conduct observational assessments, but almost all include some type of overt or covert participant observation. Patton (1990) describes a number of variations of participant observations that a program may use singly or in combination. The observer's activities may be concealed, a participant observer may be identified as an observer but not as a participant, the observer's activities may be publicly known, or the observer may act as a participant and not as an observer. Lofland notes four concerns in conducting observations:

First—the qualitative methodologist must get close enough to the people and situation being studied to be able to understand the depth and details of what goes on.
Second—the qualitative methodologist must aim at capturing what people actually say: the perceived facts.
Third—qualitative data consist of a great deal of pure description of people, activities, and interactions.
Fourth—qualitative data consist of direct quotations from people, both what they speak and what they write down. (1971:136)

Unobtrusive measures (e.g., discarded cigarettes at a school ground or work site) may also provide appropriate data (Webb et al., 1966). It is essential to identify beforehand what is to be observed,

Table 4.6 Item-Total Correlation for Instructor Evaluation Form

Item	Item-Total Correlation Coefficients
1. The instructor puts high priority on the needs of the class participants.	.51
2. The instructor makes a lot of mistakes in class.	.52
3. The instructor gives directions too quickly.	.52
4. The instructor helps me feel that I am an important contributor to the group.	.55
5. A person feels free to ask the instructor questions.	.61
6. The instructor should be more friendly than he/she is.	.58
7. I could hear what the instructor was saying.	.65
8. The instructor is a person who can understand how I feel.	.57
9. The instructor focuses on my physical condition but has no feeling for me as a person.	.65
10. Everyone who wanted to contribute had an opportunity to do so.	.57
11. There was too much information in some sessions and too little in others.	.52
12. Just talking to the instructor makes me feel better.	.60
13. The purposes for each session were made clear before, during, and after the session.	.50
14. Covering the content is more important to the instructor than the needs of the class.	.60
15. The instructor asks a lot of questions, but once he/she gets the answers she/he doesn't seem to do anything about them.	.62
16. The instructor held my interest.	.68
17. The instructor should pay more attention to the students.	.69
18. The instructor is often too disorganized.	.67
19. It is always easy to understand what the instructor is talking about.	.61
20. The instructor is able to help me work through my problems or questions.	.62
21. The instructor is not precise in doing his/her work.	.60
22. The instructor understands the content he/she presents in class.	.68
23. I'm tired of the instructor talking down to me.	.60
24. The instructor fosters a feeling of exchange and sharing between class participants.	.58
25. The instructor is understanding in listening to a person's problems.	.72
26. The instructor could speak more clearly.	.60
27. The instructor takes a real interest in me.	.62

SOURCE: Miller and Lewis (1982:56–66).

how, where, and the frequency and duration of the observations. The observation process may range from a casual period of personal observation of a session to video- or audiotaping or full sessions. The evaluator should carefully examine the interaction between participants and staff can be performed. From this, the evaluator can assess what information was presented, how, and the quality of interactions between presenter and audience. This method, commonly referred to as *interactive analysis* (Bales, 1951; Flanders, 1960), is often beyond the capability of the evaluator of an ongoing service project. Roter (1977) provides an excellent example of an interactive analysis study of patients and physicians.

Conducting program observations with limited resources is possible. Observations provide insights into what people do in a program, how they experience it, the organization of activities, and the behaviors and interactions of participants. A program may routinely apply a quality assurance system in which all instructors are evaluated by consumers.

Miller and Lewis (1982) report on a 27-item instructor assessment form that was administered to 150 program participants in the Puget Sound HMO Group Health cooperative. The instrument was developed by the health education department to offer feedback to its more than 70 facilitators per year from a sample of 3000 program enrollees. The form was used to assess technical and interpersonal competence. Table 4.6 presents the items and the strength of the correlation of response to each. An overall alpha reliability of .94 with all individual items having high ($>$.40) correlation was reported. This confirmed an excellent level of item-to-total correlation coefficient reliability (internal consistency). Information on observation skills and methods are available in the education, business, communications, and social–behavioral sciences literature.

PRACTICE STANDARD: Health promotion programs should document the quality of communicating (interaction) between program staff and consumers.

Process Evaluation: Implementation Assessment

Data in Table 4.7 represent hypothetical results of a process evaluation. This example applies to a work site with 500 employees. The first procedure entailed conducting a brief survey screening all 500 employees, to identify the proportion with specific behavioral or disease risk factors that made them eligible participants. Of the 500, 150 were found to be at high risk. These 150 employees were notified by the health education program (HEP) staff about participating in a spe-

Table 4.7   Hypothetical Process Evaluation of Employee Participation in a Health Promotion Program

Procedures	Eligible Partic- ipants (A)	Partic- ipant Exposure (B)	Percent- age Reached (B/A = C)	Perfor- mance Standard (D)	Implemen- tation Index (C/D = E)
1. Risk screening of employees	150	100	67	80	.84
2. Educational diag- nosis/health-risk assessment	100	88	88	90	.98
3. Health behavior counseling	100	84	84	90	.93
4. Group session 1	100	81	81	90	.90
5. Behavior monitoring	100	76	76	90	.84
6. Group session 2	100	72	72	90	.80
7. Behavior contract	100	62	62	90	.62
8. Group session 3	100	60	60	90	.67
9. Follow-up 1	100	56	56	90	.62
10. Follow-up 2	100	50	50	90	.55

cial program to help them deal with this particular risk factor. Over a 6-month period, 100 of the 150 contacted by the HEP enrolled. As noted in Table 4.7, this represents 67% of the eligible population. For this and the remaining nine procedures, the HEP established a set of performance standards for implementation.

For procedure 1, the HEP decided that the standard would be to enroll 80% (120 of 150) of employees identified as high risk (e.g., high blood pressure) in the screening survey. Only 100, or 67%, en-rolled, however, producing an implementation index of .84. Of the 100 enrollees, 88 received procedure 2, the educational diagnosis/ health-risk assessment. Following assessment, 84 participated in pro-cedure 3, the one-to-one health behavior counseling. An increasingly smaller proportion participated in the three health education and risk-reduction sessions conducted with groups of 5 participants each (procedures 4, 6, and 8). As part of the series, each participant was expected to complete two principal procedures: a self-assessment ex-ercise between sessions 1 and 2 (procedure 5), consisting of recording and monitoring the frequency and sites of their smoking behavior, and discussion and signing of a behavioral contract with a significant other (procedure 7), between sessions 2 and 3. As noted in Table 4.7, 76 percent and 62 percent of the participants participated in these two processes, respectively. Two follow-up assessments and counseling sessions (procedures 9 and 10) were required of all participants, 3 and 6 months after the program; 56 participants were exposed to follow-up session 1 and 40 to session 2. This program reported a 20% behavior-change rate—20 successes out of 100 initial enrollees for each procedure.

A Program Implementation Index (PII) can be computed by dividing the proportion reached for each procedure by the program standard: $C/D = E$. Compute PII by adding all indexes and dividing the total by the number of procedures:

$$PII = \frac{.84 + .98 + .93 + .90 + .84}{10}$$

$$+ \frac{.80 + .69 + .67 + .62 + .55}{10} = .78$$

A high-quality HEP should specify in advance and confirm levels of exposure to each program procedure. A program should specify the expected PII for individual procedures and a projected total PII. This approach enables a program evaluator to plot individual and group exposure and to make clear statements about the level of implementation success. It suggests that the program is being managed well or not so well. The PIIs and indexes pinpoint problem areas.

PRACTICE STANDARD: Health promotion programs should provide documentation of what proportion of eligible participants were served, the extent of participation of each individual, the program completion rate, and the effect of the program on participants' behavior. A PII should be reported for all health promotion programs.

Case Study: Smoking-Cessation Programs for Pregnant Women

R. A. Windsor, M. Dalmat, T. Orleans, and E. Gritz, *The Handbook to Plan, Implement, and Evaluate Smoking Cessation Programs for Pregnant Women* (White Plains, N.Y.: March of Dimes Foundation, 1990), pp. 44–45.

Information presented in Table 4.8, a process evaluation of the Jefferson County Health Department (JCHD) Smoking and Pregnancy Project, involving 309 patients provides an application of the process evaluation methods discussed in the previous section. For this patient education project, 16 procedures were specified. The anticipated number of JCHD patients (eligible = A) to receive these procedures was enumerated and percentage of exposure documented (B). A performance standard (D) was chosen that reflected an absolute (100%) or superior level (>90%) of staff performance. With this information, the implementation of a process

Table 4.8 A Process Evaluation of the JCHD Smoking and Pregnancy Project

Procedures	Eligibles (A)	Exposed (B)	Completion Rate (B/A = C)	Performance Standard (D)	Implementation Index (C/D = E)
1. Conduct external review	N/A	N/A	N/A	Completed	1.00
2. Survey participants	200	200	100%	100%	1.00
3. Survey staff	86	80	93%	90%	1.00
4. Pretesting component— instruments	100	100	100%	100%	1.00
5. Pretesting component— health education methods	50	50	100%	100%	1.00
6. Observe sessions— three sites	3	3	100%	100%	1.00
7. Screen participants	1800+	1863	100%	100%	1.00
8. Recruit smokers	460	368	82%	80%	1.00
9. Collect baseline data	309	309	100%	100%	1.00
10. Collect baseline SCN[a]	309	300	96%	100%	.96
11. Apply intervention	102	102	100%	100%	1.00
12. Collect midpoint data	309	281	91%	95%	.96
13. Collect midpoint SCNs	309	278	90%	95%	.95
14. Collect final data	309	247	80%	95%	.84
15. Collect final SCNs	309	232	75%	95%	.79
16. Prepare final report	N/A	N/A	N/A	Completed	1.00

PII = 1.00 + 1.00 + 1.00 + 1.00 + 1.00 + 1.00 + 1.00 + 1.00 + 1.00 + .96 + 1.00 + .96 + .95 + .84 + .79 + 1.00 = .97

SOURCE: Windsor, et al. (1990:44–45).
[a]SCN = Saliva thiocyanate, a metabolite of nicotine.

evaluation requires that the number of health promotion and education participants (schoolchildren, patients, workers, or community participants) be documented (exposed = *B*). With the specification of the number of eligible participants for each procedure and documentation of exposure, a completion rate (*C*) can be computed. A comparison can be made with the performance standard (*D*) and then an implementation index (*E*) can be computed. An implementation index documents the extent to which the program has successfully implemented critical procedures. It is presumed that peers who might review these procedures (an EPR) would concur that these procedures were critical components of the JCHD.

Using this process, the program evaluator can compute the PII. The PII provides a general statement of the extent to which program managers can confirm that participants have been exposed to each part. Procedures 1–6 represent planning steps, and 7–16 represents program steps. Data in Table 4.8 confirm successful implementation of the patient education program. With the exception of the end of pregnancy follow-up, procedure 15, all completion rates were high. This project used a computerized system for each clinic to document monthly, quarterly, midyear, and annual reports to monitor implementation of the program.

By conducting the process evaluation using a systematic and empirical methodology, we documented successful implementation of the program. For another detailed discussion of how to conduct a process evaluation see Lowe et al. (1989). Finnegan et al. (1989) also provides alternative methods, as part of a process evaluation to track program implementation.

Focus Group Interview

A focus group interview is a group session method to explore insights of target audiences about a specific topic. This method is discussed in greater detail in Chapter 7. Market researchers and advertisers use this method to derive the perceptions, beliefs, language, and interests of an audience to whom the product or service would be marketed. The focus group interview usually involves eight to ten people. Using a detailed discussion outline, a moderator keeps the group session within the appropriate time limits but gives considerable latitude to participants to respond spontaneously. The moderator has the opportunity to probe and gain in-depth insight from the interviews. These sessions are often video- or audiotaped.

Particularly used in the concept development stage of the communications development process, focus group interviews help health communications/media planners identify key concepts that may trigger awareness and interests in participation. This method is often used to complement population-based, representative-sample surveys on specific topics. Qualitative information is used in combination with the survey data to make judgments about the perceptions, beliefs, and behaviors of the target population and subgroups within it.

To implement a focus group discussion, individuals with the characteristics of the target group are recruited 1 week to 1 month in advance. Ideally, participants would not know the specific subject of the session in advance, nor would they know one another. The total number of focus groups needed is not absolute, but four groups are likely to be the minimum. It will depend on the needs, resources, and time that a health promotion and education program has. The group moderator must be experienced and capable. A bachelor's- or master's-trained specialist who has had courses in group dynamics, group process, and community organization could capably handle such a task. Several sequential steps include warm-up and explanation, introductions, assessment of general attitudes, general knowledge dealing with the disease, major sources of information and program assistance of services, and attitudes toward proposed programs. Other categories could be added as appropriate to the topic and to the health promotion and education program. Krueger (1988) and Basch (1987) are excellent resources for using this method.

Component Pretesting

Pretesting, a quality control method used by health educators and health communicators, documents needs and perceptions of target audiences. All programs should have their selected intervention elements pretested prior to their application. Good pretesting is a continuing problem in the field because it requires technical skill from the staff, resources, and time often not available. The importance and utility of pretesting cannot be overstressed. The three most common program elements that should be pretested are instruments, media, and materials, both written and visual. The following sections discuss the purposes and methods of pretesting these elements.

Instrument Development and Pretesting. In conducting a process evaluation, the quality of the evaluation instrument (questionnaire) should be determined. In the literature, a well-documented deficiency is the failure of many health education program planners to establish the reliability and validity of their instrument data. Examine all instruments to determine their relevance to the specified objectives of the program. In the development and pretesting of an instrument, program planners must demonstrate concern for the consumer. The instrument should be a manageable length—the shorter, the better. Collect only essential information from participants.

Pretest instruments for such characteristics as time of administration, ease of comprehension, readability, sensitivity, reactivity of questions, organization of questions, and standardization of administration and scoring. First, select a sample of individuals who are representative of the population for whom the instrument is prepared. Then test the instrument under conditions comparable to those in which it will be applied in the program setting. The following are common procedures for developing instruments (Windsor, Roseman, et al., 1981):

1. Formulate program objectives—review the literature.
2. Define objectives in behavioral or performance terms.
3. Review existing instruments and record-keeping systems.
4. Identify by internal review essential cognitive, affective, and psychomotor skills and descriptive information needs.
5. Construct a draft instrument and agree on procedures.
6. Identify measurement methods and coding and interviewer training.
7. Pilot-test with 30 to 50 people from the target group to determine essential characteristics of the instrument—validity, reliability, adequacy of questions, ease of administration, degree of standardization, and efficiency (the time required).
8. Repeat the internal review and modification; perform an external review.
9. Conduct a formal instrument testing with 100 target group members; reexamine the characteristics in step 7.
10. Repeat an internal review; revise and finalize the measurement process and the instrument for routine application.

As a preliminary step (before a formal pilot test), to eliminate glaring problems of omission or commission, four or five people from the target group can be asked to review and complete the instrument. The target group should identify issues such as ambiguous questions, lack of clarity, or insensitivity in word choice.

To ensure distribution of responses across characteristics, usually 30 to 50 people participate in a pilot test. If the pilot test is self-administered, provide a set of written instructions on how to complete the form. Respondents should be able to provide reactions and suggestions for changes.

Instrument pretesting is a critical first step to ensure data quality. Rely heavily on instruments used by comparable programs; no program planner should develop a new instrument unless absolutely necessary. If, for example, the program is attempting to change the participants' personal health practices or beliefs, the staff should adapt forms identified in the literature or available from national agencies for surveying health risk factors, practices, knowledge, and beliefs.

Use the preceding procedures to modify an existing instrument to fit the objectives of the program. After applying these procedures, program planners are in an excellent position to modify the instrument. In its final form, the instrument should facilitate the aggregation of data for hand tabulation or data entry and processing. Information in Chapters 6 and 7 will expand the technical discussion related to data completeness and data quality.

PRACTICE STANDARD: Health promotion programs should document the pretesting of their instruments, providing information on data accuracy (validity) and reproducibility (reliability).

Media and Messages. Pretesting systematically gathers target audience reactions to written, visual, or audio messages and media. In assessing the quality of media, program staff should document their having followed procedures that meet professional standards. Program planners who do not pretest media lose the opportunity to gain valuable insights into the quality of those methods of communication (Bertrand, 1978). A thorough review of formative evaluation methods for media is provided in "Making Health Communication Programs Work" (U.S. Department of Health and Human Services, 1989). It is important to follow well-established steps to create media (see Figure 4.3).

The ultimate purposes of pretesting media—formative evaluation—are to improve means of communication before their diffusions and to predict which alternatives will be most efficient and effective in the field. The concept of pretesting is simple; it involves measuring the reactions of a group of people to the object of interest, for example, a film, booklet, radio announcement, or poster. Pretesting should be done not only with members of the target audience but also in-house staff. Obviously, the sophistication and budget that can be applied to conducting a pretest are almost unlimited. The resources expended by the advertising industry each year confirm this fact.

In developing health information programs and revising existing messages and media, pretesting is an essential tool to assess ease of comprehension, personal relevance, audience acceptance, ease of recall, and other strengths and weaknesses of draft messages before they are produced in final form. A pretest should establish a target audience baseline and help determine if there are large cognitive, affective, perception, or behavioral differences within the target audience.

Program planners should design pretests of media to provide information on the following components of effectiveness (Bertrand, 1978; U.S. Department of Health and Human Services, 1989):

Attraction: Is the presentation interesting enough to attract and hold the attention of the target group? Do consumers like it?

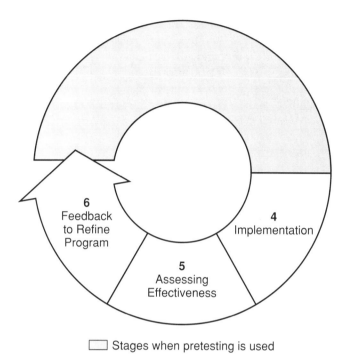

☐ Stages when pretesting is used

Figure 4.3 Stages in Health Communication

Which aspects of the presentation do people like most? What gained the greatest share of their attention?

Comprehension: How clear is the message? How well is it understood?

Acceptability: Does the message contain anything that is offensive or distasteful by local standards? Does it reflect community norms and beliefs? Does it contain irritating or abusive language?

Personal involvement: Is the program perceived to be directed to persons in the target audience? In other words, do the consumers feel that the program is for them personally, or do they perceive it as being for someone else?

Persuasion: Does the message convince the target audience to undertake and try the desired behavior? How favorably predisposed are individuals to try a certain product, use a specific service, or initiate a new personal health behavior?

No absolute formula can be used to design a pretest or field trial. A pretest should be tailored to your objective and consider time, cost, resources, and availability of the target audience. Planners may have to decide which media will be formally pretested and which may undergo only internal staff review. This decision must be tempered by the risk of creating active opposition to a program by not assessing beforehand audience or organizational responses.

Hecht (1978) makes the following general suggestions to planners of instructional media:

1. State briefly the program topic.

2. List the primary and secondary program audiences.

3. State why a program is important.

4. Specify expected objectives for consumer and provider.

5. Specify what the viewer should know and do from media exposure.

6. State belief changes the media are attempting to influence.

7. Prepare a 10- to 30-minute instructional program.

8. Choose the medium—provide information on why this is an important health information source.

9. Prepare script content based on characteristics of the audience.

10. Plan visual materials.

11. Develop a storyboard.

12. Describe the evaluation procedures to assess cognitive, belief, skill, and behavioral impact.

13. Conduct the program.

14. Evaluate the program.

15. Revise the product.

All ongoing programs need to have their media examined carefully before using them with the audience. A wide range of simple or highly technical and costly methods and procedures are available. The acceptability and memorability of selected media and products may often be improved, however, without a major allocation of time or resources. Flay (1987) is a good source of methods to evaluate the total health communication campaign.

Written Materials. Written materials are almost always used in health promotion and education programs. The major concern is, Can people read and understand the material? Written materials should serve as aids to information transfer and should clarify and reinforce the principal messages specified in the program objectives. Using written materials as principal behavior-change elements of your program is, however, archaic. Many professionally developed and field-tested written materials are available for most health problems and risk factors. To assess program materials, use a three-step process: (1) assessment of reading level, (2) content analysis, and (3) review by content and health education specialists.

The program staff must first gather materials and review them thoroughly to determine which ones might serve program objectives best. Some can be modified for the target audience. Design written materials for efficient, low-cost distribution. They must be capable of capturing the interest of the audience and be presented in an imaginative yet simple fashion. It is important that terms, word choice, and other characteristics be chosen to promote reading. Use pretesting to gather words, phrases, and vernacular from target audiences, so that appropriate language can be used in materials, and to determine the most effective method for communicating information. Manning (1981) offers the following suggestions for preparing written materials:

1. Use one- and two-syllable words if appropriate.

2. Write short, simple sentences with only one idea per sentence.

3. State the main idea at the beginning of each paragraph.

4. Break up parts of narrative with subheadings and captions.

5. Use the active voice.

6. Highlight important ideas and terms—boldface or italic type.

7. Leave plenty of "white space" on the printed page.

8. Add the phonetic pronunciation of key technical terms.

9. Define difficult words.

10. Summarize important points in short paragraphs.

To assess the quality of materials, program evaluators should ask the following major questions:

What are we trying to accomplish?

Why are we using this particular medium to communicate this information?

For whom are the written materials intended?

Under what circumstances will people read it?

What languages or ethnic perspective do we need to consider in preparing our materials?

These issues must be resolved during the development of written material before significant resources are spent. In constructing materials, the writer must select a succinct title, prepare a written text in some format, and consider the number and type of illustrations to be used. The staff also must reach agreement on when, how, and how often the written materials will be introduced to participants in the health promotion program. Programs should have a mechanism to document the distribution of written materials, for example, monthly or quarterly by type. "Making Health Communication Programs Work" (U.S. Department of Health and Human Services, 1989) provides current information on the content and methods, to assess printed materials.

If a program uses written materials extensively as aids or reinforcement to its educational efforts, staff may want to assess whether participants are using the information. In a study by the Rand Corporation for the Food and Drug Administration on informing patients about drugs, participants were asked seven questions to determine their behavioral responses to a written insert in a medication package (Winkler et al., 1981:32):

1. Do you remember a leaflet that came with your prescription?

2. Did you read it before you started taking erythromycin?

3. (If no): Did you get a chance to read it later?

4. After you read it, did you ever go back and read it again?

5. (If yes): Why did you read it again?

6. Did you keep the leaflet, did you throw it away, or what?

7. Did anyone else read the leaflet from your prescription?

The results from 879 men and women using 69 pharmacies in Los Angeles County in 1979 and 1980 provide evidence refuting the myth that "no one reads those things." As Table 4.9 indicates, a very large proportion of subjects read the leaflet before starting to take their prescription, a significant proportion read it more than once, a majority kept the leaflet, and approximately one in four showed it to someone else. Many ongoing programs that use written information could use the questions, documentation, and formative evaluation design applied in this study. They determine in a formative fashion how effective written components of a program are in communicating information to program participants.

Although many other questions were examined in this study (e.g., variations in format, length, content, and style), the basic process was to determine what type of document worked best. The study

Table 4.9 Behavioral Responses to Leaflets, Study 1

	Experimental Condition			
Response	Low Explanation, No Instructions	Explanation	Instructions	Explanation and Instructions
Read leaflet	77.6%	84.6%	70.3%	80.6%
Read before starting medication	67.2%	65.3%	64.1%	59.7%
Read more than once	36.2%	32.7%	31.3%	33.9%
Kept leaflet	53.4%	63.5%	51.6%	61.3%
Showed leaflet to someone else	22.8%	25.0%	29.7%	27.4%

SOURCE: Winkler et al. (1981).
NOTE: Based on the responses of 236 men and women who received leaflets in study 1. Cell sample sizes ranged from 44 to 64. Effective sample sizes were slightly lower because of missing data.

used methods that have broad applicability to health programs. It conducted a qualitative effectiveness assessment of participants' reactions to the package insert using a semantic differential scale. Individuals were asked to rate different pamphlets on the basis of their thoroughness and clarity of explanation, degree of stimulation, simplicity or complexity, level of reassurance, and factuality. Wilkie (1974), Ligouri (1978), Dwyer and Hammel (1978), and Hladik and White (1976) have also performed such studies. Doak et al. (1985) is a good source of information on how to teach patients with poor reading skills.

Visual Materials, Radio, and Television. In pretesting visual aids (e.g., posters), a principal aim is to assess their ability to attract. In general, they should be attention getters, conveying one single idea. The extent to which they are comprehensible, educationally and ethnically acceptable, and promote audience involvement should be assessed. If a major fiscal expenditure is being made, multiple samples from the target audience at different locations may be needed. To pretest a poster, however, a small number of people may be sufficient—five to ten. Although many questions can be asked, ten are presented here that are often used by an interviewer or in a self-administered questionnaire to determine an individual's response to a visual aid:

1. What is the most important message presented?
2. Is this visual aid asking you to do something?

3. Is there anything offensive to you or other people who live in your community?
4. What do you like about it?
5. What do you dislike about it?
6. In comparison to others you have seen before, how would you rate it?
7. Is the information new to you?
8. Are you likely to do what the visual aid asks?
9. Do you think the average person would understand it?
10. How would you improve it?

These questions and others that staff may consider appropriate should be asked as the visual is shown to the individual. The responses will provide insight into the attractiveness, comprehensibility, and acceptability of the visual aid (U.S. Department of Health, Education and Welfare, 1980a; U.S. Department of Health and Human Services, 1980b).

The pretesting of radio and television announcements follows the general principles outlined for other categories of media. One difference, however, is the need to produce and pilot-test an announcement. Cost is a major factor to consider. A radio announcement can be easily taped on a recorder and a poster designed in rough form, but producing a TV announcement or program, even in preliminary form, can be expensive. Figure 4.4 is an instrument used to pretest a radio announcement and illustrates the questions that might be asked.

Health Message–Testing Service. For programs on a number of specific health problems (e.g., smoking cessation, breast self-examination, physical fitness), the staff may choose to use a commercial health message–testing service. This type of service provides a standardized system to assess audience response to radio and television messages about health to gauge the communication effectiveness of these messages (U.S. Department of Health, Education and Welfare, 1980a). The system informs program planners of the audience's message recall, comprehension, and sense of the personal relevance and believability of the message, as well as identifying strong and weak communication points. In testing a message, the major concern is its appropriateness for its intended subgroup. To measure communication, a testing service examines the attention-getting ability of the message and audience recall of the main idea. Overall, a health message–testing service can provide invaluable insights to refine draft message an-

---

Case number: _____
Radio spot (identification): _____

Code

1. In your own words, tell me what the spot said. ⬜

   _____

2. Was the spot asking you to do something in particular?
   1. ____ Yes   2. ____ No   9. ____ Don't know   ⬜
   2a. If yes: What? _____

3. Did the spot say anything that you don't think is true?
   1. ____ Yes   2. ____ No   9. ____ Don't know   ⬜
   3a. If yes: What? _____

4. Did the spot say anything that might bother/offend people
   who live here in _____ (name of community)?
   1. ____ Yes   2. ____ No   9. ____ Don't know   ⬜
   4a. If yes: What? _____

5. Do you think this spot is intended for someone like yourself, or is it for other people?
   1. ____ Self   2. ____ Others   9. ____ Don't know   ⬜
   5a. If "others": Why? _____

6. Was there anything about the spot that you really liked?
   1. ____ Yes   2. ____ No   9. ____ Don't know   ⬜
   6a. If yes: What? _____

7. Was there anything about the spot that you didn't like?
   1. ____ Yes   2. ____ No   9. ____ Don't know   ⬜
   7a. If yes: What? _____

8. In comparison to the other spots on the radio these days,
   how would you rate this spot on _____ (topic)?
   1. ____ Excellent   2. ____ Good   3. ____ Fair   ⬜
   4. ____ Poor   9. ____ Don't know

9. What do you feel could be done to make it a better spot? ⬜

   _____

Figure 4.4 Questions for Pretesting Radio Announcements

nouncements, choosing between alternative messages and planning future health promotion campaigns. It is, however, very expensive.

Television Program Evaluation and Analysis by Computer. A recent advance in the evaluation and research of television productions has been the application of microcomputer technology. Electronic analyses can be made of the effects of a TV presentation, documenting an audience's reaction second-by-second. With this technology, observing the effects of minute changes in presentation on the audience's attitudes, knowledge, and skill is possible. This information gives program personnel the opportunity to manipulate covertly what audience members see and to analyze their responses instantaneously. It allows program personnel to collect instant feedback data on an infinite number of visual, graphic, verbal, and other configurations.

Although most service programs are not capable of applying this highly sophisticated method of assessing audience response, it is a new, useful, and powerful technique for conducting formative evaluations of media during the production stages. Given the increased impetus to use television as a major medium in health promotion and education via the Public Broadcasting System and cablevision, this technology may be of particular relevance to national or multisite efforts where considerable formative evaluation of products is essential. Before investing in production costs that easily could run into six or seven figures, agencies will need to perform careful preliminary assessments.

PRACTICE STANDARD: Health promotion programs should conduct pretests of their media and materials for the following effectiveness components: (1) attraction, (2) comprehension and readability, (3) acceptability, (4) audience involvement, and (5) persuasion.

Readability Testing

Readability is another important aspect of pretesting written materials. Interpreted pretests for readability are available and easy to apply. Readability tests essentially determine the reading grade level required of the average person to understand the written materials. Readability estimates provide evidence of only the structural difficulties of a written document, that is, vocabulary and sentence structure. They indicate how well the information will be understood but do not guarantee the effectiveness of the piece. Many readability formulas exist (Dale and Chall, 1948; Flesch, 1948; Fry, 1968; Klare, 1974–1975), but the SMOG grading formula for testing the readability of educational material is one of the most commonly applied (McLaughlin, 1969). Generally considered the best method of assessing the grade level that a person must have reached to understand the text, it requires 100% comprehension of the material read. To calculate the SMOG reading-grade level, McLaughlin (1969:639) advises program personnel to use the entire written work that is being evaluated and to follow these four steps:

1. Count off 10 consecutive sentences near the beginning, in the middle, and near the end of the text.

2. From this sample of 30 sentences, circle all words containing three or more syllables (polysyllabic), including repetitions of the same word, and total the number of words circled.

3. Estimate the square root of the total number of polysyllabic words counted—find the nearest perfect square and calculate the square root.

4. Add a constant of 3 to the square root to calculate grade (reading-grade level) that a person must have completed if he or she is to fully understand the text being evaluated.

Sentence and word length and difficulty affect the readability score. The SMOG formula ensures 90% comprehension; that is, a person with a tenth-grade reading level will comprehend 90% of the material rated at that level. This procedure can be applied to all texts prepared by a program for public consumption. "Making Health Communication Programs Work" (U.S. Department of Health and Human Services, 1989) presents useful discussions of readability in general and in health-related literature.

Content Analysis

The following discussion, by Glanz and Rudd, represents an excellent example of how to assess the readability and content of printed materials. The purpose of this case study, a condensed version of the article, was to review available print cholesterol education materials and to examine their readability and content.

Case Study: Cholesterol Education Materials

K. Glanz, and J. Rudd. "Readability and Content Analysis of Print Cholesterol Education Materials," *Patient Education and Counseling* 16 (1990):109–118.

Readability Testing and Content Analysis

Readability testing examines the linguistic and structural qualities of written text, but it does not assess the content, difficulty of concepts, or appropriateness for a target audience. Content analysis is a systematic, quantitative description of a communication's content. The use of content analysis and readability assessment permits a more meaningful profile of the characteristics of currently available cholesterol education materials.

Methods: Criteria to Include and Identify Materials

Inclusion Criteria. This analysis focused on print educational materials that met five criteria:

1. Materials that focus on low-fat, low-cholesterol eating and/or those used by cholesterol education programs.

2. Materials that are generally available to the public or patients from government, voluntary health agencies, professional associations, universities, or the public education units of proprietary health and laboratory organizations. Materials could be distributed through health professionals or patient educators.

3. Materials that are patient "give-aways"; there may be some costs to providers but should not involve a patient charge. Commercially available books were excluded.

4. Materials that can stand alone as educational materials—not be intended for use only in combination with other educational media or delivery modes, for example, slides, tapes, lecturers, individual counseling.

5. Materials that are available by July 1989.

Identification of Materials. The first source of materials involved items received by the authors in their prior work in nutrition education. Materials and sources were identified through the Abstract Book of the National Cholesterol Conference (November 1988). Requests were also made directly to organizations known to be involved in public and patient cholesterol education. These methods of identification produced an incomplete list of materials: 38 items. [See article for materials analyzed.]

Analysis of Materials

Analysis of materials was completed in three steps: characterization of materials, assessment of readability level, and content analysis.

Characterization of Materials. Each item was cataloged by title, sources, date of publication, and primary intended audience (general public, public and screening participants, those identified with elevated cholesterol, and patients in treatment). Size was measured from unopened dimensions of the brochure or pamphlet. Length was assessed by word count and by number of pages (based on one page in an unopened state). Appearance was assessed by presence of blank ("white") space between text (space of two or more lines between blocks of text) and use of visual images and print size.

Readability Analysis. Readability was assessed using two methods. The first, the SMOG grading formula, predicts the grade of a written passage correctly with a standard error of predication of 1.5 grades. Because

Table 4.10   Mean Readability Levels of Cholesterol
Education Materials

	Audience			
No. of items	General 11	Screening 10	Hi Chol 17	Total 38
SMOG grade level	11.5	10.3	10.9	10.8
FOG grade level	11.4	11.0	10.9	10.9

SOURCE: Glanz and Rudd (1990:109–118).

the SMOG is based on 100% comprehension of materials, we also use the FOG formula, which is based on 50%–75% comprehension of the written material. Both formulas give estimates of grade level of education required to understand the text.

Content Analysis. For each educational brochure or pamphlet, we assessed the presence or absence of nine content elements. Four were related to diagnosis of elevated cholesterol and related cardiovascular risk factors, discussion of HDL/LDL lipid fractions, the physiology of cholesterol elevation, other heart disease risk factors, and weight control or reduction. Five elements were related to instrumental information about dietary behavior change and food—choice mention of types of foods to emphasize or avoid, use of brand names, information on food preparation methods, portion size, and the distinction between saturated fat and polyunsaturated or other types of fats.

Analysis Procedures

The analysis and coding procedure was pilot-tested on a sample of materials. An independent analysis of a subsample of materials was completed, followed by resolution of any discrepancies by agreement among raters.

Results

Readability Assessment. The mean readability levels of the materials was grade 10.8 (S.D. 1.50), SMOG grading formula, and 10.9 (S.D. 1.99), FOG grading formula. Approximately 70% of all items were written at a reading level of grade 10 or higher.

As Table 4.10 shows, readability levels were uniform across audience categories. No significant correlation existed between reading level and length of the item, defined either in terms of word count or number of pages. There was a strong, significant, and positive correlation ($r = 0.78$) between SMOG and FOG readability level. This adds confidence about the accuracy of the reading levels.

Table 4.11   Percentage of Items Containing Content Elements by Audience Category: Diagnosis and Risk-Related

	Percentage with Content Element*			
Audience	HDL/ LDL	Physiol	CHD Risk	Wt Control
General (n = 11)	36.4[b]	54.5	45.5[b]	36.4
Screening (n = 10)	70.0[a]	90.0	90.0[a]	40.0
Hi Chol (n = 17)	47.1[b]	64.7	64.7[b]	58.8
Total (n = 38)	52.8	68.4	65.8	47.4

SOURCE: Glanz and Rudd (1990:109–118).
*Explanation of content elements: Mention/discussion of HDL/LDL = HDL/LDL lipid fractions; Physiol = physiology of cholesterol elevation; CHD Risk = other heart disease risk factors; Wt Control = weight control/reduction. Within content elements, percentages with different superscripts indicate $P < 0.05$ by Mann–Whitney U-test (a's indicate significantly higher percentages than b's).

Content Analysis. Table 4.11 presents the findings for diagnosis and risk-related content elements, audience category, and complete sets of materials. Statistically significant differences (Mann–Whitney U-Test [23]) in the percentage of mentions within content elements across audience categories were determined. Approximately half the materials explained the meaning of HDL/LDL lipid fractions. Fewer than half addressed weight control and its role in cholesterol management. Mentions of HDL/ LDL and other heart disease risk factors were slightly more frequent in materials for screening audiences. A similar but nonsignificant trend was evident for the elements of cholesterol physiology. Weight control was most often discussed for those identified with elevated levels (hi chol).

The results of the content analysis for dietary behavior appear in Table 4.12. Nearly all the materials addressed types of foods, food preparation, and the distinction between saturated and other types of fat (87%, 82%, and 87%, respectively). Fewer than two-thirds (60.5%) discussed portion size. Only 7.9% included brand names when recommending desirable food choices. The materials designed specifically for patients (hi chol) were significantly more likely to include types of foods and food preparation information. A similar but nonsignificant trend was evident for portion size and saturated–unsaturated fats.

Discussion

The recency of publication of most of the cholesterol education materials identified and analyzed attests to the rapid expansion of information on

Table 4.12   Percentage of Items Containing Content Elements by Audience Category: Dietary Behavior Change, Food Information

Audience	Percentage with Content Element*				
	Food Types	Brands	Food Prep	Portion	SatFat
General (n = 11)	72.7[b]	0.0	72.7[b]	63.6	90.9
Screening (n = 10)	80.0[b]	20.0	70.0[b]	40.0	80.0
Hi Chol (n = 17)	100.0[a]	5.9	94.1[a]	70.6	88.2
Total (n = 38)	86.8	7.9	81.6	60.5	86.8

SOURCE: Glanz and Rudd (1900:109–118).
*Explanation of content elements: Mention/discussion of Food Types = food groups/types; Brands = uses brand names; Food Prep = preparation methods; Portion = portion size; SatFat = types of fat (saturated/unsaturated). Within content elements, percentages with different superscripts indicate $P < 0.05$ by Mann–Whitney U-test (a's indicate significantly higher percentages than b's).

Table 4.13   Implications for Practice: Providing Readable and Relevant Cholesterol Education Materials

Know your audience and audience segments
  Racial, ethnic, age, and socioeconomic background
  Reading ability
  Lifestyle patterns
Design, locate, and/or request materials at lower reading levels
Pretest materials for understandability and appeal before printing or ordering large quantities
Create materials that are easy to carry
Use larger print (at least 12 points) for older and visually impaired audiences
Address other CHD risk factors and weight control
Consider use of brand name lists of lower-fat food items

SOURCE: Glanz and Rudd (1990:109–118).

this subject. This assessment suggested that the majority are aimed at well-educated, middle-class, middle-aged, nonminority populations who are highly motivated to translate abstract concepts into food choices. There appears to be a need to develop materials to reach important but underserved segments of the population, to tailor messages and materials to the needs of potential users, and to design materials with attention to the consumer's or patient's lifestyle. The implications of this study for practice are presented in Table 4.13 and discussed in greater detail in the original article. [See article for references.]

SUMMARY

Numerous quality control methods, standards, and guidelines are available to use in conducting a qualitative-process evaluation of an ongoing health promotion and education program. Standards exist in the fields of health education, promotion, and communications that apply to all elements discussed in this chapter. Program planners, evaluators, and administrators must know these established methods and be able to apply them.

5

Evaluating Program Effectiveness

"How do we choose the best design to evaluate our program?"

"My health officer said he wants us to evaluate our hypertension program. I don't know how many people we will need to do a good evaluation."

"When I read or hear evaluation reports, I'm not sure what to look for or what questions to ask."

"Our evaluation consultant really helped us. She made sense, and she managed to explain the important problems with internal validity."

Professional Competencies Emphasized in This Chapter

• Selecting an evaluation design

• Identifying factors affecting internal and external validity

• Applying a standard notation system

• Determining sample size

• Describing strengths and weaknesses of common designs

• Establishing a control or comparison group

• Applying meta-evaluation and meta-analysis methods to critique the results of evaluation reports

Although program evaluations are essential, they are often neglected because of lack of time, resources, and staff. Even when resources are available, program staff may lack the technical expertise or experience to plan an evaluation. Despite these problems, federal, state, and local agencies that support health education/health promotion programs require that evaluation be a component of the planning and delivery of services. Before expending significant fiscal resources on new or ongoing programs, all organizations need to establish an evaluation system to examine the extent to which they have delivered services and/or produced desirable changes among participants. Realistically, however, every intervention program and/or component cannot and should not be evaluated.

You need a number of components to begin a discussion of evaluation of a program's effectiveness, including written program plan objectives, specification of the intervention and program methods, measurement and data-collection procedures, and a description of methods to pilot-test and to document program implementation (Cook and Campbell, 1983; Rossi et al., 1979; Windsor and Cutter, 1981; Windsor et al., 1980). Experience and the literature suggest that these components cannot be assumed. Evaluation consultants are often asked to help evaluate programs for which one or several of the above components are lacking or not well defined. So, before you can design an evaluation of program effectiveness, you may have to go back to step 1 to specify program elements and methods and address related methodological issues.

You will need to gain competence and confidence in selecting, applying, and adapting program evaluation designs and methods. You should be able to choose from among alternatives, basing your decisions on factors such as (1) the objectives of your program, (2) the purposes of the evaluation, (3) the availability of evaluation resources, and (4) the characteristics of your health and behavior problems, setting, and population-at-risk. Before preparing an evaluation plan, be aware of and attempt to control for the numerous possible sources of bias that will affect the interpretation of impact data. You need to determine what is and is not possible for your particular setting, time period, and resource constraints.

You must address a number of methodological issues to conclude that your program has been effective. You will need an appreciation of evaluation principles and methods described in the literature, to answer two questions commonly asked about a program: Did it work? Can the observed impact (if any) be attributed to the program intervention(s)? To answer these questions, consider two broad issues: What design will be used? What is its purpose?

Often, the setting and type of a program may make it difficult to conduct an evaluation of high methodological quality. A common constraint is the challenge of applying the experimental model: a randomized design with an experimental group and control group(s). Although you should continue to stress the value of the experimental model when planning evaluations, this design may not be feasible for some programs. You can usually make methodological adjustments to the constraints of a given situation. The literature confirms that several good designs can be adapted to special circumstances. The adaptation of these designs and methods to your setting is one of the most creative exercises an evaluator will face (Cook and Campbell, 1979; Green and Figa-Talamanca, 1974; Kenny, 1975; Rubin, 1974; Shortell and Richardson, 1978; Weiss, 1972; Windsor et al., 1980).

TYPES OF EVALUATION DESIGNS

A design is a guide to specify when, from whom, how, and by whom program procedures will be applied and measurements will be made during the course of program implementation and evaluation. A blueprint for a well-organized evaluation, a design allows you to draw conclusions with varying degrees of certainty about the impact of a program: Program results can be judged within an appropriate context for magnitude and programmatic importance. It also helps you estimate, with varying degrees of confidence, what outcomes are produced if the participants had not been exposed to the program (Fitz-Gibbon and Morris, 1978; Spector, 1981).

Three types of design are important for this discussion: experimental, quasi-experimental, and nonexperimental.

An *experimental design* includes random assignment, a control (C) and an experimental (E) group, and observations of both groups, usually prior to and always after application of the intervention. Results derived from an experimental design usually yield the most interpretable, definitive, and defensible evidence of effectiveness. Designs of this type assert the greatest degree of control over the major factors that influence the internal validity of results.

A *quasi-experimental design* includes the establishment of an experimental (E) group and a comparison (C̲) group by methods other than random assignment. Such designs include observations of both groups, both prior to and after application of the intervention. Results from this design may yield interpretable and supportive evidence of program effects. Quasi-experimental designs exercise varying degrees of control over several biases but usually not all that affect the internal validity of results.

A *nonexperimental design* does not include random assignment or a control group and asserts little or no control over the major factors that confound interpretation of an observed effect.

FACTORS AFFECTING VALIDITY OF RESULTS

Internal validity is the extent to which an observed effect (e.g., improved cognitive, skill, behavioral, economic, or health-status indicators) can be attributed to a planned intervention. In selecting a design to evaluate a program, a major question is, Did the planned intervention *A* produce the observed impact *B*? Did *A* cause *B*, or was the observed change produced by other factors?

External validity is the extent to which an observed impact can be generalized to other settings and populations-at-risk with similar characteristics (e.g., workers in a similar business, patients using a comparable clinic, or high school students in another county school system). External validity, as noted in Chapter 1, is an issue addressed by evaluation research. Selection bias is one of the most critical biases to external validity. If results are valid, to which population can you generalize? Although program personnel should be concerned with both internal and external validity, generally speaking, ongoing health education programs and services should be more concerned about internal validity. External validity is frequently beyond their scope or capability. Attempts to create a program that has broader applicability (e.g., statewide) may dissipate the unique characteristics and synergy of program personnel and participants at a given site, so that little or no impact is produced. Moreover, improving the internal validity of results should be the major focus of an ongoing program because it enables the program staff to make optimal use of resources, time, facilities, and personnel to maximize the opportunity to produce a desired change among program participants.

FACTORS AFFECTING INTERNAL VALIDITY

Several common factors influence the internal and external validity of an observed program outcome. In selecting an evaluation design, you need to consider eight common factors that bias the internal validity of an observed result. Each factor may confound or bias interpretation of program efficacy or effectiveness by independently producing all or part of an observed impact or outcome. The factors are the following:

1. *History* is the significant, unplanned national, state, local, or internal organizational events or exposure occurring at the program site during the evaluation study period that result in change by participants. EXAMPLE: A principal and school board impose a schoolwide smoking ban on school grounds.

2. *Program or participant maturation* is the natural, biological, social, behavioral, or administrative changes occurring among the participants or staff members during the study period, such as growing older, becoming more skilled, or becoming more effective and efficient in program delivery. EXAMPLE: A 10-year-old child matures socially and psychologically to an adolescent of 13 years old in an urban setting where peers encourage drug use.

3. *Testing or observation* is the effect of taking a test, being interviewed, or being observed on outcomes. EXAMPLE: An adult in a screening program is interviewed by a nutritionist about her amount of fiber intake; she may be prompted to give socially and programmatically desirable responses and might change her fiber-intake behavior over a short period of time.

4. *Instrumentation* is a bias produced by changes in the characteristics of measuring instruments, observation methods, or data-collection processes, that is, factors affecting the reliability and validity of instruments. EXAMPLE: Evaluators use a carbon monoxide method of ascertaining smoking levels at baseline and a behavioral report at follow-up.

5. *Statistical regression and artifacts* is the selection of an experimen-

tal, control, or comparison group on the basis of an unusually high or low level or characteristic that may yield changes in subsequent measurements. EXAMPLE: A program is used to select and study a group of employees at least 30% overweight at the beginning of a weight-reduction program.

6. *Selection* is the identification of a control or comparison group not equivalent to the treatment group because of demographic, psychosocial, or behavioral characteristics. EXAMPLE: A group of 100 adult-smoking community residents is chosen as a comparison group to 100 adult-smoking university employees.

7. *Participant attrition* is a bias introduced in outcome data by nonrandom or random and/or excessive attrition (10% or more) of the treatment or control group participants. EXAMPLE: In a stress-management course, 20 of 100 participants from the control group and 6 of 100 from the intervention group drop out of the program; those experiencing high stress levels drop out in greater numbers because they cannot devote time to the program, due to other commitments.

8. *Interactive effects* are any combination of the previous seven factors (Campbell and Stanley, 1966; Cook and Campbell, 1983; Kerlinger, 1973; Windsor and Cutter, 1981; Windsor et al., 1980).

You need to become thoroughly familiar with these factors that confound evaluation results and learn how best to control for each. With increased competence and confidence, you can select an appropriate design to help you rule out other plausible, alternative explanations for an impact. Problems with any of the confounding factors will limit your ability to observe an impact or attribute it to the program interventions.

The literature and our experience confirm that factors 4, 6, and 7—instrumentation, selection, and attrition—are the most frequent major compromisers of evaluation results (Bernstein, 1976; Porter and Chibocos, 1975; Windsor and Cutter, 1981).

A NEW EVALUATION DESIGN PARADIGM
FOR THREATS TO INTERNAL VALIDITY

Contemporary evaluation thinking demands a reassessment of the traditional discussion and schematic presentation of the eight threats to validity. Bias (threats) to the internal validity of program results should be condensed into the three categories which confound attribution of causation to an intervention: historical bias, measurement bias, and selection bias (Table 5.1).

Table 5.1 Biases to Attribution of Causation: Internal Validity

Type of Bias	Dimensions	Issues
History	External events ($\underline{H}$) Internal events (I) Treatment (X)	Exposure: Frequency and duration of stimulus
Measurement	Validity (V) Reliability (R)	Procedures Type of data
Selection	Eligibility (Participation rate) (P) Refusals rate (R) Dropout rate (D) Attribution rate (A)	Representativeness: Sample vs. defined population

Attribution of Causation to an Intervention

The first bias to attribution is *history*, which has three dimensions. First is the external events ($\underline{H}$) that may, either in a transient or more extended way, be plausible cause(s) of the changes in an impact or outcome rate. Second is the internal programmatic, historical events (I) that may have occurred in either the natural history of a behavioral risk factor or structural, staffing, and administrative changes in a program. Third is treatment effects (X). The concern here is the extent to which exposure to a program (X)—intensity, duration, and frequency of exposure to specific behavioral or educational elements— has occurred (process evaluation) and the degree of standardization and replicability of intervention methods. Addressing this dimension gives the evaluator an idea of when exposure occurred, what occurred, and how observed changes were produced.

The second bias to attribution is *measurement*, which has two dimensions. These dimensions include the empirical evidence, collected prior to and during an evaluation, to confirm that your impact or outcome rates are valid (V) and reliable (R). The two issues of concern are (1) the process or methods used to collect the data and (2) the type and variations of the different types of data. The critical concern here is the extent to which methods are standardized and replicable and data are provided to empirically document reliability and validity characteristics. Resolution of these critical dimensions must occur before an evaluator can accurately assess if and how much change has occurred.

The third bias to attribution is *selection*. How representative is your evaluation study sample? Can the results of your evaluation be applied to the defined population in your setting (internal validity) for a behavioral risk factor or health problem rate? The key issue is representativeness. Describing the eligibility criteria for an evaluation of a program and enumerating the total number of eligible participants (denominator) are critical. Selection bias comprises four dimensions. First are those individuals who are eligible (P) to participate in a program and your evaluation—the defined population-at-risk. Second are those individuals who are eligible and accept (numerator) or refuse (R) to participate. Third are those individuals who initially agree to participate but decide to drop out (D). Fourth are those individuals (attrition) who did not drop out but were lost to follow-up (A). Each of these four dimensions will produce serious selection biases to internal and external validity. Thus, your ability to generalize evaluation results to a defined population may be severely limited or impossible, if you do not address these issues in your planning and formative evaluation.

These three biases play a direct role in explaining the degree of attribution of causation: Did your program produce changes? It should be apparent that an evaluation design does not always "control" for these major biases. The purpose of a design is to create E versus C (or $\underline{C}$) group equivalence at baseline and follow-up. Keep this in mind: An experimental design attempts to distribute (in equal proportions) samples of participants and the individual variability (bias) of each. An experimental design and randomization tries to equally distribute (known and unknown) variance for multiple characteristics that are predictors of change, independent of external ($\underline{H}$), internal (I), or treatment (X) exposure. An evaluator must, in the planning and formative evaluation phase, address these biases to attribution of causation to have any confidence in the results the evaluation produces.

EVALUATION DESIGN NOTATION

Learning the hieroglyphics of evaluation design is necessary for effective communication. A small, specialized number of notations, representing different elements of a design, will be used in discussions in other sections of this chapter:

R = random assignment of an individual (or unit) to a group.
E = experimental, or intervention, group; it may be expressed as E_1, E_2, E_3, to portray exposure of a group to different elements or types of treatment.
C = control, or equivalent, group established by random assignment; this group is not exposed to an intervention or exposed to only a minimum or standard intervention.

$\underline{C}$ = comparison group established through any method other than randomization.

X = treatment of intervention methods applied to an E group; $X_1, X_2, X_3, \ldots, X_n$ signifies that the interventions consist of different elements.

N = number of subjects or participants in an E, C, or $\underline{C}$ study group.

O = observation to collect data; methods include tests, interviews, visual or audio ratings, or record reviews; $O_1, O_2, O_3, \ldots, O_n$ signifies multiple observations at different times.

T = time; it specifies when an observation, assignment to a group, or application of a treatment or program element has taken place; $T_1, T_2, T_3, \ldots, T_n$ describes the period time between observations.

EVALUATION DESIGNS

There are numerous designs that you might select to evaluate your program. The number of designs that are administratively feasible and produce valid, interpretable results, however, are few. Five designs are frequently used to evaluate programs. Each design will allow you to assess the degree to which you can attribute observed outcomes to the application of your program. More complex designs (e.g., multifactorial designs) are possible, but they are almost always beyond the resources of an ongoing program. More complex designs are also likely to fall within the domain of evaluation research, which has increased expertise, resource, and time demands.

In the following section, we describe the methodological and analytical issues in selecting these five designs and their strengths and weaknesses in interpretability and internal validity. Table 5.2 presents information on the internal validity and potential independent sources of bias of these five common evaluation designs. As noted in the table, the nine potential biases to internal validity and the tenth (Σ), the interactive effects of any or all of the nine, represent ten possible sources of bias all program evaluations must address. Each factor may be a plausible explanation for an observed impact. To control for a factor, select a design appropriate for the purposes of your evaluation and adapt the design to what is possible.

Program staff often do not select more rigorous, more powerful, and methodologically stronger evaluations. Start with the most rigorous design possible and then, if necessary, adapt it to your situation. The assumption is that, if you start off in a compromising mode, you may lose an opportunity to examine the total program or

Table 5.2 Biases to Internal Validity of Selected Designs

	(1) H	(2) I	(3) X	(4) V	(5) R	(6) P	(7) R	(8) D	(9) A	(10) Σ
	(H)[a] History			(M)[b] Measure- ment		(S)[c] Selection				Synergistic Effects[d]
Design										
1. One group pre-test and posttest: E O X O										
2. Nonequivalent comparison group: E O X O C O O										
3. Time series: E OOO X OOO										
4. Multiple time series: E OOO X OOO C OOO OOO										
5. Randomized pretest and posttest with a control group: R E O X O R C O O										

[a]H = External Events; I = Internal Program Events; X = Program.
[b]V = Validity; R = Reliability; P = Eligibility.
[c]R = Refusals; D = Dropouts; A = Attrition.
[d]Σ = Sum of $H + M + S$.

program elements before you have thoroughly explored all possibilities. The best design is one tempered with a good sense of reality, derived from a careful individual and internal peer review process.

Design 1: One Group Pretest and Posttest

Design 1 is the simplest design (nonexperimental) for a program evaluation. It should not be your choice to assess program *impact* or *effectiveness*. A number of factors may prevent you from attributing an observed change among program participants to the intervention. This design has many problems of inference and may control for few or none of the ten biases that threaten interpretation of observed changes. Although you might be tempted to attribute an observed change that occurred between O_1 and O_2 to the intervention (X), a number of alternative explanations might be equally plausible. For example, other historical events, unplanned exposures, or unexpected activities involving program participants between O_1 and O_2 may have played a role in producing the observed change. The longer the time period between O_1 and O_2, the more probable it is that historical events or other such factors will influence program results. This design, then, has multiple weaknesses (Campbell and Stanley, 1966; Windsor and Cutter, 1982).

Design 1, however, though not ideal, may be useful in conducting a formative evaluation of a program if the interval between observations is short and if you can reasonably rule out other significant selection, historical, or measurement biases. It may be useful to assess the immediate educational or instructional impact of an information skills or in-service training program. It is important to know that a pretest may have a modest impact on participants. If the baseline observation is minimal and occurs prior to the intervention (e.g., 1 week earlier), it may not pose a plausible threat to the interpretation of short-term program impact. To control for this threat, regardless of the size or purpose of your evaluation, routinely asserts maximum control over measurement quality and the data-collection process. You must conduct reliability and validity checks.

The weakness in Design 1 is the extent to which participants selected for the program are comparable to users of the typical organization, community, school, work site, or clinic—selection bias. By determining the comparability of those who do and do not participate in the formative evaluation, you can examine the extent to which selection biases result.

EXAMPLE: A maternal–child health (MCH) program conducts a smoking behavioral assessment of patient smoking status. The staff observes a 3% quit rate between the onset of pregnancy and childbirth. On entry into a maternity clinic, 50 smokers are interviewed (O_1) on their level of smoking knowledge, health beliefs, and practices. They also receive a new health education program (X): a 10-minute, one-to-one counseling session plus a self-help cessation manual. A follow-up interview of the 50 patients (O_2) is performed at the participants' next monthly visit, using the same instrument. A saliva thiocyanate test is performed on all self-reported quitters. The following impact is reported: (1) increased health belief score—60% to 95%; (2) decreased smoking prevalence—50 smokers to 45 smokers. This level of immediate effect, a 10% quit rate (5/50) versus the normal 3% quit rate from the existing program, with biases to validity acknowledged, provides the program with encouraging immediate feedback on program feasibility and impact. Two examples of this design are presented by Dial and Windsor, (1985) and Windsor, (1981).

Design 2: Nonequivalent Comparison Group

Design 2 builds on Design 1 by adding a comparison group ($\underline{C}$). This design may improve your chances of attributing observed effects to the program. The dashed line in Table 5.2 between the intervention group (E) and the comparison group ($\underline{C}$) confirms that the groups were established by a method other than randomization. A comparison of the strengths and weaknesses of Designs 1 and 2 suggests that the comparison group often improves your ability to rule out some alternative explanations of the cause of an impact.

The extent to which this design may control for selection is always an issue. This can be partially dealt with by ensuring that neither the comparison nor the experimental group is selected because of an extreme trait. Careful matching of individuals in the two groups or units is critical. As noted, baseline (O_1) and follow-up observations (O_2) are necessary for both groups. The observation must have high measurement quality.

A continuing problem with Design 2 is the difficulty of selecting the most appropriate method for statistical analysis of results. There is still much discussion in the literature about what analytical technique is the most appropriate for results produced by nonequivalent comparison group designs (Kenny, 1975; Rubin, 1974; Cook and Campbell, 1979; Windsor et al., 1980). A good example of the application of this design is presented in Case Study 2 in this chapter.

Design 3: Time Series

You might select Design 3 if your program allows you to:

1. Establish the periodicity and pattern of the outcome variable being examined.
2. Establish the degree of stability of the outcome measurement.
3. Collect outcome data unobtrusively.
4. Observe at multiple data points, typically 1 to 2 years before and after the intervention.
5. Introduce an intervention that can be applied in a specific time period and, if desirable, withdrawn abruptly.

In using a time-series design (TSD), many data points increase the power of the design so that you can make causal inferences. Thus, a principal need for application of a TSD is that an adequate number of observations has been made to document trends for your outcome. Some recommend a minimum of 50 data points for assessing an effect

(Glass et al., 1975; Ostrom, 1978). The observation points must occur at equal intervals and must cover a sufficient time period to confirm preintervention and postintervention variations for the outcome variables.

Although you should be sensitive to the statistical issues in choosing a TSD, you may use one with fewer data points. Observation and analysis of a behavior-change trend over time, even with fewer than 50 data points (for example, two or three baseline and two or three follow-up), represent a significant gain over Design 1. Because the principal issue in applying a TSD is to determine the significance of a trend, the treatment must be powerful enough to produce shifts in the dependent (impact) variable considerably beyond the variation you would normally expect in your setting (Campbell, 1969; Cook and Campbell, 1983; Windsor and Cutter, 1981, 1982).

If you apply a TSD, you must still examine the extent to which you can control for the major biases to internal validity—history, selection, and measurement. Did external or internal historical, non-program events or activities confound the observed results? The plausibility of the effects of factors such as weather, seasonality, shifts in personnel, and changes in resources must be examined. The threat of extraneous historical effects increases with the duration of the evaluation. You need to establish the pattern of the program impact variables being used.

Design 3 may provide evidence of effects ranging from suggestive to very good. It may not produce definitive evidence about intervention effects. Only through replication of an evaluation using a TSD and reports of consistently significant evidence of impact over time can you make conclusive statements about effectiveness (Windsor and Cutter, 1981, 1982). An example of the application of this design is included in Case Study 1 in this chapter.

Design 4: Multiple-Time Series

The quasi-experimental Design 4 can be more powerful than the non-experimental Design 1 and quasi-experimental Designs 2 and 3. A multiple-time series (MTS) describes a design in which outcomes are studied at different times for an experimental group (E) and a comparison group (C). The addition of the comparison group strengthens the program's control over possible historical effects. The MTS design is particularly appropriate in situations where retrospective and prospective databases are easily accessible or where an organization can periodically observe rates for program participants (e.g., each month).

The MTS design may improve your control over the major factors that confound or compromise interpretation of observed program results. A major inhibitor to the use of this design is the need for multiple observations of the comparison group before and after the program. These observations are time- and resource-intensive. Like the simple TSD, the MTS design demands a number of baseline and follow-up observations, depending on what factors affect these observations. Your main concern is to be able to say with reasonable assurance that, before the program, a stable pattern of outcome measurements was confirmed for both the comparison and the treatment groups. Time-series analytical techniques, as noted for Design 3, require a large number of data points to produce sensitive statistical analyses. You need to be concerned about this trade-off and choose the number of observations to optimize your ability to rule out extraneous factors that may bias your results (Cook and Campbell, 1983; Spector, 1981; Windsor and Cutter, 1982). Windsor (1986) provides a useful synopsis and multiple case studies of the application of TSDs.

Design 5: Randomized Pretest and Posttest with a Control Group

There are several methods to conduct an experimental study of program efficacy or effectiveness. A common approach is to evaluate an existing program (X_1) by comparing it with a hypothetically more effective program (X_2). If you have a large number of participants interested in your program, you usually can assign them by random selection (R) to different intervention groups. A common mistake made by the inexperienced evaluator is to assume the comparison ($\underline{C}$) or control (C) group receive nothing. What the C or $\underline{C}$ group receives is up to the evaluator.

Random assignment may be done all at once if participants enter the program together, or you may assign persons randomly as they sign up and enter the program over time. Assuming no major implementation problems, this design may produce good control over the biases that confound interpretation of program impact—selection and history. The principal concept behind this experimental design is that the evaluator establishes two groups that are not significantly different for any salient outcome characteristic at baseline (e.g., E_1 has 33% smokers, and C_1 has 31% smokers). Programs that use random assignment may assert control over the biases to internal and external validity. Confirmation that the randomization process has established equivalent groups, however, is critical (Cook and Campbell, 1979).

In selecting a design, considering what is possible within the constraints of time, resources, and characteristics of the situation is crucial. The designs we have discussed form a hierarchy, in ascending order from Design 1 to Design 5, representing an increasing ability to provide defensible evidence of program efficacy and effectiveness.

provide defensible evidence of program efficacy and effectiveness. Even when a randomized design such as Design 5 is used, however, the evidence may not be conclusive. Case Study 4 in this chapter (and all case studies in Chapter 9) is an example of the use of Design 5.

DETERMINING SAMPLE SIZE

Two questions frequently asked in planning an evaluation are, How large should the control (comparison) and experimental groups be? How should we select each group? Knowledge of what the sample size should be for each study group is of paramount importance to ensure sufficient statistical power in data analysis and interpretation. Prior to implementation, estimate the minimum number to be recruited in each group. Two types of error need to be considered: Type I and Type II. A Type I error is the probability of rejecting a null hypothesis (H_0) when it is true. A null hypothesis is an hypothesis of no significant differences between the E and C groups. Because the objective of a program is to have an impact (i.e., to reject H_0), you must establish large enough E and C groups to have the opportunity to do this. Regardless of the total number in a group, the groups should be approximately the same size (e.g., $E = 77$, and $C = 80$).

You must define certain components to determine the most efficient sample size for each study group. One of the first steps is to select a level of statistical significance. An accepted convention for step 1 is $\alpha = 0.05$. This level (or 0.01) should be used for efficacy and effectiveness evaluations. In other words, if $\alpha = 0.05$, you are willing to reject a null hypothesis when the probability of being wrong is less than 5%. (NOTE: In a formative evaluation, you can use $\alpha = 0.10$ as an adequate level to test statistical significance and to estimate sample size.) The use of 0.10 versus 0.05 can be justified because you are trying to get a good preliminary estimate of "promising new intervention methods." If your meta-evaluation and formative evaluation results confirm a consistent effect size, and you are not concerned about harm, you may choose a one-tailed test to estimate sample size.

Having specified the α level, in step 2 you must consider the β level, the probability of accepting a null hypothesis when it is not true (committing a Type II error); in other words, you conclude that a program could not produce a significant effect when it can. The literature suggests that

$$\beta = 1 - (4 \times \alpha) \qquad \text{or} \qquad 1 - \beta = 4 \times \alpha$$

Thus, where $\alpha = 0.05$, power $(1 - \beta) = 0.08$ (Cohen and Cohen, 1975).

Given these two conventions, in step 3 you estimate expected effectiveness—either from the literature or, better, from your program data (a natural history study or formative evaluation)—the current level of documented effectiveness: the effect size (ES). The process of estimating ES can be described by using a smoking-cessation example. The literature indicates that the self-initiated cessation rate (P_1) annually for a 12-month period among smokers is approximately 10% (or $P_1 = 0.10$). Available evidence also confirms that a reasonable expectation of impact for a smoking-cessation program (P_2) at a 6- to 12-month follow-up is approximately a 25% cessation (or $P_2 = 0.25$). With these four parameters, $\alpha = 0.05$, power $= 0.80$, $P_1 = 0.10$, and $P_2 = 0.25$, you can use standard sample size tables to find out how many participants you need in both E and C groups to test the significance of a difference (Fleiss, 1981).

Data presented in Table 5.3 for a two-tailed test on proportion specify the sample sizes needed for an experimental and control group for various α, power, P_1, and P_2 statistics. Using the statistics from our smoking cessation example, the data in the table indicate that the program would need 113 participants *per group* to confirm as statistically different the hypothesized difference between P_1 and P_2. The data refute the common statement that 30 or 50 individuals are needed per group. The use of 71 and 50 subjects per group, respectively, would require a program to produce an impact of at least a 35% or 30% cessation to statistically confirm the effect as significant. The likelihood, then, of finding a statistically significant difference between the E and C groups with sample sizes of $N = 50$ each, where $P_1 = 0.10$ and $P_2 = 0.25$, is a little higher than chance (50/50)—not very good odds.

The underlying steps in deciding on sample sizes is to determine what level of impact you expect. If the literature and empirical evidence suggest that your program will have a small effect size (e.g., $P_1 = 0.10$ vs. $P_2 = 0.20$) and if a small impact is programmatically or organizationally important, then using the data in Table 5.3 and the same α, power, and P values, each of your study groups (E and C) will need approximately 219 people. If the evidence suggests that the impact of your program will be large (e.g., $P_1 = 0.10$ and $P_2 = 0.40$), then a sample size of 38 per group may be sufficient. There is limited discussion in the health promotion/education literature on the logic and methods used to determine experimental and control group size. Consideration must be given to this major methodological issue to improve the quality of future evaluations. It also has serious fiscal implications—the number of people to recruit over a period of time. Because of the complexity of determining sample size and selecting appropriate analytical methods, you may need to seek biostatistical consultation (Anderson, 1976; Cohen and Cohen, 1975; Fleiss, 1981; Windsor et al., 1980).

Table 5.3   Sample Sizes per Group for a Two-Tailed Test on Proportions Where $P_1 = 0.10$

P_2	α	Power 0.95	0.90	0.80	0.50
0.20	0.01	471	397	316	189
	0.05	348	286	219	117
0.25	0.01	238	202	162	98
	0.05	117	146	113	62
0.30	0.01	149	126	102	63
	0.05	111	92	71	40
0.35	0.01	104	88	72	45
	0.05	77	64	50	29
0.40	0.01	77	66	54	34
	0.05	58	48	38	22

SOURCE: Adapted from Fleiss (1981), p. 262.

META-EVALUATION AND META-ANALYSIS: ESTIMATING POSSIBLE IMPACT

One of the first steps all evaluators should take in the development of an intervention and evaluation plan is a thorough review of the literature. This review will help estimate effect size and sample size for different types of intervention. In reviewing the literature, there are two methods to use: meta-evaluation (ME) and meta-analysis (MA). Both ME and MA are methods that the contemporary evaluator must understand and be able to apply. The distinction between the two methods rests primarily with the degree to which the literature base is mature or not. In the early stages of a literature, documentation of the efficacy of an intervention is usually limited. Often, only a few published evaluation studies exist to provide insight about the estimated impact of intervention methods or programs for a defined population and a risk factor. In this case, only an ME is performed.

Meta-Evaluation

Meta-evaluation assesses the methodological rigor of published intervention studies by rating five methodological areas using standard criteria to assess internal validity (efficacy):

1. Type of research design.
2. Sample size and representativeness.
3. Specification of population characteristics.

Table 5.4 Methodological Ratings of Completed Smoking-Cessation Intervention Research for Pregnant Women[a]

	Criteria					
Investigators (years)	1: Design	2: Sample	3: Characteristics	4: Measurement	5: Intervention	Rating Score
1. Baric et al. (1975)	4.0	3.0	2.0	1.0	0.0	10.0
2. Donovan et al. (1972–1973)	4.0	3.0	1.0	0.0	1.0	9.0
3. Loeb et al. (1979–1981)	4.0	3.0	2.0	0.0	1.0	10.0
4. Ershoff et al. (1980–1981)	2.0	2.0	3.0	1.0	4.0	12.0
5. Bauman et al. (1981)	4.0	3.0	4.0	1.0	3.0	15.0
6. Burling et al. (1983)	4.0	2.0	1.0	2.0	2.0	11.0
7. Sexton and Hebel (1979–1983)	5.0	3.0	3.0	3.0	3.0	17.0
8. Windsor et al. (1982–1984)	5.0	5.0	4.0	3.0	5.0	22.0
Range	1–5	1–5	1–5	1–5	1–5	5–25

SOURCE: Windsor and Orleans (1986):131–161.
[a] Includes only studies that have used quasi-experimental or experimental designs.

4. Measurement quality.

5. Appropriateness and replicability of E and C procedures.

Windsor and Orleans (1986) discuss the application of the ME method. Only eight evaluation studies of smoking-cessation programs for pregnant women were available at the time of the review in 1985. To be included in this ME, only studies with a quasi-experimental or experimental design were included. Table 5.4 presents the overall methodological ratings for each criterion area and a total rating score for the eight studies critiqued. From this review, the following minimal standards were recommended for future program evaluations:

1. Use randomized control group design only with an inception cohort of at least 80% of the smoking patients at all sites.

2. Confirm representatives of study participants at all sites.
3. Specify sample size and documented effect size needs based on power = .80, including at least 100 subjects in each study group.
4. Provide complete, demographic, behavioral, and clinical assessments with definitions—minimal exclusionary criteria.
5. Use self-reports based on patient knowledge of test combined with independent biochemical tests–cotinine (COT)/thiocyanate (SCN) measures using specified cutoffs at baseline, midpoint, and end-of-pregnancy (and ideally at the first postpartum visit).
6. Document 90% or more follow-up rate for all patients at each observation point.
7. Provide a complete intervention description—specification of cessation methods to permit replication and documentation of pilot testing of procedures and training of treatment groups.
8. Conduct an ongoing process evaluation to document intervention exposure, including exposure by type, frequency, and duration for each cessation component and program procedure.

The preceding synthesis confirms the importance and utility of a thorough review of all primary resource material from completed evaluation studies. It is essential to systematically apply well-established standards of evaluation to determine the extent to which the literature provides insight—a meta-evaluation. Boyd and Windsor, (1993), provide an additional example of meta-evaluation.

Meta-Analysis

Meta-analysis is a statistical analysis of the results of completed empirical research. MA differs from ME in that it presumes a large number of completed quasi-experimental or experimental evaluation studies with sufficient rigor to rule out major biases to validity. The first step is to review the literature to identify published studies. At this stage, a serious bias may occur if an incomplete review of the literature is performed. An explicit set of ME rules should be established to screen out studies with serious methodological flaws: For example, inclusion of studies (1) with only a comparison or control group, (2) that had sample sizes in both the experimental and control groups in excess of 100 subjects, and (3) that only provide confirmed evidence of measurement validity and reliability of the impact or outcome rate used to document change.

This step in the MA (the ME) should provide an accurate and impartial quantitative description from completed studies of the impact of an intervention for samples of populations for a specific risk factor and setting. Besides the information on sample size, the intervention used in a setting and the effect size (ES) are specified for each evaluation study. ES, as previously noted, refers to the difference between the E and C groups on the outcome or impact variable.

The MA aggregates prior studies into a quantitative estimate of the impact of an intervention. It is a weighted average of the individual results, providing more weight for larger studies and less weight for smaller. The methodology for combining findings from studies is not new, and the techniques are straightforward. The primary difficulty of the MA is the selection of the studies to be used. Information from one study is rarely a replicate of another: Populations, research procedures, and comparison groups differ. The use of published literature can also lead to biased results. Often, journals choose not to publish negative results. Thus, performing the MA on the basis of published literature alone may produce results with a biased effect.

Some MA techniques merely combine the results of studies based on whether they were successful (statistically significant). The implicit assumption when performing this type of summarization is that lack of significance is equal to a zero effect; this may not be valid. In addition, just counting statistical significance can also cause problems. If two studies have the same significance level but opposite results, concluding there is an effect might be misleading, especially in view of an overall estimate that might be zero. Fleiss and Gross (1991) provide four principal uses of properly performed MAs:

1. To increase statistical power for important endpoints and subgroups

2. To resolve controversy when studies disagree

3. To improve estimates of effect size

4. To answer new questions not previously posed in the individual studies

These rules cover several situations. A situation for use of rule 1 might be to estimate whether the intervention was effective among women in a work-site smoking-cessation study. In a single study, there may be insufficient numbers of women to demonstrate a statistically significant result, but pooling results by performing the MA for several studies may provide an answer or conflicting results. Performing a sound MA may enable the answer to be more clearly seen.

Rule 3 is used in planning studies and/or interventions. Basing sample size decisions and estimated impacts on a single study, however, is risky. Even though an effect may be real, there is a chance that what was observed was an overestimate. The MA may serve to refine an estimate, providing a better estimate, with increased assurance that the study design will answer the basic question.

In some situations, the use of available data related to a new question may bring some insight into previously unspecified questions. For example, suppose you are interested in the potential for vitamin supplements to aid in increasing birth weight. From studies of smoking cessation among pregnant women where birth weight or percentage low birth weight is reported and whether vitamins were taken are recorded, estimating the impact of vitamin-supplement use from recorded data might be possible. If this information were available from a variety of sources, the MA of this information might be used to infer potential benefit for future studies. Performing the MA is a valuable exercise. Too often, researchers and evaluators fail to adequately use available information, continuing the proverbs—"history repeats itself," or "rediscovering the wheel." Even though an MA is a sophisticated analytic process, much can be learned with this method. For a thorough discussion of MA, two excellent references are Glass et al. (1981) and Hunter and Schmidt (1990).

Mumford et al. (1982) provide an excellent discussion of the application of the MA methods to studies of the impact of health counseling on surgical or coronary bypass patients. Among a review of 13 studies, a health-counseling intervention, on average, reduced hospitalization below the control group average by approximately 2 days. This review provides a detailed discussion of the characteristics of the patient population, the health-counseling intervention, the sampling methods and sample size, outcome indicators, and effect size. Bruvold (1993) presents another excellent discussion and example of MA.

Staff must have a clear idea of the potential impact of the intervention and establish realistic objectives. This is accomplished in two ways: (1) performing an ME and/or MA, depending on the maturity of the literature, and (2) conducting a formative evaluation that represents an application of the best intervention and evaluation methods synthesized from the ME and program experience by staff. The application of these two procedures—ME, MA—and a formative evaluation will provide the best evidence to initiate a program evaluation. Windsor, et al. (1994), provide an example of both ME and MA.

ESTABLISHING A CONTROL GROUP

The key question in establishing a C group is, Does it adequately control for the effects of factors (known or unknown), such as age or education, that might produce or explain part of an observed impact?

An equivalent C group is used to assert control over the independent variables so that extraneous or bias from **H-M-S** are minimized. It does this by distributing individuals with particular characteristics equally between E and C groups. An E group is used to determine whether program participants have improved as a result of exposure to the intervention by comparing them to those not exposed or to those exposed to something else. An assumption in making a comparison between E and C groups is that the groups were equivalent before introduction of the intervention. Equivalence must be documented and tested; random assignment does not always produce equivalent groups at baseline. Ideally, E and C are identical for all dependent (impact or outcome) variables and independent variables associated with the dependent variables.

In selecting a design, you face the immediate problem of identifying and selecting a C group. As noted, a control group refers to a group established only by random assignment, whereas a comparison group ($\underline{C}$) refers to a group established by any nonrandom assignment method. A major constraint in designing an evaluation may be the availability of individuals who can be used as C or $\underline{C}$ subjects; this varies by the characteristics of each situation.

An issue, which at times has limited C group establishment, is that program staff do not want to withhold the intervention from participants. This may seem an insurmountable problem at first glance, but in practice it need not be. Because human nature and all programs are fallible, program improvements are usually needed. Although you cannot withhold the standard-minimum program, you can vary the intensity and duration of methods and materials or the frequency of program elements to see which are most effective; or, you can compare the standard program (X_1) to $X_1 + X_2$ (where X_2 is systematic reinforcement or additional sessions). Or, you can devise other alternatives. Ask practical questions. The central issue is, How effective is the existing program, and what practical methods could be applied that might increase that level of effectiveness? Can you reduce the existing intervention time by 50% and be as effective?

Random Assignment

Randomization of participants into E and C groups is the best method to establish groups for evaluation purposes and to control for the biases to internal validity. Multiple computer programs are readily available to generate a random assignment list. If participants are randomly assigned as they are recruited, assignment may take a number of forms. If the numbers of confirmed participants are large (e.g., 200), then simple random assignment may be adequate to establish equivalent groups. To achieve greater precision, however, a program planner may choose a stratified system of randomization. Individuals with selected demographic characteristics are grouped by an important demographic characteristic (e.g., age-gender-race) with other individuals with similar characteristics, matched or clustered, and then randomly assigned to the *E* or *C* group.

Delayed Treatment

A common misinterpretation of classical experimental design is that the administration of an intervention (*X*) is an all-or-nothing affair. In the simplest of delayed approaches, about half the individuals from an applicant pool are randomly selected to serve as a *C* group. The rest of the applicants are exposed to the program initially, while the group is delayed in its participation (e.g., 1–3 months). In this way, eligible candidates are randomly assigned to immediate or delayed treatment, with each having an equal opportunity to participate. Randomization may be the fairest and most equitable method of selecting initial program participants in a case where all who are interested in participating cannot be served at the same time.

Table 5.5 shows how a delayed-treatment method can be diagrammed. At T_1 a group of individuals agree to participate in a program. Using the parameters $\alpha = 0.05$, power $= 0.80$, $P_1 = 0.10$, and $P_2 = 0.30$, a sample size of 75 per group is chosen (see Table 5.3). Of 150 individuals who agree to participate, 75 are randomly assigned to group *E* and 75 to group *C*. A baseline observation (O_1) is performed during the recruitment period prior to the start of the program. At T_2 those assigned to group *E* are exposed to the program (X_1); those assigned to group *C* are not exposed. Observations (O_2) are made of both groups. At a predetermined time in the future (3 months), T_3, those in group *C* are exposed to the program (e.g., 30–60–90 days). This approach is particularly useful in confirming immediate and

Table 5.5   Establishing a Control Group
for a Delayed-Treatment Program

Time 1 (T_1): Recruitment—Baseline Observations	Time 2 (T_2): Program 1 Starts	Time 3 (T_3): Program 2 Starts	Time 4 (T_4): Follow-Up
O_1 R E ($N = 75$)	X_1 O_2	O_3	O_4
O_1 R C ($N = 75$)	O_2	O_3 X_1	O_4

Table 5.6 Establishing a Control Group
for a Multiple-Component Program

Time 1 (T_1): Recruitment—Baseline Observations	Time 2 (T_2): Program 2 Starts	Time 3 (T_3): Program Ends	Time 4 (T_4): Follow-Up
O_1 R E_1 ($N = 75$)	X_1 X_2 X_3 O_2	O_3	O_4
O_1 R E_2 ($N = 75$)	X_1 X_2 O_2	O_3	O_4
O_1 R C_1 ($N = 75$)	X_1 O_2	O_3	O_4

short-term (1–3 months) estimates of program effectiveness. It typically cannot be used to assess intermediate or long-term impact and impacts after 6 months or 1 year or more because people who expect to receive the program are usually unwilling to wait much longer than 1–3 months. This design is very useful in conducting formative evaluations of different program elements in the early stages of program development (Boruch, 1976; Campbell, 1969).

A Multiple-Component Program

You may choose to apply combinations of different interventions to some individuals and withhold them from others. In other words, if you have many individuals who want to participate in your program, you may elect to conduct a randomized, factorial study in which selected program elements are applied or withheld. You might examine factors such as duration, reinforcement, and intensity, to determine which individual or combined elements are the most effective.

You may be interested in determining the differential effects of elements of the program. To do so, establish an applicant pool and design the program with multiple components; then expose subsamples to different components. As indicated in Table 5.6, the initial pool of 225 recruited applicants can be randomly assigned to three "equivalent" groups ($N = 75$). Equivalence should be tested, not assumed. Participants in each group may be exposed to single or combinations of parts of a program. The C group might receive nothing or, a minimum standard intervention (see Case Study 4).

A New Program

If your organization has an opportunity (or is required) to develop or present a totally new program or a new version of an ongoing program, you could randomly assign participants to be exposed to either the standard program (X_1) or the new, enriched program (X_2), for

Table 5.7 Establishing a Control Group for a New Program

Time 1 (T_1): Recruitment—Baseline Observations	Time 2 (T_2): Programs Start	Time 3 (T_3): Programs End	Time 4 (T_4): Follow- Up
O_1 R E_1 ($N = 100$)	X_1 O_2	O_3	O_4
O_1 R E_2 ($N = 100$)	X_2 O_2	O_3	O_4

purposes of comparison of impact. An evaluation of which program was the most effective can then be made. As indicated in Table 5.7, having recruited and established baselines for a pool of 200 participants, you randomly assign each to participate in program X_1 or program X_2. Follow-up observations are conducted as in other group designs.

ESTABLISHING A COMPARISON (C̲) GROUP

The opportunity to perform randomized experimental studies occurs far more often than the literature suggests. In a number of program evaluation situations, however, an experimental design may not be feasible. This is particularly true in a field setting where a program does not have easy access to a "captive audience." It may then be necessary for an evaluator to select a comparison group. Where a comparison group (C̲) and not a control group (C) is established, the potential level of effect size (P_2) of a program is likely to be reduced (Boruch, 1976). To the extent that the randomized experimental design is compromised, the study's results and conclusions are usually weakened.

The definition of a C̲ group, as noted, is any group not formed by random assignment. The goal then is to identify a comparison group(s) that is highly comparable to the E group exposed to the program. In essence, in using a nonequivalent C̲ group, you are attempting to replicate an experimental study in every way with the exception of randomization. In establishing a C̲ group, you must document at baseline the similarities and differences between the C̲ and the E groups. The following methods are suggested for selection of the C̲ group to improve your chances of identifying your program's effectiveness.

Matching by Unit

You may have the opportunity to match program data in your area to program data in a comparable area where the intervention you are applying will not be introduced. This design is most feasible in a situation where a uniform database exists or can be introduced at alternative locations. Examples include public health clinics, hospitals, schools, or work sites. In identifying subjects to serve in a C group, you should seek approximately the same number of individuals as you have in the E group. If the C site already has a monitoring system, you may be able to identify a number of units whose participants have highly comparable demographic traits to your E group. The greatest difficulty in using this method is gaining the cooperation of intact groups in other settings. Some type of longitudinal design, often a time series, is the most appropriate evaluation method to use with this type of C group (Windsor and Cutter, 1982). An example of the method of matching by unit is presented in Case Study 2 in this chapter.

Participant- or Peer-Generated ($\underline{C}$) Groups

One useful method is to have individuals match themselves with a friend. In the participant-generated method, a participant identifies one or two friends or neighbors very much like himself or herself in age, sex, race, socioeconomic status (SES), and so on. You request participants to provide the names and phone numbers of these people to be contacted by the program staff. This method, used to establish the $\underline{C}$ group reported in Table 5.8, may create a nonrandomized comparison group at little cost (Wang et al., 1975; Windsor, 1973; Windsor et al., 1980). One problem with participant generation, as observed in Table 5.8, may be the failure of a significant proportion of treatment group participants to identify a comparison friend. Using this method may also result in interaction between E and $\underline{C}$ subjects, increasing the potential for contamination of $\underline{C}$ subjects. This possibility should be monitored.

COMPARABILITY OF EVALUATION STUDY GROUPS

Establishing the baseline comparability of E and C or $\underline{C}$ groups in a quasi-experimental or experimental evaluation cannot be over-stressed. Although randomization is the best choice, a nonequivalent $\underline{C}$ group may represent the only reasonable alternative in your circumstances. In identifying a C or $\underline{C}$ group, give considerable attention to selecting individuals or groups who are as similar to the E group as possible. The rationale for identifying individuals, units, or groups to serve as a C or $\underline{C}$ group must be well thought-out and described in detail. The objective of comparing baseline data on the E and C or $\underline{C}$ groups is to confirm that no major differences exist between these

Table 5.8   Baseline Data for Treatment and Comparison Groups

Variable	Group Experiment (E) ($N = 280$)	Comparison (C) ($N = 170$)	Significance Level (P)
Age (years)	45.7	44.1	NS[a]
Annual income	$9077	$8776	NS
Years in school	11.3	11.5	NS
Black female	25%	28%	NS
White female	75%	72%	NS
Has a family doctor	79%	84%	NS
Has had uterus removed	24%	23%	NS
Has had a physician's visit in the last six months	74%	77%	NS
Mean cognitive score	71.8	70.9	NS
Mean belief score	1.45	1.47	NS
Breast self-examination practices in the last three months			SIG[b], 0.01
None	33%	23%	
One	20%	23%	
Two	19%	14%	
Three or more	27%	40%	
Pap smear practices			
None	22%	14%	NS
Fewer than 12	55%	56%	
More than 12	23%	30%	

SOURCE: Windsor et al. (1980):203–218.
[a]NS = not significant.   [b]SIG = significant.

groups prior to program exposure. Data in Tables 5.8 and 5.9 portray the comparability of E, $\underline{C}$, and C groups participating in two published studies.

Table 5.8 presents baseline statistics for 450 female participants in a rural cancer control program (Windsor et al., 1980). Randomization was not possible in this program. The $\underline{C}$ group was identified using a peer-generation method—female participants were asked to identify a nonparticipant friend of the same age and sex. The data indicate that the two groups were relatively comparable at baseline for sociodemographic factors, physician utilization, cognitive and health belief scores, and behavioral reports. The noted exception was the higher level of breast self-examination reported by the $\underline{C}$ group at baseline. Another small problem, but not a major flaw, was the difference in sample size between the E and $\underline{C}$ groups.

Table 5.9 Mean Values of Selected Variables Among MRFIT
Participants Assigned to Special Intervention (SI) and Usual Care (UC)

	Units	SI (N = 6428)	UC (N = 6438)
Values at first screen			
Serum cholesterol	mg/dL	253.8	253.5
Diastolic blood pressure	mm Hg	99.2	99.2
Cigarette smokers	%	63.8	63.5
Cigarettes/day smoked	No.	33.7	34.2
Framingham 6-year risk of CHD death	%	3.12	3.15
Values at second screen			
Age	years	46.3	46.3
Diastolic blood pressure	mm Hg	91.2	91.2
Systolic blood pressure	mm Hg	136.0	135.8
Percentage on blood pressure medication	%	19.6	19.1
Weight	lb	189.3	189.1
Height	in.	69.2	69.3
Drinks/week	No.	12.5	12.7
Serum Fasting glucose	mg/dL	99.5	99.3
Thiocyanate	μmol/L	131.0	131.1
Plasma Total cholesterol	mg/dL	240.3	240.6
HDL cholesterol	mg/dL	42.0	42.1
LDL cholesterol	mg/dL	159.8	160.3
Triglycerides	mg/dL	194.7	193.9
Values at third screen Diastolic blood pressure	mm Hg	90.7	90.7
Cigarette smokers	%	59.3	59.0
Cigarettes/day smoked	No.	32.4	32.8
Flat or downsloping ST depression ≥0.5 mm post-exercise	%	2.48	2.35

SOURCE: Sherwin et al. (1981):402–425.

Table 5.9 presents data on the Multiple Risk Factor Intervention
Trial (MRFIT) (Sherwin et al., 1981). This national trial effort established two groups, one to receive a special intervention (SI) (or *E*
group) and one to receive usual care (UC) (or *C* group). Three screening procedures took place before the program intervention began.
The data confirm that the mean values of the quantitative measures
performed for the SI and UC groups were almost exactly the same.
No significant differences were noted for the screening variables.

These two studies—a small demonstration project in a rural community with limited resources and a randomized clinical trial of national significance with resources over $125 million—confirm that program resources, scope, and duration play a significant role in the ability of investigators to establish comparability of study groups. The amount and type of data collected will vary dramatically according to a program's purpose and resources, but all programs must establish the baseline characteristics of *E*, *C*, or *C* group participants and their comparability.

CASE STUDIES: THEORY INTO PRACTICE

We present four case studies to illustrate the strengths and weaknesses of the quasi-experimental and experimental designs discussed in this chapter. They have been selected because they are part of the current literature and represent programs with different purposes and samples of subjects: adults and youth and community, school and work-site settings. Case Study 1 and Case Study 2 include a methodological critique.

Case Study 1: Rural Cancer-Screening Program

SOURCE: R. A. Windsor, G. Cutter, and J. Kronenfeld, "Communication Methods and Evaluation Designs for a Rural Cancer Screening Program," *American Journal of Rural Health* 7(3) (1981):37–45.

Background and Objectives

In 1974 the Alabama Department of Public Health established a cancer-screening program (CSP), initially with National Cancer Institute support, to remove barriers to service use in local rural communities: availability, accessibility, acceptability, and cost. At the end of 1981, this project had 50 clinics in operation and had screened approximately 110,000 women, 90% of whom were members of families below the poverty level. Of those newly screened, 57% reported that they either never had a Pap smear, had not had one within the last 2 years, or did not remember ever having one. The CSP has a continuing interest in determining methods to increase service utilization, particularly by women who have never used the program.

In 1978 a collaborative effort with representatives from the University of Alabama–Birmingham faculty, the Alabama State Health Department, and the Cooperative Extension Service was initiated to develop, implement, and evaluate a community-based Cancer Communications Program. The objective of the program was to increase, during the second quarter of 1979 and 1980, the number of women using the CSP in Alabama. The Hale County screening program was selected as a demon-

Table 5.10 Selected Demographic Characteristics of Hale County
and Alabama

Location	Estimated Population (1977)	Percentage Black	Percentage Rural	Population per Physician
Hale County	15,500	63	79	3972
Alabama	3,600,000	26	42	1860

Location	Percentage Below Poverty Line	Percentage Without Adequate Plumbing	Socioeconomic Status Index
Hale County	55	51	50
Alabama	25	16	100

SOURCE: Southern Regional Council (1974); (1979).
NOTE: U.S. mean = 100; standard deviation (SD) = 20.

stration site because it had a large pool of high-risk women over 35 years
of age (approximately 3500), it was similar to a number of counties in
south central Alabama, and it had been operational since 1977. As indicated in Table 5.10, residents in this county were predominantly black,
poor, and rural, with limited access to primary health care services and
personnel.

Intervention

As shown in Table 5.11, five elements were identified as the principal
components of the community intervention. A multiple-component intervention was used because the literature and the experience of the investigators strongly confirmed that no single source of exposure could be
expected to have an appreciable behavioral impact on the target group.
Combinations of messages from multiple salient channels, particularly
interpersonal sources at repeated intervals, were applied.

Two community health education programs were implemented separately in Hale County during the second quarter, April–June 1979 and
1980. The principal messages communicated by the programs during the
3-month interventions were (1) women over age 35 years who had never
had a Pap smear were at higher risk for cervical cancer and therefore
should contact the CSP and (2) cervical cancer was highly curable if detected in its early stages. The first intervention, element 1 in Table 5.11,
was applied in 1979. This community organization effort recruited and
trained 39 female lay leaders, 21 white and 18 black, from existing community groups. The leaders were trained to conduct programs for wom-
en's groups throughout the county. They held 45 cancer communications
meetings with about 15 to 20 participants each. Approximately 750
women were documented as having been directly exposed to the Cancer
Communications Program. Considerable emphasis was placed on word-

Table 5.11 Elements, Channels, and Purposes of the Hale County Intervention

Element	Channel of Communication	Purpose
1. Community organization (X_1)	Local lay and professional leaders	Increase acceptance and support Demonstrate and increase program credibility
2. Mass Media (X_2)	Electronic and print media: radio, local newspaper, church and club newsletters, posters, and bulletin boards	Increase awareness of and interest in program message Reinforce program message
3. Lay leadership (X_3)	Leadership training— standardized package	Increase assumption of responsibility by locals in community or group Decrease misinformation Increase program acceptance by groups through peer participation and pressure Increase standardization of messages
4. Interpersonal group sessions (X_4)	Group process: 1- to 2-hour standardized cancer education program session	Increase efficiency of networking Increase adaptability to personal evaluation and responsibility Increase motivation and social support Increase personalization of messages Increase legitimacy of at-risk role
5. Interpersonal individual sessions (X_5)	Individual word-of-mouth diffusion	Increase persuasion Increase efficiency of diffusion Increase salience of messages Increase trial and adoption

SOURCE: Windsor, Cutter, and Kronenfeld (1981): 37–45.

of-mouth diffusion by participants to friends. The second intervention, in 1980, used elements 2 and 5.

Evaluation Design

A time-series design (TSD) with a repeated treatment was chosen to evaluate the behavioral impact of the Cancer Communications Program.

The computerized data system of the CSP of the Alabama Department of Health was used to unobtrusively confirm the pattern of new users by quarterly report. These data were examined to determine the extent to which the two interventions increased CSP use by new users beyond what one would normally expect. In applying a TSD, this project (1) established the periodicity of the pattern of behavior being examined, (2) collected outcome data unobtrusively, (3) confirmed multiple data points 1 year prior to and 1 year following the intervention, and (4) applied and abruptly withdrew the intervention during a specific time period. This design was used because it was the highest quality quasi-experimental design that was feasible to evaluate a program of this type in a field setting.

Program Impact

Figure 5.1 illustrates the frequency (number) of new users by quarter and by year for Hale County. A new user was defined as an individual who

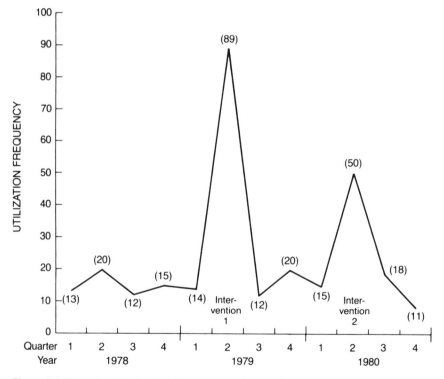

Figure 5.1 Frequency of New CSP Users by Quarter and Year

SOURCE: R. A. Windsor and G. Cutter, "Methodological Issues in Using Time Series Designs and Analysis: Evaluating the Behavioral Impact of Health Communication Programs," in *Progress in Clinical and Biological Research*, vol. 83: *Issues in Screening and Communications*, ed. C. Mettlin and G. Murphy, 517–535 (New York: Alan R. Liss, 1981).

had not previously used the Alabama CSP. A look at the pattern of Figure 5.1 for the 3-year period suggests a significant difference in CSP use during the two intervention periods. The frequency of CSP new users for the five baseline quarters prior to intervention 1 was relatively stable, although the increase in the frequency of new users in the second quarter of 1978 suggested a seasonal variation. An increase of 345% in new users, from 20 to 89, was observed for the second quarter of 1979, the intervention quarter. In other words, 89 new clients used the service during this period, compared with an average of 15 in 1978 and a maximum of 20 for the second-quarter baseline in 1978.

As noted in Figure 5.1, another increase in client use, from 20 to 50 (approximately 150%), was observed during the second intervention period. In the aggregate, an estimated 100 more new users were motivated to use the CSP than would be expected from the pattern observed during the nonintervention periods in 1978 and 1979. Throughout the 3-year period, the demographic characteristics of the new users remained relatively stable, suggesting that the two interventions had an effect on similar women. An analysis of the new-user increase using a linear regression model found that the observed frequencies for the intervention quarters were significantly higher ($P > 0.01$) than the observed frequencies for the nonintervention quarters. An examination of utilization data from a contiguous, matched county revealed no changes in CSP use by new users of the magnitude noted in Hale County. From the available evidence, it was concluded that the increases in new CSP users in Hale County were *primarily* due to the two interventions.

Internal Validity of Results

As noted in previous discussions in this chapter, program evaluators should consider the plausibility that a number of factors, other than the intervention, produced an observed impact. Using the Hale County project data, each of the major factors noted in Table 5.2 is examined with regard to the plausibility that it produced the increases observed. The main question to ask for each factor is, Could this factor have produced the observed change?

Historical Bias. Because a TSD was applied, historical effects represented a large threat to the internal validity of the results. In examining the possibility that historical events caused the observed increase, the evaluators found that no local, countywide, area, state, or national cancer communication program or cancer event had occurred during the 3-year demonstration project period. Local organizations that might have had an independent effect on CSP use were collaborators with or supporters of the project. No changes in CSP use of the magnitude noted in Hale County were evident in several adjacent counties. Although a seasonal variation was observed in the spring, even considering this fluctuation, the magnitude of program impact was 3.5 times more than the baseline use in 1978 (89 users vs. 20). The fluctuation in the spring baseline quarter of 1978 was most likely due to American Cancer Society fund-raising and screening–promotion efforts introduced each spring throughout Alabama. From this evidence and statistical analyses, it was concluded that history represented an implausible explanation for the increases observed.

Measurement Bias. Because the data observed were unobtrusive measures of behavioral impact (CSP use), this factor could not be a plausible explanation for the observed change during the intervention periods. No direct contact occurred between study personnel and clinic users. The TSD controlled for the effects of multiple observations by using unobtrusive measurement.

An examination of the instruments and data-collection procedures used by the CSP confirmed a high degree of standardization. No documentation errors were apparent to the investigators during the 3-year observation period. CSP instruments and personnel remained constant, and the endpoint (i.e., increased service utilization by new users) was easy to confirm. All CSP users were confirmed as Hale County residents. No significant administrative or staffing changes occurred during the study period. It was concluded that instrument and measurement errors did not represent a plausible explanation for the observed behavior changes.

Selection Bias. No $\underline{C}$ group was used in this study. In addition, the demographic characteristics of those motivated to use this service were comparable to new and previous users. The age distribution and racial makeup of the new users were also very stable. The information available suggested that selection did not play a significant role in producing the observed change.

The evaluators assessed the extent to which the observed change was a statistical artifact. The demographic characteristics of the users for the 3-year period were very stable. Although it was confirmed that more women used the service, those new users were not significantly different from previous new users. The level and type of new CSP users were relatively stable during the nonintervention period. Hale County was selected because it is generally comparable to a number of counties in south central Alabama and not because of any extreme characteristic or screening problem. The evidence suggested that the observed impact was not due to a regression effect.

Because the impact variable of this study was CSP use by new users, attrition by study participants was not an issue. Although this factor frequently represents a problem in studies and might have represented a problem in this study if a concern had been repeat-user attrition (missed appointments), it could not have compromised the internal validity of the observed results in the present study.

New CSP users throughout the county were all women with similar socioeconomic characteristics. An examination of the age and racial characteristics of the county population and CSP users confirmed a high degree of demographic stability and homogeneity. The Hale County CSP was selected because it had been operating for 2 years and was considered a stable and mature program. No significant social, biological, or psychological changes among female residents of this county were apparent. A maturation effect, therefore, was thought to be an implausible explanation for the noted impact.

Summary

Considering the discussion of the case material relating to the principal threats to internal validity, it was thought that the observed behavior changes in CSP use were produced by the Cancer Communication Program applied in the spring of 1979 and 1980. This conclusion was strengthened by the replication included in this field experiment. The observed increases were statistically and programmatically important in that the methods and issues examined were useful to ongoing community health education efforts (Windsor, 1983; Windsor and Cutter, 1982).

Case Study 2: The Class of 1989 Study

SOURCE: C. Perry, S. Kelder, D. Murray, and K. Klepp, "Communitywide Smoking Prevention: Long-Term Outcomes of the Minnesota Heart Health Program and the Class of 1989 Study," *American Journal of Public Health* 82(9) (1992): 1210–1216.

Background and Objectives

The Class of 1989 Study was designed to test the efficacy of a smoking-prevention program as part of a larger effort to reduce heart disease in entire communities. It was a substudy of the Minnesota Heart Health Program (MHHP), a population-based, communitywide cardiovascular disease prevention program. It was hypothesized that the impact of the school-based smoking prevention program for adolescents would be maintained if the program was part of a 5-year effort implemented within the schools and within the communities.

Evaluation Methods

The design of the Class of 1989 Study was determined by the parent project: the MHHP. Two of six MHHP communities were selected: North Dakota (C) and Minnesota (E). A quasi-experimental design was used to assess the impact of the school health education program provided as part of the communitywide cardiovascular disease prevention program in Moorhead, Minnesota. All sixth graders enrolled in public schools in both an experimental (E) and comparison communities (C) were invited to participate in a baseline survey in 1983. This cohort was surveyed annually each April until graduation in 1989. The annual survey was a cross-sectional sample of all students. Cohort data were also analyzed due to the availability of identifying information from the cross-sectional samples.

The behavior impact data for this project was derived from the annual cross-sectional and cohort surveys. A test–retest correlation for smoking intensity for this population was $r = .99$. Saliva thiocyanate samples were obtained to validate self-reports from a random sample of 50% of the classrooms. A cutoff of ≤ 79 micrograms per milliliter was used. A nonequivalent comparison group design was implemented to evaluate the impact of the intervention in the 13 grade schools and 7 high schools in the Moorhead community.

Intervention

The smoking intervention, the Minnesota Smoking Prevention Program, was implemented in 1984 at the beginning of the seventh grade. The primary focus of the intervention was to prevent tobacco use by attempting to influence the social and psychological factors that encourage smoking initiation. Detailed discussions of the intervention are presented in the full report of this case study and other sources referenced in the case study. The MHHP intervention was applied in 1983, 1984, and 1985, in addition to the school-based adolescent smoking-prevention program. Thus, all students were indirectly exposed to the larger communitywide MHHP behavioral intervention over the 5-year period. The adolescent cohorts in the intervention community were also exposed to the seven strategies of the MHHP: (1) population-based screening; (2) food-labeling education; (3) community organization citizen task force; (4) continuing education of health professionals; (5) mass media; (6) adult education at work sites, churches, and the like; and (7) youth education. The purpose of this MHHP was to restructure the adult social and physical environment related to cardiovascular disease prevention.

Program Impact

The cross-sectional and cohort smoking impact data were analyzed to assess differences between the two communities for each year from 1983 to 1989. No significant baseline differences were documented between the two communities. Data are presented in Figure 5.2 on the smoking prevalence cohort sample by grade, reflecting significant differences for the experimental and comparison cohort for each observation year. At the end of high school, 14.6% of the cohorts sampled from the experimental (E) community were smoking, compared with 24.1% from the comparison ($\underline{C}$) community. The saliva sample confirmed the self-reported data, indicating a false-negative report in the E community of 9.8% and 6.5% in the $\underline{C}$ community.

Internal Validity of Results

In assessing the quality of this study and its reported results, examining the plausibility of alternative explanations for the behavioral impact data reported is important.

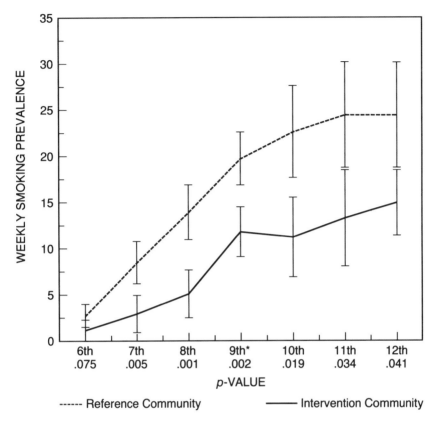

Figure 5.2 Smoking Prevalence of the Cohort Sample, by Grade

SOURCE: C. Perry, S. Kelder, D. Murray, and K. Klepp, "Communitywide Smoking Prevention: Long-Term Outcomes of the Minnesota Heart Health Program and the Class of 1989 Study," *American Journal of Public Health* 82(9) (1992):1210–1216.

*Smoking prevalence adjusted for false-negatives in 9th grade.

Historical Bias. When a nonequivalent comparison group design is used, particularly where the unit of analysis is an entire community, and when the evaluation study is conducted over an extended period of time (5 years), examining the role that historical events may have played in producing behavior change is important. Information presented in the case study through documentation of events over the study period in both communities provides convincing evidence that the impact of historical events was minimal. Independent surveys in the general area confirmed that the rates of smoking in a comparison adolescent cohort were comparable to those observed in independent surveys. Thus, it would appear that the ongoing activities at the national, state, and local levels relating to adolescent smoking cessation affected both the *E* and *C* communities equally.

The observed gradual rise in the *E* and *C* community is consistent with the expected annual increases in the incidence and prevalence among adolescents observed in the literature.

The psychosocial changes occurring among the two adolescent cohorts on the basis of information provided, and noted in the literature, reflect anticipated rates of experimentation and adoption of new behaviors. The maturation of the class of 1989 from sixth grade to twelfth grade occurred equally in both adolescent cohorts. The design asserts good control for this threat to validity.

Measurement Bias. The baseline equivalence of the two communities for the larger MHHP study and the adolescent smoking-prevention studies were well documented. The smoking prevalence rates for the sixth grade for both communities were comparable. In addition, the self-report data on smoking status were confirmed by saliva thiocyanate tests. A thorough discussion of the methods used to analyze the cohort and cross-sectional data are presented. The discussion of the analyses presents convincing information of the comparability of groups and assessment of changes over time.

This study used both self-reports and saliva thiocyanate levels to confirm smoking behavior. Data presented document a very high quality of instrumentation and measurement. Any error in measurement or classification is likely to have been small. Measurement of smoking behavior was accurate and stable.

Selection Bias. The selection of the communities and the schools was based on the larger cardiovascular disease prevention study. They reported demonstrated E versus C group "equivalence." Presentation of data on the two communities would, however, have been preferable. Although it is likely that some differences existed between the two communities, the use of both cohort and cross-sectional samples and having the capacity to thoroughly characterize community and parent characteristics lend support to the hypothesis that selection bias, if any, was very small. The sophistication of the sampling frame, statistical analyses, thoroughness of measurement, and follow-up procedures also provides evidence that selection was an unlikely threat to the validity of the reported results.

The issue of attrition and attrition analysis is dealt with directly by this case study. The magnitude of any intervention differences associated with attrition was examined by the investigators and found to be small. Thus, although some attrition occurred, it was well documented. The characteristics of students lost to follow-up were considered in the assessment of the efficacy of the smoking-cessation program. This issue was addressed by the discussion.

Summary

This evaluation study is an excellent example of the application of evaluation principles and intervention methods for school- and community-based studies. The evaluation was well designed, reflecting a high level of quality and methodological rigor. The conclusions reported by the investigators reflect a high level of internal validity. The results are likely to be generalizable to other midwestern communities and other areas of the country with comparable community demographics. The observed differences between the *E* and *C* communities were large and enduring. In contrast, other evaluation studies of the impact of adolescent smoking-prevention programs have found no impact or substantially diminished impact over time. This evaluation study documented a large impact (50%) for a cohort representative of the population-at-risk in these communities. The optimism reflected in the Class of 1989 discussion on efficacy is well grounded.

These results indicated that a smoking-prevention program integrated into an existing school health education curriculum and strongly maintained and reinforced over time, by a communitywide multiple-risk factor cardiovascular prevention trial, can produce large, sustained, lower rate of smoking initiation among adolescents. This case study represents an excellent follow-up of an earlier formative evaluation by Perry and colleagues (1980) to field-test the efficacy of school-based smoking-cessation interventions.

Case Study 3: AIDS/HIV Education

SOURCE: R. Stevens, T. Feucht, and S. Roman, "Effects of an Intervention Program on AIDS Related Drug and Needle Behavior Among Intravenous Drug Users," *American Journal of Public Health* 81(5) (1991):727–729.

This case study presents a discussion of a "formative evaluation" to assess the impact of a one-to-one health education session and risk-reduction strategies for AIDS. It provides insight about the adaption of evaluation methods to this problem and population.

Methods

Intravenous (IV) drug users, recruited between February 1988 and August 1989, were paid a nominal fee to participate in an AIDS education program. Baseline and follow-up assessments were conducted for most subjects between 3 and 5 months after the intervention. Pretest and posttest data were available for 402 subjects of 560 pretested. Subjects were street addicts not under treatment. Included in the impact analysis were 322 subjects—80 were dropped because they were not considered at risk for HIV infection.

Measurement

Pretest and posttest interviews assessed two major risk factors for HIV infection caused by IV drug use: measures of risks for needle behavior and drug-use behavior. Two scales measuring the frequency of using drug works of the others and use of cleaning of works were also used. Measures of risks associated with the more general issue of drug use were assessed. The baseline assessments were done 2 months prior to the interview as a referent for the risk behaviors.

Intervention

The intervention consisted of a one-to-one 45-minute session provided by a trained health educator. Four modules were presented: a film (*AIDS— A Hard Way to Die*), basic information about HIV, modes of transmission and progression of disease, and methods to reduce risks associated with sexual behavior. Methods to assess the risks associated with drug behaviors were also presented. Condom use was demonstrated, and risks of sexual practice were discussed. Subjects in the experimental group (*E*) were also provided with a kit to sterilize needles. Subjects were told about HIV testing and results.

Design

A pretest, posttest, one-group design was used to determine the immediate impact (3 months plus) of the intervention among the group. A nonequivalent comparison group (*C*), composed of subjects interviewed for the pretest at approximately the same time as those interviewed for the posttest was also used. The *E* groups reported a significantly lower risk versus the posttest *C* groups for 19 or 21 measures of risks associated with a needle behavior.

Results

Data presented in Table 5.12 document the short-term impact of the intervention. As noted, six of the seven needle-behavior risk behaviors decreased in frequency at the posttest. A major reduction was reported in sharing works and cleaning works with bleach. All 12 measures of risks associated with general drug behavior recorded a significant reduction. An additional analysis was performed to determine the lasting nature of the impact of the intervention. Subjects were regrouped by those interviewed within 111 days, between 122 and 154 days, and in 154 days or later.

Critique of Internal Validity of Results

An assessment of the internal validity of the results reveals that attribution of the observed changes to the intervention should be approached with caution. The investigators were forthright in their discussion of the limitations of this study. The measurement of risks based on self-report, use of convenience samples, and the lack of a control or true comparison

Table 5.12   Needle and Drug-Related Behavior, Pretest–Posttest Comparisons 2 Months Prior to Interview

	n[a]	Pretest	Posttest	Difference (95% CI)
Needle Behavior				
Scale means				
Using others' works	317	2.28	1.61	43.1 (36.0, 50.2)
Cleaning with bleach	315	1.86	1.87	—
Sharing works (%)	304	67.4	24.3	43.1 (36.0, 50.2)
Using others' works (%)	317	92.2	67.1	25.1 (19.4, 30.8)
Sharing cooker (%)	305	70.3	20.3	50.0 (44.5, 55.5)
Using drugs IV (%)	322	92.2	70.5	21.7 (16.1, 27.3)
Cleaning with bleach (%)	278	33.5	62.2	28.7 (21.0, 36.4)
Drug Behavior				
Means				
Number of drugs used	322	4.53	3.30	1.23 (1.13, 1.33)
Number of drugs used IV	322	2.24	1.43	0.81 (0.70, 0.92)
Heroin IV scale	278	4.24	3.32	0.92 (0.77, 1.07)
Cocaine IV scale	311	4.43	3.67	0.76 (0.63, 0.89)
Heroin use scale	322	3.49	2.15	1.34 (1.16, 1.52)
Cocaine use scale	322	4.47	3.27	1.20 (1.04, 1.36)
Speedball use scale	322	1.91	1.06	0.84 (0.70, 0.98)
Using heroin (%)	322	65.5	45.7	25.9 (18.4, 33.4)
Using heroin IV (%)	278	74.5	50.3	24.2 (16.4, 32.0)
Using cocaine (%)	322	83.9	67.2	16.7 (10.8, 22.6)
Using cocaine IV (%)	311	80.4	60.5	19.9 (13.8, 26.0)
Using speedball (%)	322	40.7	27.3	13.4 (6.2, 20.6)

SOURCE: Stevens et al. (1991): 727–729.

[a]The sample n varies from 322 due to missing values.

were acknowledged. Although the interview schedule used to collect data appeared to be fairly complicated and may have guarded against misrepresentation and self-report biases, the validity of self-reports represents the most critical methodological issue. Payment to participants (although nominal), also adds a bias to the reported results. Because of the probable bias to measurement validity, the reported changes presented in Table 5.12 are partially and possibly mostly attributable to the social desirability of the response and/or poor recollection of users.

The issue of selection—attrition of 160 subjects (560 to 401)—further complicates the interpretation of the results. The large reduction of subjects decreases the degree of attribution of impact to the intervention. Given the relatively short duration between the first and second observation, it would seem unlikely that external history played a role in producing the observed impact. The intervention was standardized and applied to all subjects. It also appears that there was limited opportunity for internal historical events to produce the impact. It is unclear whether any external events (i.e., any major police or media campaign), may have occurred over the 3–6 months covering the period of the evaluation. This seems unlikely and would have been noted in the evaluation report.

Summary

This evaluation presents one example of how to intervene with and conduct a formative evaluation of the impact of a health education program for adults at high risk for AIDS/HIV. The development of a standardized intervention, which appeared well grounded in the methods and theories of AIDS education and provided the means by which the risk behavior can be dealt with, was a strength of the study. Documentation of the exposure to the intervention and the assessment of multiple risk factors and behaviors reflected a good understanding of this population; good support for feasibility of program (appropriateness-implementation) was demonstrated. The use of a nonequivalent C group (historical comparison) added some strength to the design and interpretation of results. The relatively short period of time between baseline assessment, intervention, and follow-up assessments provides some support for attributing part of the observed impact to the intervention. The consistently high level of follow-up, although problematic because of its spreading out over an extended period of time beyond the plan of 3 months, 86%–100% (278 over 322) of the posttest data was commendable. To evaluate the efficacy of this intervention, however, it will be necessary to include at least a nonequivalent C group with pretest and posttest data or an experimental design, using a minimum or basic intervention versus the intervention provided to determine efficacy. Both designs would address the issue of the ethics of withholding education. The validity and reliability of the needle- and drug-related behaviors need to be significantly improved.

Case Study 4: Employee Health Promotion

SOURCE: R. Windsor, J. Lowe, and E. Bartlett, "The Effectiveness of a Worksite Self-Help Smoking Cessation Program: A Randomized Trial," *Journal of Behavioral Medicine* 11(4) (1988).

Background

At the onset of the project in 1983, the University of Alabama at Birmingham (UAB) had 10,000 employees, 8000 full-time and 2000 part-time. It is the largest employer in the city of Birmingham, with a wide range of occupations such as physicians and nurses, senior and junior administrators, faculty, secretaries, clerical staff, skilled labor, and custodial staff. In 1988 it employed 12,000 people and had a budget of $500 million.

As part of the planning process, a Senior Advisory Committee (SAC) was established. Meetings were held with the SAC—president, University of Alabama at Birmingham; senior vice-president for Health Affairs; and senior vice-president for University College—to discuss the employee program and to present updates by the principal investigator twice yearly. In addition to the SAC, an Employee Advisory Group (EAG) was established with representation from all major employee constituents in-

Table 5.13 Strategies of Recruitment Effectiveness

Strategy	Percentage Reporting as Source
UAB Report (employee newspaper) (articles, advertisements, etc.)	44.0
Memorandum from the president of the university	30.4
"Word of mouth" (nurses' competition, other participants, etc.)	19.3
Contact by staff (those who stated interest during surveys, etc.)	4.5
Memorandum from the University Hospital administrator	0.5
Other/missing	1.3

SOURCE: Windsor, Lowe, and Bartlett (1988).

cluding medicine, university hospital staff, nursing, public relations, administration, secretarial, and others.

Recruitment

Publicity to the employees about the Quit Smoking Program (QSP) began on March 1, 1983, approximately 1 month prior to the initiation of the program on April 2, 1983. An "enticement" message, "QSP Is Coming," appeared in the *UAB Report,* a weekly newspaper distributed to all UAB employees. This announcement and a press conference by the president of UAB initiated the program on April 2, 1984. The president sent a letter to all employees, encouraging each of them to use the service. Articles also appeared in that week's *UAB Report,* other UAB bulletins and newspapers, and local newspapers. The QSP established its own telephone extension and offices. The QSP was provided free of charge and during working hours, 8:00 A.M. to 5:00 P.M. All QSP health educators were trained to provide the smoking-cessation intervention methods. Our training methods were described by Bartlett et al. (1986).

Table 5.13 includes a summary of the activities conducted during the 18-month recruitment period and the percentage of participants reporting the sources from which they became aware of QSP.

Smoking Prevalence Surveys

Smoking prevalence surveys among full-time employees were conducted at 6-month intervals. A computer-generated 5% sample (440/8000) stratified by employee classification was provided by the university personnel department. The first survey forms, and each thereafter, were sent to 440 individual employees through the campus mail. Those not returning the survey within 1 week were sent a second letter and survey form. All nonrespondents to the second request were contacted by phone. All prevalence surveys exceeded a 90% response rate. These surveys continue to be conducted to monitor the incidence of this behavior for this population over time.

Approximately 24%, or 1920 (.24 × 8000), of this population smoke cigarettes. Approximately 60% of the smokers (1192) expressed a positive interest in participating in an employee smoking-cessation program during working hours. Reliability checks confirmed a 5% subsample of employee respondents, with a stability coefficient of $r = .89$.

Enrollment–Data Collection

Enrollment was provided from 7:00 A.M. to 6:00 P.M., Monday through Friday. A telephone appointment was made with the QSP clerk. Employees who enrolled in the QSP were informed that they would be scheduled to be interviewed at baseline, 6 weeks, 6 months, and 1 year. The following information was collected at baseline: (1) name, (2) address, (3) home phone number, (4) current occupational status, (5) current brand smoked, (6) number of cigarettes smoked daily, (7) estimated degree of difficulty to give up smoking, (8) main reasons for smoking, (9) number of times attempted to quit in the last year, (10) number of individuals in household who currently are smokers, (11) number of friends or co-workers who are smokers, and (12) estimate of the confidence (self-efficacy) that the person will be successful in quitting within the next 12 months and next 5 years.

A saliva sample to test for thiocyanate (SCN) was collected from each employee at enrollment (baseline). Prior to saliva collection, each employee was told the SCN would improve our ability to detect their levels of smoking exposure. The QSP staff (health educator) demonstrated the collection process, using a cotton dental roll, plastic test tubes, and stopper. The cotton roll was placed in the buccal cavity of the employee, who saturated it with saliva for at least 3 minutes. Saliva samples were also collected and tested for SCN at 6 weeks, 6 months, and 1 year *only* for employees who stated that they had quit. All self-reports of smoking status agreed with the SCN total for the sample of our 600 SCNs.

A SCN value of ≤100 g/mL was used as the cutoff to corroborate the self-report of smoking status. All employees for whom a follow-up was not performed were counted as failures. A total of 37 employees of the recruited 378 employees were lost to follow-up; all were counted as failures—still smokers, in our analyses. These were distributed equally among each group. However, a minimum of seven quitters from groups 2 and 4 (five at 6 weeks and two at 6 months) was reported as smokers because they could not be followed up.

Self-Help Interventions

Cessation Method 1: Self-Help Manual. After a review of available manuals based on behavioral self-management principles, the American Lung Association (ALA) manual was selected because of its low-cost, attractive format and because some evaluation data on its effectiveness were available. The *Freedom from Smoking in 20 Days* manual (ALA, 1980a) provides a structured, daily plan to cessation, including such techniques as behavioral contracting, behavioral self-monitoring, stimulus control, contingency management, imagery, and stress management. On the smoker's quit date (day 17 after the initial visit), he or she received a maintenance manual, *A Lifetime of Freedom from Smoking* (ALA, 1980b). This maintenance manual encourages continued cessation, emphasizes the self-control techniques presented in the cessation manual, and stresses the development of new behavioral and thought patterns consistent with being a nonsmoker.

These two manuals represent the minimum self-help intervention and were presented to all employees. Employees who received this intervention only (group 1—*C* group) were told that the manual provides the smoker with proven techniques to be used daily through the cessation date, day 17. The smoker was asked if he or she had additional questions. The discussion that followed, taking approximately 10 minutes, was unstructured, with no emphasis on practicing specific quitting skills. It varied according to the employees and covered topics such as motivation for quitting, common antecedents of the smoker's behavior, and concerns about weight control.

Cessation Method 2: Skill Training Plus Enhancement of Social Support. Method 2 used three behavioral approaches: (1) learning and improving cessation skills (e.g., learning to keep a diary and practicing deep-breathing techniques), (2) enhancing commitment to cessation through a quit-smoking contract and defined activities, and (3) increasing social support by developing a quit-smoking buddy and reinforcing through buddy education.

Each employee was taught these behavioral approaches in a one-to-one counseling session that took approximately 20–30 minutes to be conducted. The intervention was structured, allowing ample time and flexibility for the employee to ask questions and have his or her needs met. During the intervention, the health educator discussed the individual's perceived ability (self-efficacy) to quit smoking. In addition, personal instructions in how to deep breathe and use other methods in the manual specifically relevant to that individual were discussed.

A quit-smoking buddy system was set up between the employee and a nonsmoker or ex-smoker friend of the employee's choice. Although not measured directly, no employee responded negatively to the cessation buddy idea or procedures.

An educational prescription-contract was signed at the conclusion of the intervention between the health educator and the employee. This contract specified (1) a quit date, (2) an agreement about calling buddies, and (3) an agreement to perform deep-breathing exercises during urges to smoke. The contract also provided the employees with a telephone number to call if they should need additional information. The employees received a copy of this prescription-contract, and the health educator kept a copy. Employees were then given an opportunity to ask questions and deal with any other concerns that they had in attempting to quit smoking.

Cessation Method 3: Monetary Incentives. Consistent with our knowledge that relapse is most likely to occur during the first few weeks after cessation (National Center for Health Statistics, 1979), the first monetary incentive of $25 was awarded following 6 weeks of cessation. An additional $25 incentive was awarded at the end of 6 months of cessation. We wanted to determine the effect of a monetary incentive in the amount that an employee might be willing to pay. The monetary reward was mailed within 2 days after confirmation of cessation by saliva thiocyanate. This information was explained to the participant in about 3 minutes.

Experimental Groups

Group A received cessation method 1 only. Group B received cessation methods 1 and 2. Group C received cessation methods 1 and 3. Group D received cessation methods 1, 2, and 3.

Evaluation Design

A randomized, 2×2 factorial pretest–posttest control group design was employed to evaluate the individual and combined effects of the interventions. Randomization using a computer-generated assignment system to group occurred before the baseline interview. Prior to the initiation of the trial, 400 employee group assessment labels were placed in separately sealed envelopes. After informed consent and completion of the baseline questionnaires, the health educator used the next sequentially numbered envelope to confirm the employee group assignment. As presented in Table 5.14, employees were randomly assigned to one of four treatment conditions. All employees received a self-help manual. The two other intervention components, (1) cessation skills training/social support and (2) monetary incentives, were applied in a factorial fashion.

Table 5.14   Self-Help Smoking Cessation Study Design[a]

	Phase 1	Phase 2	Phase 3	Phase 4
Group A	R O_1 X_1 $(A + B)$	O_2 $(A + B)$	O_3 $(A + B)$	O_4 $(A + B)$
Group B	R O_1 $X_1 + X_2$ $(A + B)$	O_2 $(A + B)$	O_3 (A,B)	O_4 $(A + B)$
Group C	R O_1 X_1 $(A + B)$	O_2 X_3 $(A + B)$	O_3 X_3 $(A + B)$	O_4 $(A + B)$
Group D	R O_1 $X_1 + X_2$ $(A + B)$	O_2 X_3 $(A + B)$	O_3 X_3 $(A + B)$	O_4 $(A + B)$

SOURCE: Windsor, Lowe, and Bartlett (1988).

[a] O_1 = baseline observation; O_2 = follow-up (6 weeks); O_3 = follow-up (6 months); O_4 = follow-up (12 months); R = random assignment to group; X_1 = self-help cessation/maintenance manuals (American Lung Association); X_2 = commitment enhancement, social support, and skills training; X_3 = monetary incentives; A = smoking practices questionnaires; B = saliva thiocyanate.

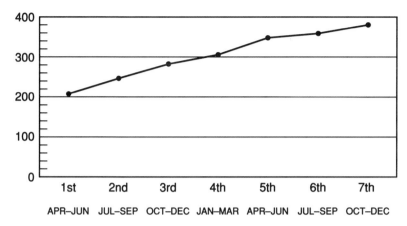

Figure 5.3 Recruitment of UAB Employees into the Quit Smoking Program

Program Impact

Participation–Penetration Rates. Figure 5.3 presents the recruitment pattern of the UAB employees into the QSP by quarters. As indicated by the graph, the majority (54%) was recruited during the first 3 months of the project. The program provided them with an immediate opportunity to try to quit by reducing the barriers of cost and availability. Recruitment of 378 employees occurred over a 21-month period. This represents a penetration rate of 19.7% (378/1920) among at-risk smoking employees. If you divide the 380 who enrolled by the estimated 1152 who expressed verbal interest in participating in the QSP (.60 × 1920), it confirms that a high penetration rate, 33% among the "ready-to-act" smoking employees, was produced.

Comparability of Study Groups. Data in Table 5.15 confirm the equivalence of the four employee study groups at baseline by employment categories. In addition, a comparison of the groups by smoking characteristics is presented. The four groups were comparable by smoking characteristics, number of cigarettes, initial SCN value, and years smoked. Other studies have found these variables to be predictors of quitting smoking. There was also no difference among the age, quit attempts, and self-efficacy of quitting by employees in each of the four groups.

Figure 5.4 confirms that QSP participants were similar to the typical UAB employee smoker. The difference in cigarettes smoked per day appears to be produced by a digit preference by employee rather than a real difference in number of cigarettes smoked. In addition, we believe that QSP participants' reports may be more accurate due to the physiological measure (SCN) taken at the time of self-report. No such measure was taken on the surveyed UAB employees. At best, QSP smokers smoked a little more. These data also provide good evidence of the level of penetration among a wide range of employee classifications.

Table 5.15 Comparison of Groups by Employment Categories

	Groups				
	A	B	C	D	Total
Admin/faculty	20 (21%)	21 (22%)	18 (19%)	21 (22%)	80
Sec/clerical/ maintenance	33 (35%)	28 (30%)	38 (40%)	30 (32%)	129
Professional nonfaculty, includes residents, nurses	24 (25%)	28 (30%)	18 (19%)	25 (27%)	95
Technical/skilled crafts	18 (19%)	17 (18%)	21 (22%)	18 (19%)	74
Employees in group ($n =$)	95 (100%)	94 (100%)	95 (100%)	94 (100%)	378
Number of cigarettes smoked daily	25	24	23	27	
Initial SCN level	180	188	187	177	
Years smoked	17	16	18	18	
Age	37	37	36	37	
No. of quit attempts	02	01	01	01	
Belief in being able to quit (0 = low, 100 high)	68	68	65	71	

SOURCE: Windsor, Lowe, and Bartlett (1988).

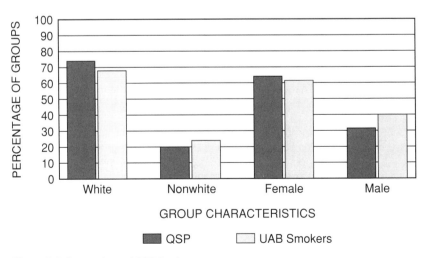

Figure 5.4 Comparison of QSP Participants and UAB Employees Who Smoke

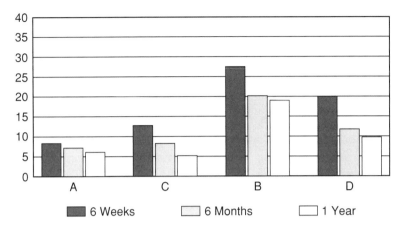

A = Self-Help Manual Only
C = Self-Help Manual + Monetary Incentive
B = Self-Help Manual + Social Enhancement
D = Self-Help Manual + Social Enhancement + Monetary Incentive

Figure 5.5 Success by Group at 6 Weeks, 6 Months, and 1 Year

Quit Rates by Group. Figure 5.5 presents continuous quit rates at 6 weeks, 6 months, and 1 year by groups A–D. The criterion on slippage by an employee was predetermined. If an employee smoked more than two cigarettes more than one time during the follow-up period, he or she was considered a smoker. The information was collected at the end of the follow-up period. The criterion for success or failure was not made known to the employee. We think that, although these are self-reported data of slippage, even employees who slipped considered themselves still a nonsmoker and were not reluctant to report this information. Employees lost to follow-up were counted as smokers. The data indicate that these individuals were equally distributed among groups. A chi-square analysis comparing rates of 1-year abstainers in each group revealed that the skills training plus social support intervention (group B) and the skills training plus social support plus monetary incentive (group D) were significantly more successful ($P < .05$) than the manual-only (group A) or manual plus monetary incentive (group C).

Effect of Monetary Incentives. One of the aims of this project was to determine if monetary incentive had an effect on smoking status. Although a difference between group A and group C quit rates was observed, suggesting that a monetary incentive might have had a behavioral impact, examination of groups B and D data created an inconsistent picture. A level and direction similar to those of groups A and C would be expected in groups B and D if monetary incentives were having an effect. This was not observed. Monetary incentives in these groups appear to have a

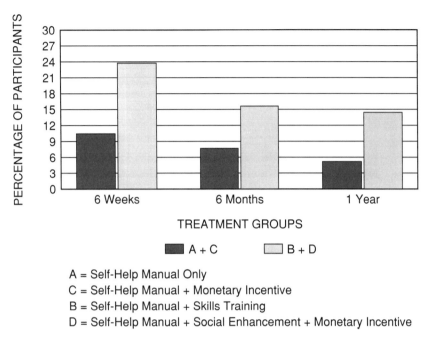

A = Self-Help Manual Only
C = Self-Help Manual + Monetary Incentive
B = Self-Help Manual + Skills Training
D = Self-Help Manual + Social Enhancement + Monetary Incentive

Figure 5.6 Success at 6-Week, 6-Month, and 1-Year Follow-Up by Treatment Group

negative effect on quitting smoking. Because an inconsistent pattern was observed at 6-week follow-up, we concluded that the monetary incentives would not have an effect at 6 months.

One can only speculate on why the monetary incentive was not effective. At 1 year, none of the participants stated that money was the main reason for quitting or attempting to quit. The motivation induced by offering only $50 to employed individuals was small. Employees stated that they never had the money, so they did not lose it by continuing to smoke.

A chi-square analysis revealed no significant difference between group A and group C ($P = .347$) or group B and group D ($P = .306$) at a 6-week follow-up. The four study groups were reconstituted, A + C (group AC) and B + D (group BD), for further analysis.

Figure 5.6 is a summary of the quit rates at 6 weeks, 6 months, and 1 year of cessation by reconstructed treatment group—AC versus BD. A chi-square analysis revealed a significant difference ($P < .001$) at each follow-up period. The observed group BD quit rate was significantly higher than the group AC quit rate at all three observation points.

Conclusion

The results of this evaluation indicate that if you simply give a self-help smoking-cessation manual and provide a 10-minute general smoking discussion to an employee at the work site, you may achieve a quit rate of approximately 5%. This result was consistent with one of the results of the study by Davis et al. (1984). They found that, although 20% of the individuals given the cessation manual and maintenance manual quit initially, only 5% of that group remained abstinent after 12 months. The provision of a standardized training session designed to enhance cessation skills of approximately 20 minutes increases cessation rates twofold. This level of impact was also consistent with the results reported by Prue et al. (1983). They found that self-help methods with a structured but limited duration of phone calls resulted in 23% abstinence. With additional structured effort, additional gains in cessation rates can be achieved while still adhering to the concept of a minimal-contact smoking-cessation program.

In this study, a monetary incentive was not effective in getting employees to quit. This may be attributable to two factors: (1) $50 to an employee population in the 1980s was not much money, compared to the effort the employees must make to quit smoking; (2) the employees could not "miss something they never had." If the employees had lost their own money, this may have been more of an incentive to quit.

This type of self-help program, when provided at the work site, appears to be successful. High levels of employee acceptance and utilization of this type of program were evident. However, self-help programs may be only one option an employee may want. Some employees may select a multicessation group process cessation program.

SUMMARY

In evaluating the efficacy or effectiveness of health promotion and education programs, there are a number of critical methodological issues to address. The time frame, resources, and capabilities of your program must be considered prior to making a final decision about the specific design or methods you will propose and implement. In making a decision about a design, you must consider the potential factors that affect internal validity—factors that will compromise or bias estimates of program impact. A number of designs exist, but only a few are really useful for program evaluators. The five designs identified in this chapter—a one-group pretest and posttest, nonequivalent comparison group, time series, multiple-time series, and randomized pretest and posttest with control group—are the most likely choices. In deciding what design to implement for your program, you need to fully appreciate the strengths and weaknesses of each.

Because designs play a prominent role in increasing the probability of a demonstrable effect and in determining significant observations, you must estimate an effect size and decide on the needed sample size during the planning of an evaluation. There are a few good ways to establish a control or comparison group. You must consider what problems will arise in implementing an evaluation that includes two or three study groups. Although, at first glance, using a randomized design may seem impossible, more careful thought about the key questions to be answered, combined with a consultation and literature review, may provide insight into the use of a control group instead of a comparison group in evaluating a program. Regardless of the type of design or group that is used, you must establish the baseline comparability of study groups. In summary, the theory and applications discussed in this chapter represent an essential body of information that you must know and be able to apply to plan, manage, and evaluate a health promotion and education program.

6

Measurement Issues in Data Collection

"Of course, this measures what I want; just read the sentences, and you can tell."

"I don't have the time to assess reliability. Let's assume it's reliable."

"I don't care how the program works, as long as it produces changes in outcomes."

"We'll collect all the measures we can and figure out what to do with them later."

"I want all the best measures collected, but we only have a very limited amount of money."

Professional Competencies Emphasized in This Chapter

• Identifying and providing mechanisms to assess selected educational methods

• Establishing the scope of a program evaluation

Selecting the right approach to measurement for your evaluation can be a confusing task. A person looking at the smoking-cessation literature will find self-reports of the number of cigarettes smoked per day, measures of attitudes toward smoking, measures of serum thiocyanate (a by-product in the blood that varies with the number of cigarettes smoked), or possibly even tests of knowledge about smoking. A person looking at the weight-loss literature will find measures of weight, calories consumed, and energy expended. A person looking at the sex education literature will find measures of knowledge, self-reports of frequency of sexual intercourse with and without contraception, and measures of attitudes toward certain erotic topics. In evaluating practically every aspect of a health promotion and education program, you will have to select what to measure from alternatives.

Along these lines, the initial Role Delineation Project (U.S. Department of Health and Human Services, 1980a) identified two skills:

The health educator must be able to provide mechanisms to assess selected methods.

The health educator must be able to establish the scope for program evaluation.

You must consider a variety of issues in establishing the scope of and developing mechanisms for program evaluating. The selection of endpoints should be based on the objectives of a program. If a program has been designed to promote weight loss, weight should be measured by a standard calibrated scale. If a program has been designed to promote positive attitudes toward heavy people among spouses of the obese, an attitudinal measure is appropriate. If a program attempts to influence what a person is *able* to do (as opposed to what a person actually does), a measure of the ability to perform the behavior—that is, a skills or capability test—is appropriate.

Almost all health promotion and education programs attempt to influence the frequency of a particular behavior. Methods to measure a targeted behavior may not be readily available. For example, an explicit goal of your sex education program might be to reduce the number of teenage pregnancies in your community by promoting either sexual abstinence or effective contraceptive behavior. The primary effectiveness indicator is the number of teenage pregnancies in a geographically defined area (community). A lack of reduction in the pregnancy rate, however, does not necessarily mean that your sex education program was ineffective. The incidence of teenage pregnancies may have been rising over the last 5 years, and your program may have slowed the level of increase; or the program may be reaching only a segment of the population of sexually active teenagers who are abstaining or using contraception while the rest are not; or the program may have unintentionally misinformed the teenagers. In either of the latter two cases, you may want more behavioral data from the teenagers. Because following all the teenagers 24 hours a day to observe their sexual habits and contraceptive practices is not feasible, you might ask for self-reports of these practices. Alternatively, the teenagers might be asked to demonstrate effective contraceptive techniques on a plastic model. Although these latter two methods are reasonable approaches to collecting data, who can say that the self-reports are accurate or that the teenagers practice what they can demonstrate in the classroom?

As this example shows, the area of measurement is fraught with complexities and pitfalls. In this chapter, we review in general terms the possible measures and issues in selecting variables, including development of an intervention model, assessing the validity and reliability of instruments, secondary selection criteria, threats to measurement validity, and a procedure for developing multiitem scales.

CONCEPTS AND VARIABLES, INSTRUMENTS AND MEASURES

Evaluation is most useful when based on a conceptual foundation. You cannot understand a program or evaluate its efficacy unless you have some conceptual basis for understanding how it is supposed to work. *Conceptual basis* means that a theory or, at a less formal level, a model hypothetically explains how the program and its parts are supposed to work. Any theory or model has variables. Variables define specific concepts. A model proposes that the variables are related in specific ways. Variables in your model can then be measured.

Someone new in the field may ask, Why is a theory or model necessary? There are several reasons. First, our programs and our evaluations should be based on what is known about theories of human behavior. Many behavioral and social scientists have conducted extensive basic and applied research to improve our understanding of human behavior and how it might be changed. Behavioral theory provides a medium in which findings across many studies can be integrated to improve our understanding of human behavior. If theoretical ideas hold up in many kinds of basic and applied research, then we can have some confidence that it embodies valid insights about behavior. One program or evaluator will not likely have completely new and more accurate insights into understanding behavior and its change, than the combined work of many professionals. Programs therefore will have the greatest likelihood of being effective if they are based on the latest and most useful theories and models of health behavior and its change. Creativity enters in trying to design interventions that most effectively implement or put into operation the underlying theoretical constructs.

Second, in many cases, a program may not have been theory-based or may have been based on intuition. The evaluator can serve a useful function for the program staff by generating a model that makes explicit the underlying theoretical ideas and relationships. Comparing and contrasting the intuitive model with what is known in behavioral and social science may lead to sharper critical thinking on the part of program staff. This may lead to changes in program activities to conform more to what is known about human behavior and effective practice.

Third, if the program is based on a theory or model, then it should be evaluated against the underlying theory or model. The theory identifies what variables should be measured. This is helpful because the evaluation may reveal that changes did not occur in one or more key mediating variables, thereby precluding behavior changes. This finding would give guidance to the program staff to change their training program to increase the odds of changing the mediating variables and thereby increase the likelihood of changes in impact.

Fourth, an evaluation can contribute to our knowledge about human behavior. If a rigorous evaluation obtains patterns of results inconsistent with the underlying theory, then the theory needs to be modified to account for these findings. This happens by publication of the evaluation.

Consider, for example, a model that identifies how people learn to lower the amount of salt in their diet. At a simple level, a model based on social learning theory (Bandura, 1977; Baranowski, 1989–1990) proposes that the likelihood a person will reduce salt in his or her diet is directly related to three mediating variables: the person's preference for low-salt foods, behavioral capability (knowledge and skills) to do so, and self-efficacy (or perceived self-confidence) at being able to act (Figure 6.1). The initial patient outcome is early efforts by patients to lower salt in the diet. The model specifies four relationships (all positive) among these variables. The positive sign indicates that the higher the level of one variable, the more likely you will ob-

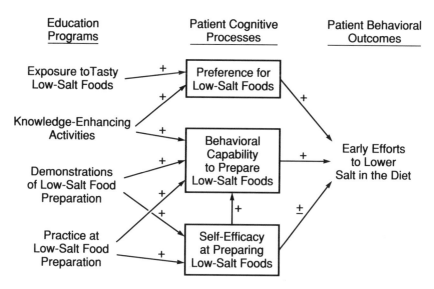

Figure 6.1 A Simple Social Learning Theory Model for Reducing Salt in the Diet

serve a higher level of the other variable. According to this model, a program interested in reducing salt in a target group's diet would attempt to increase preference, behavioral capability, and self-efficacy for salt reduction among members of the target group. Working with these three variables, we present four components of an education program that should affect these mediating variables and thereby have impact on outcome.

The direct approach to evaluating the efficacy of a program based on this approach would be to measure dietary salt consumption (e.g., from a food-frequency questionnaire) of a target group and the initial behaviors participants may use to lower salt intake (e.g., removing the salt shaker from the table, buying no-salt bread). If you want to know whether the program was working according to the hypothesized model, you would also need to measure the group's preferences, behavioral capability, and self-efficacy for lower-salt foods. Measuring these variables requires instruments and measurements.

The word *instrument* has been used to identify something that produces a measure of an object. In the physical sciences, instrument usually refers to a machine (simple or complex) designed to produce meaningful, accurate numbers—for example, in the form of degrees Fahrenheit or Celsius pertaining to the heat in some object. A flame spectrophotometer produces numbers in the form of percentages of the volume of one type of chemical contained in a solution.

Although at times behavioral and social scientists and health promotion and education program evaluators use machines as instruments to obtain measures, they more commonly have some sequence of questions (usually with precoded response alternatives) to measure a concept (construct). These sets of questions are also instruments. The numbers that come from applying the instrument to a person are called *measures*. Two or more instruments may produce or attempt to produce the same measure. To produce the measure, the instrument includes not only the specific questions but also instructions to an interviewer in asking the questions or in probing initial responses and procedures for taking the responses and producing numbers. The terms *instrument* and *measure* are often used interchangeably in discussions of categories of measurements. In this chapter, *instrument* will be used primarily to refer to the questions and procedures used to obtain measures on individuals.

Figure 6.2 shows the stated relationships among models, variables, measures, and instruments. A model and variables exist in the conceptual world. *Variables* are ideas that exist in the mind: verbal or written abstractions about human experience. Referring to Figure 6.1, no one has ever seen behavioral capability or self-efficacy to reduce salt in a diet. They are useful concepts, however, to organize our understanding of what may explain why some people are able to reduce salt in their diet. A *model* is based on one or more theories that describe expected relationships between two or more variables.

An instrument and measures exist in the operational world: They reflect the procedures, terminology, and methods professionals use. Under the best of circumstances, there will be a close correspondence or agreement between the variables in the model and the measures produced by the instrument. Sometimes, however, there is not good agreement, as if there were refraction through a lens. How to achieve the highest degree of this agreement (accuracy) is the subject of validity, discussed later in this chapter.

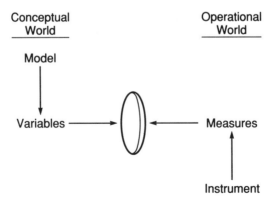

Figure 6.2 Relationships Among a Model, Variables, Measures, and an Instrument

TYPES OF VARIABLES

Many types of variables exist. In the "human factors" area, Alluisi (1975) has described psychobiological, psychophysiological, sensorimotor, and performance variables. In the personnel counseling area, there are ability, performance, and sociopsychological adjustment variables. Obviously, in each area of inquiry, certain kinds of variables are more appropriate than others. In health education and promotion programs, the following variables seem to be most frequently used: (1) demographic, (2) informational, (3) cognitive, (4) value or motivational, (5) attitudinal (belief), (6) personality, (7) capability (skill), (8) routine performance (behavioral), (9) health service utilization, (10) environmental, (11) clinical–biological, and (12) cost. Because cost is discussed in detail in Chapter 9, it is not presented here.

Demographic

Demographic variables are used to describe social characteristics such as age, sex, race-ethnicity, occupation, and education. These data are useful for characterizing the people in a program and comparing them with groups in other programs or to the population-at-risk (through census data). Who has your program reached? Demographic variables separate people into common groups that are useful to test for differences in program efficacy or to define the population to which an evaluation's results can be generalized (effectiveness). For example, the percentage of mothers breast-feeding their infants (an important health-promoting behavior) upon departure from the hospital varies by ethnic group, income level, and family structure (Baranowski, Bee, et al., 1983).

Informational

Informational variables have usually been labeled *knowledge* variables. Measures of knowledge almost always assume that answers either are correct or incorrect. The greater the percentage of correct answers, the more knowledgeable the person is considered. Informational data are often used to confirm levels of community awareness about a problem, program, or activity. Whether people know that a service exists is an essential piece of datum in designing a public information campaign.

There has been an increased interest in how people *represent* to themselves health-related phenomena (Leventhal et al., 1984). Research has been conducted on the aspects of health or illness to which people pay attention and how people decide if they are ill or when they have recovered. Investigators have found differences between people in how they represent health and illness, with implications for how they behave. A health education program could be directed at how people mentally represent health and disease.

Cognitive

Cognitive variables measure the product of a mental process by which a person arrives at a conclusion. Cognitive processes of concern to a health education/health promotion program may include attributional processes about illness, judgmental processes about achieving health, and problem-solving processes. *Attributional processes* deal with how people infer certain characteristics about themselves or about other people or events. Attributions are involved when a person uses symptoms to infer that he or she is sick. *Judgmental processes* refer to how people use various sources of information to arrive at a quantitative estimate of some characteristic of others or events. Judgments are often made about "how sick" a person is. *Problem-solving processes* refer to how a person defines a particular problem, identifies alternative solutions to the problem, and selects the most appropriate solution. The goal of a health promotion and education program may be to improve any of these health-related cognitive processes. For example, knowing which symptoms people use and how they are used to decide to seek medical care is critical in educating patients about the appropriate solution.

Value or Motivational

Value or motivational variables represent the factors that attract or repel a person and thereby influence the person to act (Baranowski, 1992–1993). There are different levels of value and motivational data. At the most abstract level are enduring values (e.g., beauty, truth, health, religious faith), which can be major influences in a person's life decisions. At another level are more immediate motivations, that is, incentives, expectancies, and preferences. *Incentives* are good or bad things that people expect to happen soon after a behavior (e.g., wanting a reward for having lost 10 pounds or wanting to avoid a penalty imposed by a program for not having lost 10 pounds). Outcome *expectancies* are other things that people expect to occur from having performed a behavior (e.g., better health for their baby from breast-feeding) (Baranowski, Bee, et al., 1990). *Preferences* state or capture a person's desires or wishes to engage in certain behaviors (e.g., preferences for eating fruits and vegetables) (Domel et al., 1992). Motivational variables can be a health education program's primary dependent variable (e.g., increasing the concern for health in a person's life) or a mediating variable (e.g., a program may have the greatest impact on those who value health the most). Program planners are usually faced with what motivations to emphasize to get participants into a program and to maintain behavior changes (Baranowski, 1992–1993).

Attitudinal

Attitudinal, or belief, variables measure the opinions of people. Attitudes are typically considered to have three components: a belief about a particular content area, a value about that belief (good or bad), and a predisposition to behavior. Knowing whether clients like or dislike group meetings can assist in the design of an approach to smoking cessation. Whether attitudes toward overweight people change may be an important outcome for a training program for spouses of overweight people.

Personality

Personality variables measure enduring characteristics that differentiate individuals from one another. There are a broad range of personality measures, but two commonly used measures are internal–external locus of control (Lau and Ware, 1981) and type A behavior (Jenkins et al., 1974). Personality variables have been used as dependent measures (e.g., in attempts to promote internal control), as mediating measures (e.g., where a program is expected to be effective with the internally controlled, but not others), and as screening variables (e.g., to identify people who have type A personalities to participate in a stress-reduction program).

Capability

Capability, or skill, variables represent a person's ability to perform a task, that is, how well a behavior *can* be performed. In the sex education example, a teenager may or may not be capable of effectively performing a contraceptive task, such as putting on a condom. A person who cannot put on a condom correctly in a measurement session is very unlikely to do so at the height of passion. Persons with diabetes need to know how to monitor sugar in their urine and how to inject their insulin. Capability measures are useful because people cannot effectively perform the behavior or task routinely in other settings unless they can demonstrate the skill in an assessment setting. Just because they know how, however, does not necessarily mean they usually do the task routinely.

Routine Performance

Routine performance, or behavioral, variables represent whether or how frequently people perform one or more behaviors or tasks in their daily life. Most programs are concerned with specific health-related behaviors. Is the hypertensive patient consuming fewer high-salt foods? Is this family doing more exercise? Although these data are crucial for measurement in evaluations, they present many problems. Of greatest concern is that not all of a person's behaviors are readily available to outside observation.

Health Service Utilization

Health service utilization variables are used to describe patterns among clients in the use of a health or medical service. This is a subcategory of behavioral measures, that is, whether and what kinds of people use particular services.

Environmental

The environments in which health behaviors are performed have become increasingly important in health education (Baranowski, 1989–1990; McLeroy et al., 1990). For example, physical proximity to fitness facilities encourages physical activity (Sallis et al., 1990); aspects of social support can either encourage or inhibit health behaviors (Baranowski, Bee, et al., 1983); parents can influence whether their children engage in physical activity (Taylor et al., 1992); life events may occur that may affect a person's ability to perform the desired health behavior (Baranowski, 1989–1990). A program evaluator may wish to measure changes in environments as outcome (e.g., increased social support) or as factors moderating outcomes (e.g., absence of fitness facilities as a limit to the amount of exercise that may result from a program).

Clinical–Biological

Clinical–biological variables may be used for several purposes: an outcome measure, a check on whether a person is performing a desired behavior, or a change in an aspect of health or health risk. For example, blood pressure is often used as the primary outcome measure of patient hypertension education programs. Urine sodium tests approximately measure the amount of salt consumed by an individual and thus can be used as a check on a person's self-report of eating salt. High levels of high-density lipoprotein (HDL) cholesterol in a person's blood protect against heart attacks and reflect the amount of exercise the person habitually gets. An evaluator may want to assess serum HDL cholesterol as a screen for whether a person should get an exercise intervention.

SELECTING VARIABLES: A MODEL

Given this vast array of variables, how do you know which are most appropriate? The first step in selecting measures is to have a conceptual model. Three kinds of models may be useful: A model explaining how (1) the behavior occurs, (2) the health education service is produced, or (3) the service affects or interacts with the ongoing behavior to promote change.

Model of Behavior

A model of behavior should identify the important variables related to a behavior and how they relate to one another and to the behavior. The variables and relationships in a model should reflect the latest understanding of the behavior available in the literature. For example, in a weight-loss program, a model is needed of the variables affecting the weight of obese people. Figure 6.3 shows a simple weight-loss model. Weight is affected by the amount of food consumed (calories ingested) and the energy expended (calories burned). How much a person eats is, in turn, affected by several factors. There is reason to believe that people have a mechanism, perhaps like a thermostat, that is sensitive to the amount of fat in the fat cells. This mechanism can be called a *fat-o-stat*. It either decreases appetite to maintain a certain level of fat in those cells (Morley and Levine, 1982) or varies

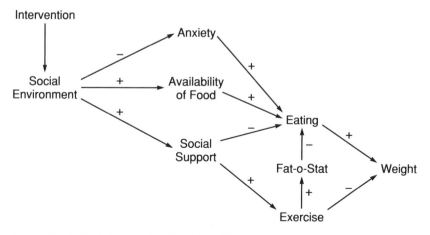

Figure 6.3 A Simple Model of a Weight-Loss Program

the rate at which energy is extracted from the food consumed (Sukhatme and Margen, 1982). Exercise may be one of the few things that can reset the regulator on the fat-o-stat. Social support may also affect eating patterns. Important people in the obese person's environment may encourage that person to overeat or to undereat. In some cases, obese people overeat when they are anxious or when food is too readily available. The availability of food and a person's anxiety level are both reflections of the obese person's social environment (family, friends, co-workers, etc.). How much exercise a person gets probably reflects, in part, the amount of social support the person receives to exercise.

This model of behavior is valuable for three reasons. First, the model identifies the basic building blocks for your program. It enables the program staff and evaluators to arrive at a common understanding of the target behavior or at least enables the evaluator to understand explicitly the basic concepts of the program staff. Second, a model describes a clear direction for action. The model in Figure 6.3 stresses the importance of the social environment in weight gain or loss and the need to design a program that at least takes the social environment into account if it does not actively involve members of the social environment, such as the family. No program can take all possible factors into account. A model thereby identifies the factors that are considered the most important for a particular program. Third, such a model identifies variables for which measures need to be found. Measures of eating, exercise, and weight are necessary to evaluate the impact of the intervention. Depending on the approach to intervention, the evaluator might also want to assess anxiety, food availability, and social support, to see if the intervention is having a desired impact on each of the hypothesized intervening variables.

Model of Service

A model of how a service is produced identifies other kinds of variables: the inputs, structures, processes, and service outputs. Figure 6.4 presents a simple conceptual model of a service system. In the inner box are the unspecified structures and processes for producing output. All programs have inputs, some of which come from the immediate environment and some from elsewhere. The output must return to some environment. The most common inputs to a program are participants, staff time, and other resources (e.g., educational and training materials). The structure for a program usually consists of the organizational structure (i.e., the positions and qualifications for positions in the organizational hierarchy) and the activity structure (i.e., the sequence of service activities provided to a participant). The process and content of a program (see Chapter 4) refer to what is

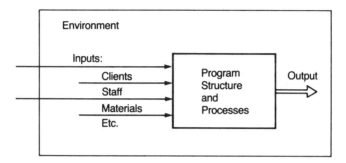

Figure 6.4 A Model of a Program as a Production System

actually done to and for a participant. The methods of a program refer to how you delivered each component of the program. The desired output of such a program (see Chapter 5) may be changes in knowledge, skills, behaviors, attitudes, or health status. The environment refers to the physical and social aspects of the surroundings within which the program operates and the participants live and work. Two questions about the environment are of particular importance: Are the necessary resources available for the program from the immediate environment? Is the output of the program, in turn, accepted by the environment? For example, developing a smoking-cessation program in an area where few people smoke would not make sense. Alternatively, producing nonsmokers who must return to groups of smokers makes little sense. They are likely to be seriously tempted and return to smoking in a short period of time.

A health promotion service model is valuable for several reasons. It describes the necessary resources, the program structures, the processes for service delivery, the desired outputs, whether the inputs are available in the environment, and whether the environment will accept the outputs. Each of these concerns could be the focus of a program evaluation. A study of the inputs to such a system is called a needs assessment (see Chapter 3 and Baranowski, 1978a, 1978b). A study of the availability of service structures can be called a resource inventory (Bosanac et al., 1982).

Model of Change

The model of how a service interacts with behavior to promote change simply shows at what points in the ongoing behavior the program would intervene and what changes would be expected as a result of such intervention. Such a model identifies points in the ongoing behavior process at which it is useful to measure or document the expected effects of program efforts. Figure 6.1 shows a model of behavior change.

SELECTING THE MOST APPROPRIATE INSTRUMENTS

Once the model has been developed, you must select the instruments to measure the specified variables. The dual issues of reliability and validity are critical in selecting and developing instruments.

Reliability

Reliability is the extent to which an instrument will produce the same result (measure or score) if applied two or more times. Imagine using an oral thermometer three times on the same person. On the first administration, a temperature reading of 105°F is obtained: a sign of serious fever. Worried, you take the temperature again, 1 minute later, and obtain a reading of 93°F: a sign of hypothermia, an equally serious problem. Still worried that something is wrong, you immediately try again and obtain a reading of 98°F: normal body temperature. If a thermometer produced measures with that much variability, it would be considered "unreliable." The instrument produced different results on each administration. These differences were so large that you could not distinguish normal from pathological states without being concerned that the results were due to chance or to a defect in the instrument rather than to a serious illness in the person.

The reason that the medicine cabinet thermometer is such a useful instrument is that it is highly reliable at what it measures. Using this instrument allows a person to decide with reasonable confidence whether the body is diseased or not. This does not mean that the medicine cabinet thermometer is reliable for all purposes; that is not the case. If you use such a thermometer three times, you may get readings something like this: 98.6°F, 98.5°F, and 98.7°F. The results are clearly different, but the differences are insignificant for the purpose for which you are using the thermometer. If, however, you need to make distinctions of one-tenth of a degree—say, between 98.4°F, and 98.5°F—or you need to measure temperature beyond one decimal place, the medicine cabinet thermometer is unreliable. Thus, one instrument can be reliable for one use, yet highly unreliable for another.

We may better understand reliability by considering the issue of error. We can think of most measures (X) as having a true score (T) component and an error (E) component:

$$X = T + E$$

What we want with any measure is a person's true score (T), but all measures have some error associated with them, and we assume that these errors are random. Random error is like "noise" on a radio. The more error, the more noise; more noise makes it harder to hear the true message on the radio.

Random errors include any effects that give something other than a true measure. For example, suppose a person takes the same test on ten different days and the scores are distributed as shown in Figure 6.5. Assume that the true response (measure) is depicted in the figure by the capital letter A. The deviations of each of the test administrations (a) from the true response are indicators of random error. Thus, errors are randomly distributed (plus or minus) around the true score. The ten measures may have varied around the true response for many reasons (e.g., the person got up late one day and was rushed, was too tired another day, and was anxious about an incident at home another day). Because of random error, the obtained scores vary around the true response. If a very large number of measures—for example, 100 were taken—the mean of the obtained measures would equal or be very close to the true response.

Figure 6.6 shows the curves from two distributions of scores. If these curves were obtained from applying an instrument many times in two different ways, we would say that the taller curve has less random error. More of the scores on that curve are closer to the true mean than those on the flatter curve. The way in which the test was

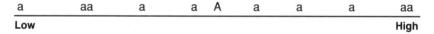

a	aa	a	a A	a	a	a	aa
Low							**High**

Figure 6.5 Distribution of Scores of Multiple Applications of a Test with Random Error

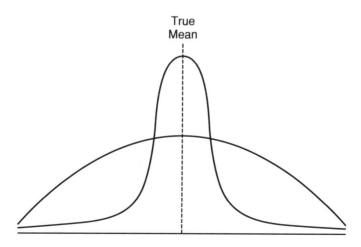

Figure 6.6 Two Distributions of Scores Around the True Mean

administered to give the taller curve is more desirable because it produces less error.

Of course, we rarely administer the same test five times to look at the distribution of scores around a true score. We never know the true score. In administering a test once, we don't know if this test is close to or far from this person's true score. We assume, however, that these errors are randomly distributed across all people being tested. Because we assume randomness in the errors, we can take the mean of the multiple administrations as our best guess of the true score. Random errors decrease reliability because they make it more difficult to detect the true score.

There may not be a constant true score for a person. The person's true score will vary from day to day. For example, how much physical activity a child gets on any day will vary, and our measure of that activity will vary around the true score. Figure 6.7 presents a child's true activity scores for each of three days (A, B, C) and the measures of those activity levels (a, b, c). These measures (a, b, c) might come from three different observers following the same child for a defined period of time. In this case, we have variability among the true scores and variability among the measures. The variability among the true scores (σ_T) is called intraindividual variability. The variability among the measures (σ_E) is error variability. The smaller we can make those errors, the less statistical "noise" there is in detecting true activity levels. Some intraindividual variability will always exist.

Another level of complexity is produced by adding more people to this system. In Figure 6.8, we have three daily activity levels for persons A and X with the true usual activity for A and X identified with vertical lines. Each of the day's estimates could come from mul-

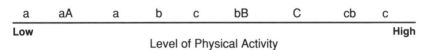

Low   **High**
Level of Physical Activity

Figure 6.7 True Activity Scores (A, B, C) for 3 Days with Three Measures (a, b, c) per ⌐⌐y

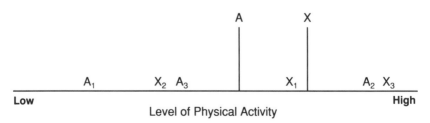

Low   **High**
Level of Physical Activity

Figure 6.8 Interindividual (A, X) and Intraindividual (A₁, A₂, A₃) Variability for Two People (A, X) in Level of Physical Activity

tiple observers, but that is not expressed here. The variability between A and X is called interindividual variability (σ_I), and variability within an individual across days is called intraindividual variability (σ_T).

Methods of Assessing Reliability. Before using an instrument to collect program data, you need to document its reliability. Reliability is an index of how much random error is in the measurement. Reliability coefficients are highest (1.0) if no error exists and lowest (0.0) when there is only error. Does the instrument you are using enable you to make distinctions between two or more behaviors with a reasonable level of confidence? For a few instruments, the reliability has already been calculated with many different groups; for most, however, it has not. There are several approaches to assessing instrument reliability. Two factors are important to consider: the type of instrument (observer or external source vs. self-report) and the times at which the instrument is applied (same time vs. different times). Figure 6.9 shows the four possibilities with corresponding types of reliability.

Interobserver Reliability. If several observers collect data at the same time, you estimate reliability by having two observers rate the same performance of a task or skill: interobserver or interrater reliability. This tells you whether two people are seeing and interpreting the same thing in the same way at the same time. Because both observers are supposed to be measuring the same actions, the perfectly reliable observer and instrument would produce reliability = 1.0. The level of error variability decreases reliability downward from 1.0. Windsor (1981) used this technique in evaluating a patient diabetes education program. If continuous variables are measured, the Pearson correlation is the common technique for measuring reliability. Because most

		Time Instrument Applied	
		Same Time	Different Time
Type of Instrument	Observer	Interobserver	Intraobserver Reproducibility
	Self-Report	Split-Half Multiple Form Repeat Item Internal Consistency Factorial	Test–Retest Reproducibility

Figure 6.9 Types of Reliability

observation scales use nominal or ordinal categories for rating, Cohen's kappa is the currently accepted statistical technique (Cohen, 1960). Kappa corrects the simple percentage agreement between two observers for chance agreement. Forms of kappa have been developed to weight deviations from exact agreement and to account for multiple observers (Fleiss, 1973).

Intraobserver Reliability. If an observer assesses the same person at two different times, comparison of the consistency of the results is called intraobserver reliability. This kind of reliability test is not frequently performed because it assumes no difference in the phenomenon being assessed (performance or whatever) between the two times. Such a technique might be used if little change is expected (e.g., on mass assembly lines in factories or about perceptions of physical environments). Because the amount of change is usually the phenomenon of concern, observer reliability is usually assessed at one time using two observers (interobserver reliability). The same statistical techniques would be used for intraobserver reliability as for interobserver reliability.

Reproducibility. An aspect of reliability for some measures is the consistency of measurement over many assessments. If more than two assessments have been done, the Pearson correlation is not appropriate. In this case, the intraclass correlation coefficient is the method of choice. Within measurement theory, total variance (σ_x^2) can be divided into variability due to the true scores (σ_T^2) (interindividual variability; see Figure 6.8) and that due to the error portion of the scores (σ_E^2) (see Figure 6.7): $\sigma_x^2 = \sigma_T^2 + \sigma_E^2$. Theoretically, reliability is the proportion of total variance accounted for by variance in the true scores:

$$R_x = \frac{\sigma_T^2}{\sigma_T^2 + \sigma_E^2} = \frac{\sigma_T^2}{\sigma_x^2}$$

where R_x = the index of reliability for test x

          σ_T^2 = the variance for the true scores

          σ_E^2 = the variance for the error portion of the scores

          σ_x^2 = the variance for the whole test

When multiple assessments are obtained per person, the error term can be further divided into variability due to raters (σ_R^2) and error (σ_E^2):

$$\sigma_x^2 = \sigma_T^2 + \sigma_R^2 + \sigma_E^2$$

This is important to show that rater variability comes out of the error term rather than the subject's term. Using mean squares within an analysis of variance, the intraclass correlation (ICC) can be estimated by

$$ICC = \frac{n(MS_B - MS_E)}{nMS_B + kMS_R + (nk - n - k)MS_E}$$

where n = the number of participants

k = the number of assessments

MS_B = the between-subject mean square (interindividual variability)

MS_E = the mean square due to error

MS_R = the mean square due to raters or times of assessment (intraindividual variability)

The ICC is sensitive both to differences in relative position and in mean values over times of assessment (k). High ICC values indicate high levels of consistency across all assessments in relative position, with little or no differences in mean values.

Multiple values or ratings may provide a more accurate estimate of a quantity (Schlundt, 1988). For example, there is much day-to-day (intraindividual) variability in what people eat (Schlundt, 1988) or in how much physical activity one participates (DuRant et al., 1992). One day's assessment is an unreliable estimate of what a person habitually or usually eats (both because of intraindividual variability and error variability). A more reliable estimate of what a person eats can be obtained by taking more than a 1-day assessment. More days of assessment will increase the reliability for a given level of accuracy or will increase the accuracy for a given level of reliability.

Several techniques are available to assess the reliability of self-report instruments applied at the same time.

Split-Half Reliability. If a large number of items measure the same concept or construct, you may conduct a split-half reliability assessment. Randomly assign items in the instrument to two sets of scores and conduct a Pearson correlation for continuous variables or Cohen's kappa for discrete variables. This correlation should be reasonably high, 0.80 or higher, because both halves are supposed to be measuring the same construct.

Multiple-Form Reliability. Another approach to assessing the reliability of self-report instruments administered at the same time is to create two instruments (or two forms of the same instrument) that theoretically measure the same thing and to have respondents answer both sets at the same measurement session (with participants randomly assigned to different sequences of administration). A correlation of 0.80 or higher should be obtained between the two sets of measures because they are supposed to be measuring the same thing. Having two equal forms is particularly valuable if you are concerned that completing the first questionnaire will increase the consistency of responses on the second administration if the same test were used (e.g., a simple knowledge test).

An extension of this idea is the repeat-item reliability. Simply repeat the same items at two points in a questionnaire, as a continuing monitor on the reliability of an instrument. If these items assess important concepts, asking the same question twice will provide a continuing monitor on how reliably a selected number of items are measured over the course of the evaluation. Because respondents may become frustrated or angry at answering the same question twice, a more common approach to this kind of reliability estimation is internal consistency.

Internal Consistency. The most commonly used method of assessing reliability is an index of internal consistency. With multiitem scales, indices of internal consistency measure the extent of interitem correlation among all items in a test. Theoretically, multiple items in one test share true variation—that is, the extent to which they commonly measure some underlying construct. The higher the interitem correlations, the more true variation is shared. This idea is so important that we provide the equation for estimating coefficient alpha:

$$\alpha_x = \frac{k}{(k-1)}\left(1 - \frac{\Sigma_i \sigma_{yi}^2}{\sigma_x^2}\right) = \frac{k}{(k-1)}\left(1 - \frac{\Sigma_i \sigma_{yi}^2}{\Sigma \sigma_{yi}^2 + 2\Sigma_{i<j}\sigma_{yi}^2\sigma_{yj}^2}\right)$$

where α_x = the alpha value for the whole test

k = the number of items in a test

σ_{yi}^2 = the variance of individual item i

σ_{xj}^2 = the variance of the whole test

This is often called Cronbach's alpha, recognizing the contribution of its originator (Lee J. Cronbach), and is used for continuous measures.

The Kuder–Richardson (KR) 20 is a form of internal consistency for continuous measures (Nunnally, 1978). As can be seen in the expression on the right, if the covariance term ($2\Sigma_{i<j}\sigma^2_{yi}\sigma^2_{yj}$) is large in comparison to the variance of the individual items, the value of the alpha will be close to 1, and the larger the number of items, the larger will be the covariance terms in proportion to the variances.

Factorial Reliability. In some ways, a more stringent test of reliability than internal consistency is factorial reliability. When multiple-item scales are used, some forms of component or factor analysis can be applied (see, e.g., Baranowski, Tsong, and Brodwick, 1990; Richards et al., 1989). If the items are supposed to measure a single underlying variable, applying factor analysis should produce a single dimension or factor. If the items are supposed to measure two or more underlying variables, applying factor analysis should produce the same number of factors with the same items loading on the same factors as in the original. Due to unreliability of assessment in individual items, the items do not always load on the same dimensions as in the original study. When they do load in the same manner, you can have greater confidence in the factors. If multiple factors are found in a set of items that should be unidimensional, the measure may respond to an intervention in unpredicted ways. Even when loading on dimensions as desired, coefficient alpha should be calculated to obtain estimates of internal consistency. Component and factor analyses are very sophisticated techniques (Nunnally, 1978), and evaluators should employ trained statistical consultants before using them.

Test–Retest Reliability. Measuring reliability by using the same test at two different times is called test–retest reliability. Reliability scores from this method are expected to be lower than the split-half or multiple-form methods because time has elapsed between the first and the second assessment. The longer this interval is, the more likely something will happen to some of the people to induce a real change in the measures the instrument provides.

Reproducibility. All the issues concerning reproducibility for observers are applicable to self-report items. In fact, the consideration of the number of items in internal consistency is similar to the consideration of the number of days of assessment in reproducibility (Bravo and Potvin, 1991).

There are many related issues in reliability assessment, and you should consult appropriate texts (Nunnally, 1978) before using one of these methods.

Managing Reliability. We have reviewed several concepts of or approaches to measuring reliability; we also need to review the sources of random errors that produce unreliability. Seven general sources of unreliability have been identified:

Natural day-to-day variability (discussed in "Reproducibility")

Instructions

The instrument

The data collector

The environment

The respondents

Data-management errors

Unreliability can enter from any and all these sources and usually does. For example, the instructions may be confusing to respondents. The target group may not clearly understand the instrument items. The person making the measurement may be sloppy in his or her use of the instrument. The environment in which the instrument is applied may be too noisy or distracting to respondents. Respondents may be suffering from hangovers, headaches, or other factors that divert their attention. Errors can be made in coding, keypunching, or editing the data.

Each of these sources of error adds to unreliability. The kinds of things that go wrong in data collecting fully support "Murphy's Law." You should assume problems will occur. Pay careful attention to anticipating possible sources of error and to developing plans to avoid or deal with them before or as they occur. Concern for and assessment of reliability should occur each time you use an instrument, regardless of past experience or existing data on psychometric properties.

Validity

In a colloquial sense, *validity* is the degree to which an instrument measures what the evaluator wants it to measure: the predictor, impact, or outcome variable. In a more formal sense, validity is the extent of correspondence between a measure and its underlying theoretical variable (see Figure 6.2). It is possible to have an instrument that measures something you do not think it does or want it to measure or that has a systematic error.

Systematic Error (Bias). Systematic errors produce a systematic difference between an obtained score and the true score. For example, assume that a person took the same tests on ten occasions and the

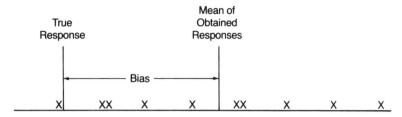

Figure 6.10 Distribution of Scores of Multiple Applications of a Test with Systematic Error

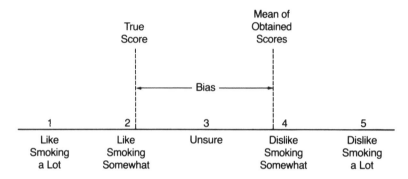

Figure 6.11 Effect of Bias on Conclusions

scores are distributed as shown in Figure 6.10. If the true response is the vertical line at the left, Figure 6.10 indicates that there was a bias in the test. The bias is the distance between the true response and the mean of the obtained responses. Of course, evaluators do not usually know what the true response is, although they may sometimes learn it from other information. With systematic errors, the mean of the obtained scores is always systematically different from the true score by one or more units: a systematic bias.

Bias threatens validity. A biased measure may lead you to conclude something completely different from a set of data than you would if you had the true measure. For example, if you were interested in attitudes toward smoking and used a 5-point scale, you might find the mean values shown in Figure 6.11. The difference between the true score and the mean of the obtained scores is only about 1.5 units. The mean of the data obtained may lead you to believe that these subjects are unsure about, or even slightly dislike, smoking. If the true score were known, however, you would conclude that they have positive feelings about smoking. Somehow a bias crept into the data and led you to an erroneous conclusion about the attitudes of this group.

Table 6.1 Definitions of Alternative Types of Validity

Type	Definition
Face	The extent to which the instrument appears to be measuring what it is supposed to measure
Content	The extent to which an instrument samples items from the full breadth of content desired
Criterion	The extent to which an instrument correlates with another more accurate (and usually more expensive) instrument (the criterion)
Concurrent	The criterion that an instrument be administered at the same time as the instrument being tested for validity
Predictive	The criterion that an instrument be administered at some time after administration of the instrument being tested for validity
Construct	The extent to which the measure of concern correlates with other measures in predicted ways, but for which no true criterion exists
Convergent	The measure that correlates with the items with which it is predicted to correlate
Discriminant	The measure that does *not* correlate with the items with which it is expected not to correlate

Invalidity or bias might happen because not enough thought went into creation of the instrument, because recent research has changed the complexity of the variable being measured, or because the instrument was not used with care and attention to detail. In many ways, the study of the validity of an instrument is more difficult than the study of its reliability. Using the same instrument at two different times or with two observers at the same time is relatively easy. Studying validity requires you to obtain or develop some more accurate measure of the variable of concern. Four general approaches to studying or assuring validity have been proposed (Table 6.1).

Face Validity. Face validity describes the extent to which an instrument appears to measure what it is supposed to measure. Thus, the question "How many minutes of running-jogging did you do today?" appears to measure one important component of a person's aerobic activity for a particular day. For most adults, this question might work fairly well. For children, however, it probably will not. Children do not usually wear watches; they have their time organized for them (e.g., by bells or buzzers at school); and they do not have a well-developed concept of time. Thus, there is little reason to believe that accurate timings of running-jogging would be assessed by asking children this question.

The question may lack validity even for adults. If you are interested in aerobic activity, which has cardiovascular benefit, a person must engage in aerobic activity for a minimum of 15 minutes at a time (without stopping), for a minimum of three times every week (American College of Sports Medicine, 1980). Furthermore, the activity must reach a certain intensity to promote cardiovascular fitness. Sufficient intensity would produce a heartbeat that is 60% or more of the person's maximum heart rate (calculated from commonly available tables for age and sex groups). You may therefore have a difficult time interpreting a response to the above question. Suppose the answer given is "20 minutes." Was the activity sufficiently intense to merit the label "aerobic"? Did the person cover 4 miles (tremendous cardiovascular benefit) or 1½ miles (less cardiovascular benefit) in those 20 minutes? Were the 20 minutes in one continuous block of time or broken into two 10-minute segments, or four 5-minute segments, or some other division without cardiovascular benefit? Each of these variations raises issues about whether the question elicits accurate data about the construct of concern. A measure therefore must be carefully written to assess the desired variable. You could create a self-report measure for adults to assess distance traveled, intensity (e.g., heart rate), and continuous duration of activity (segments in minutes). On the other hand, people may not be able or motivated to keep track of or remember all this information. In such a case, the validity of the instrument is again in question. The more complex questionnaire may work with marathon runners in training (who are highly motivated to keep such records to assess their progress) but may not work for casual early-morning joggers. The validity of the instrument thus may be high with one group (the marathon runners), but not another group (the casual joggers).

A variety of complexities in assessing face validity have been introduced in the literature (Thomas et al., 1992). The key issue in this literature is "perspective"—that is, from whose perspective is face validity being assessed? For example, a question posed by a highly trained clinician may have high validity in assessing some particular characteristic, but that validity may not be apparent to the person being interviewed. Lack of perceived relevance of an item could affect how the respondent answers the item and thereby affect its validity.

This discussion should confirm that a concern for validity requires more than attention to the face validity of the instrument. A valid measure should have other characteristics as well.

Content Validity. Another desirable characteristic is content validity. Some instruments are expected to cover several domains of content. To have content validity, an instrument must sample items from each of these content areas. For example, Windsor, Roseman, et al. (1981) developed an instrument to measure the ability of diabetic patients to care for themselves. Diabetic self-care is a complex activity requiring knowledge and skills in many areas. The Windsor team used a consulting body of experts and identified a broad variety of content areas for diabetes self-care, including foot–skin care, urine testing, diet, self-administration of insulin, safety measures, complications, and general information. Within each area, multiple knowledge and performance items were developed. Because of its comprehensiveness, this instrument has high content validity. It sampled items within each major area of concern in diabetes self-care. As the years pass, however, and more is learned about diabetes, diabetic patients will be expected to do more or different things for themselves. The content validity of this instrument will then decrease, and the instrument will need further development and refinement. Thus, the content validity of an instrument is time-limited: As the science base matures, a disease or risk factor–specific instrument must be updated.

Criterion Validity. There are instruments that produce highly accurate measures of a characteristic but are very costly or difficult to apply. The objective of the evaluator faced with this situation may be to develop a less costly measure. The less costly instrument can be assessed along with the more costly instrument. If the correlation between the two instruments is high, the criterion validity of the second instrument is considered high. Criterion validity may be assessed by using the two instruments at the same time (concurrent criterion validity) or by using the less costly measure at one time to predict the measures of the more costly instrument at the second time (predictive criterion validity).

The assessment of salt in the diet provides an interesting example. Because mounting evidence shows that salt intake is related to high blood pressure, many health education programs are interested in instruments to measure habitual salt intake. A relatively accurate measure (not subject to self-report errors and biases) is an assessment of the sodium excreted in the urine. Given the high day-to-day variability in an individual's consumption of salt and the lag time between episodes of unusually high salt ingestion and the body's achievement of sodium balance, Liu et al. (1979) estimate that an evaluator needs 7 consecutive days of 24-hour urine samples to estimate a person's habitual salt consumption. Many difficulties arise in obtaining such samples. People do not want to carry urine sample bottles to work, play, or other activities because it is embarrassing and inconvenient. People may forget to provide every sample, for a variety of reasons. It is costly to furnish the many containers necessary to collect so much urine, not allow it to become contaminated, and pick it up at intervals. Studies have been conducted to assess whether an overnight urine sample, testing for both sodium and creatinine, can obtain similar information and replace the tedious and expensive 24-hour urine samples. Other investigators have used self-report measures of dietary consumption. In both cases, however, the 7 consecutive days of 24-hour urine samples provided the criterion against which the other measures are assessed because it is the more accurate measure of the variable desired.

Construct Validity. As knowledge of a variety of phenomena increases, investigators learn more about how particular measures should relate to other measures. In part these relationships come to define the underlying construct. For example, people who are experiencing a high degree of anxiety are expected to experience a wide variety of physiological responses (e.g., more rapid heartbeat and breathing, higher blood pressure, changed galvanic skin response) and are expected to be less efficient at certain cognitive tasks (e.g., memory, judgment). If an investigator believes that the existing measures of anxiety are inadequate because they are highly related to some other variable that is not related to anxiety, she or he might decide to develop and test the construct validity of a new instrument. The investigator would expect two things. First, the new measure should correlate more highly with the physiological and cognitive performance changes (convergent validity) than the old measure. Second, it should correlate less well with the variable that is not related to anxiety (discriminant validity) than the old measure. If the new instrument demonstrates such convergent and discriminant validity, it is considered to have higher construct validity than the old measure. Such a demonstration indicates a greatly increased capacity to define and measure an important construct. If the new instrument, however, costs considerably more to use than the original measure, it may not be used frequently unless an evaluator needs to avoid the newly identified sources of error.

Relationships Between Validity and Reliability

Validity is often considered to be a more important issue than reliability. If an instrument does not measure what the evaluators think it is measuring, it hardly matters that the measurement is reliable. Reliability, on the other hand, is much easier to assess. Formulas exist for measuring various aspects of reliability. The procedures for using an instrument at two times are relatively straightforward. Furthermore, reliability sets an upper bound to validity. Thus, if r_R^2 is the reliability coefficient for a measure of a particular variable (e.g., dietary sodium) and r_V^2 is the reliability of a criterion variable (e.g., urinary sodium), the correlation (r_{RV}) between the measure and the criterion has the following limit:

$$|r_{RV}| \leq \sqrt{r_R^2} \sqrt{r_V^2}$$

(Schlundt, 1988). This makes sense. If a measure cannot be consistently reproduced from one occasion to the next, it cannot accurately measure some underlying construct. Developers and users of instruments must be concerned about both validity and reliability. A means for estimating reliability should be employed every time an instrument is used. Tests of validity should be used prior to an investigation, to confirm that the instrument is measuring the desired variable in the selected sample of participants.

Validity: Bias To Measurement

What factors might introduce bias into data-collection procedures? There are many potential sources of bias. Some authors have tried to catalog these to help develop ways of avoiding them. Webb et al. (1966) identified 12 common biases in human measurements:

1. *Guinea pig effect—awareness of being tested:* People who are aware that they are being measured may respond in uncharacteristic ways. Some experience heightened anxiety and perform a variety of otherwise irrational acts. Others become defensive and distort their behavior or reports of behavior in other ways. In some cases, the awareness of being measured is difficult to detect because the effects are so subtle. A bias will occur if awareness of being measured induces a large number of people to report answers that deviate systematically in one way or another from the responses they would have given if they were not aware they were being studied. The guinea pig effect is the basis on which instruments are divided into *obtrusive* and *unobtrusive* categories. These categories are discussed in Chapter 7. The guinea pig effect also leads to many of the following biases.

2. *Role selection:* The awareness of being measured may influence people to feel that they have to play a special role. They ask "What is expected of me in this situation?" and act accordingly. Others, angry at being measured, react by not conforming to what is expected of them and even displaying the opposite behavior. Sometimes this is called "impression management," that is, the person is managing the impression she or he wants to present to the interviewer or data collector.

3. *Measurement as a change agent:* The act of taking a measurement may affect the subsequent behavior of those being measured. For example, merely keeping track of what a person eats on a daily basis may affect what she or he eats during the record-keeping period. People who are keeping track of their intake of high-salt foods and who know that salt may have deleterious effects on their health will begin to lower their consumption of these foods for at least a short period. This may happen because the measurement instrument informs them of the many sources of salt in their diet, focuses their attention more clearly on their eating behaviors, or makes it obvious that they consume vast quantities of these foods, which they now believe they should not. The reduction in consumption is an obvious bias from the subjects' habitual, premeasurement eating.

4. *Response sets:* Several investigators have shown that people respond to questionnaires, and even interviews, in predictable ways that have little or nothing to do with the questions posed. One such response set is *yea-saying:* People are more likely to say yes than say no to any particular question in any instrument. Another response set is *social desirability:* People tend to answer a question the way they think the interviewer or tester wants the question answered, rather than according to their true feelings or thoughts about the issues. These response sets are not usually conscious strategies to distort responses; they work at a subtler level.

5. *Interviewer effects:* Characteristics of the interviewer may affect the receptivity and answers of the respondent. For example, a male interviewer may have difficulty obtaining accurate sexual information from female subjects. Interviewers of a lower socioeconomic status may elicit snide or uncharitable reactions from higher-status respondents and vice versa. You can imagine many characteristics of an interviewer that might bias responses.

6. *Changes in the research instrument:* Any time an instrument is used more than once, a learning effect is possible. Interviewers may become more proficient at implementing an interview schedule the longer they use it. They may ask more probing and sensitive questions in later interviews than in earlier ones. Or, at some point, they may get bored and ask less probing and sensitive questions. Similarly, if a respondent answers the same set of questions at different times, the later answers may be deeper and richer because the questions have greater depth of meaning from repetition, or the later answers may become more shallow and mundane because of respondent boredom.

7. *Population restrictions:* The method of data collection may impose

restrictions on the populations to which the results can be generalized. For example, telephone interviewing requires the respondent to have a telephone. Although most people have telephones, those who do not, those with new unrecorded telephone numbers, and those with unlisted numbers may be different in some characteristic from people with current telephone numbers in the public directory. Thus, estimates of this characteristic of the total population would be biased in a telephone survey because the method does not reach the total population. Other ways of collecting data may impose similar kinds of restrictions.

8. *Population stability over time:* An instrument administered at different times may be collecting the same data on differing populations. In a hypertension control project in one rural community, three random sample surveys were conducted at yearly intervals to document the impact of the program on the community. Between the second and third interviews, however, three of the five coal-mining companies in the area closed, due to difficult economic circumstances. The younger miners who lost their jobs were geographically displaced. Fewer younger miners were therefore included in the third random sample survey. These were exactly the people least likely to comply with their hypertension medication regimens and on whom the greatest amount of information was desired. Besides this sampling bias, the loss of health insurance coverage by unemployed miners may have sensitized those remaining in the area to health care issues, probably making them value the hypertension control program more and thereby biasing their responses.

9. *Population stability over areas:* The same way of collecting data in two different geographic areas may tap different kinds of people. For example, users of small clinics in rural Appalachia are different in many ways from users of small clinics in inner cities. Users of one rural clinic may be very different from users of another rural clinic in demographic, ethnic, social class, and other characteristics. Comparisons of data on clinic users in differing areas are very difficult to interpret because of these many possible biases.

10. *Restrictions on content:* Only a limited range of data can be reported by each method. Self-report questionnaires, for example, cannot be used to study the cognitive mechanisms of moving information from short-term to long-term memory. Observational data cannot be used to study relationships among a person's values. Each data-collection method has a restricted range of data

to which it can be applied. Using observational data to infer values will probably introduce several biases because of the assumptions observers make about the meaning of the observed behaviors.

11. *Stability of content over time:* If a program restricts a study to naturally occurring behavior, the content of the studied phenomenon may differ over time. For example, a study looking at the impact of health-related messages on television may find that the sophistication of these messages changes significantly over time or that certain events with higher priority (e.g., a government scandal, an assassination) force health programs off the airwaves. The content is thus not stable over time. If investigators do not take these differences in both frequency and content into account in their analyses, their estimates of the effects of exposure to health messages will probably be biased.

12. *Stability of content over an area:* A program may not be uniform in content throughout the area in which it is applied. The study of the effects of televised health messages on children's behaviors is a good example. The content and sophistication of a television message will vary in differing areas of the country, depending on what the producers perceive to be the most effective appeals to regional audiences. Comparisons across areas therefore have to take content differences into account in making inferences, or the inferences will be biased.

Any evaluation in which data are collected is subject to some forms of bias. Although controlling all sources of bias is impossible, minimizing each major source in a particular evaluation is important. From experience, you must take steps to select an instrument and method of data collection that minimize the likely biases. Other issues in selecting methods and instruments are discussed next.

CRITERIA FOR SELECTING A DATA-COLLECTION METHOD

Each instrument is based on a particular method for collecting data (e.g., interviewing, self-recording, observing, taking data from medical records). How do you select an instrument and, by inference, a method for data collection?

Thirteen issues to consider in selecting a measurement instrument and method have been propounded (Baranowski and Simons-Morton, 1991) (Table 6.2). The primary concern in selecting an instrument and method is for high reliability and validity from previous experience, especially for the groups, situations, and purposes of

Table 6.2   Specification of Issues in Selecting a Measurement Method Technique

Issues	Validity	Reliability

Prior assessment	Do previous studies or other data document that this technique:
	  Appears to measure what it purports to measure (face validity)?
	  Taps all the areas of concern (content validity)?
	  Satisfactorily predicts some "gold standard" (criterion) measure of the same variable (criterion or predictive validity)?
	  Is related to other variables in theoretically predicted ways (construct validity)?
		Do previous studies or other data document that this technique:
		  Has items that positively intercorrelate (internal consistency)?
		  Obtains similar values when administered twice in a short time period (test–retest reliability)?
		  Obtains similar values when administered twice over a longer period of time (stability)?
		  Has two or more different forms that correlate highly when administered to the same people (identity)?
		  Obtains similar values when administered by two different interviewers or observers (interrater or inter-observer reliability)?

Precision Level of detail	Does the technique obtain data in sufficient detail to specify the variable desired, such as an activity frequency will not specify energy expenditure?	Is the level of detail desired too refined given the capabilities of the collecting instrument, such as can most people recall precisely their moderate activities for the seventh day earlier?
Habitual behavior	Does the technique take into account variation by season, weekends, sick days, and holidays?	Does the technique allow for the collecting of information across sufficient repeated time periods to provide a reliable estimate of usual behavior?
Reactivity	Does the method of collecting the data affect the variable of interest, such as does having an observer present predispose the child to be more (or less) active?	
Change	Does the technique obtain data in sufficient detail to detect the level of change (from pre- to posttest) that is likely to occur in the program assessed?	How many assessments must be conducted at pre- and at posttest to detect the expected changes?
Appropriateness Developmental	Does the technique require skills or other cognitive abilities the participant is not likely to have, such as a young child's ability to estimate minutes, and if so, who can provide accurate proxy information?	Are the questions and response categories phrased and depicted in a manner appropriate to the age of the child, such as sad and happy faces for response categories for young children?

Ethnic	Does the technique include foods or activities common in a particular ethnic group, such as sausage in eastern European groups?	Are the questions and response categories phrased to respect the sensitivities of a particular ethnic group?
Regional	Does the technique include foods or activities common to a region or to all regions in a study, such as ice hockey in New England?	Are the questions and response categories sensitive to a region's usual expressions, such as "pop" instead of "soda" in parts of the South vs. the Northeast?
Implementation Procedures	Does the technique work in a manner that is theoretically sound or otherwise reasonable to collect the data of interest, such as can mothers (proxies) not at home with their very young children be expected to provide accurate reports of their children's diet?	Is there a clear and detailed protocol for collecting the data, including procedures for training the collectors, and for ensuring and assessing the quality control of the process?
Conversions	If the variables obtained need to be converted to other variables of interest, such as converting foods to nutrient consumption, is there evidence that the conversion procedure accurately produces the desired variables?	Is there a clear and detailed protocol that specifies any additional information (such as per-activity MET values) and the procedures for making the conversion?
Respondent burden	Does the method take so much of the participant's time, effort, or money that people are discouraged to participate or they systematically distort their responses, such as they provide very short answers to more quickly finish?	Does the method take so much of the participant's time, effort, or money that random error is increased, such as from fatigue?
Staff burden	Does the method take so much time or effort that staff systematically distort the procedures (intentionally or unintentionally), such as record simple synopses rather than detailed transcripts? Does the method take so much time or effort that random error is introduced by staff, such as from fatigue?	
Cost Financial	Which method provides the highest validity and reliability at a per-case cost a specific project can afford?	

SOURCE: Baranowski and Simons-Morton (1991): 195–197.

your study. Instruments without validity and reliability can produce nonfindings or even negative findings that are not warranted. Many of the other issues in selecting a method are also related to validity and reliability.

You must consider the *precision* of the instrument and method. The *level of detail* of an instrument may not be sufficient to provide the variable needed. For example, if an evaluation needs to make fine distinctions in the level of nutrients consumed, a food-frequency questionnaire may not provide sufficient detail to make that distinction. Alternatively, a measurement instrument or method (e.g., a 7-day food diary) may require a level of detail that is beyond the capability of some respondents to provide (e.g., children).

In most cases, when measuring behavior, we want to measure *habitual behavior,* that is, what people ordinarily do on a day-to-day basis. Just measuring behavior for 3 or 4 consecutive days (as is common in food or activity diaries) may miss differences in usual behavior on weekends, holidays, sick days, or season (validity issues). Recent research has shown very high levels of day-to-day variability in behavior (e.g., DuRant et al., 1992), which requires that many days be assessed (reproducibility) to get an accurate estimate of that habitual behavior.

As discussed under bias, the method of collecting data may be *reactive,* that is, induce behavior or other changes just from collecting the data. The reactivity of an instrument will likely vary by the population assessed and the situation in which the assessment occurs. The method should be selected to minimize reactivity for the population and settings to be studied.

Just because an instrument has been shown to have validity and reliability in cross-sectional research does not mean that it can detect change over time in the underlying variable (Guydatt et al., 1987). This inability will usually be due to the level of changes expected being smaller than the units meaningfully obtained by the instrument. For example, weight loss may be achieved by a consistent reduction of as little as 50 kilocalories (kcal) of consumption per day. Our methods of dietary assessment, however, are probably not precise enough to detect changes of 50 kcal. In a similar vein, a weight loss of 7 ounces may go undetected by a digital scale that reports in pounds. This is a particular problem in behavior-change programs. In selecting an instrument, a key consideration should be that it has detected change under comparable conditions.

Instruments and methods may be appropriate or inappropriate for particular populations and settings. There are considerations of developmental appropriateness. That is, are the instrument and method appropriate to the cognitive and other abilities of respondents? What can be asked of normal adults may not be developmentally appropriate for children or the mentally impaired. Examples of ethnic and regional appropriateness could include whether a food-frequency technique includes foods common in a particular ethnic group or region of the country (e.g., greens in the South) and worded in a way understandable in that ethnic group or region (e.g., "turnips" in parts of Georgia means "turnip greens").

There are many issues in the implementation of an instrument and method. The procedures for a method should be clearly and explicitly detailed in a protocol that can be reviewed to assess their appropriateness for a particular population. The protocol should include a detailed presentation of conversions that need to be made on the data obtained (e.g., from foods to nutrients consumed). The instrument and method may place undue burden on the respondent (e.g., participants may fall asleep during lengthy interviews or otherwise lose interest and provide meaningless responses just to hurry the interview along). The instrument and method may place undue burden on the staff, which also may result in error.

A common problem is cost. Cost has several characteristics: (1) dollar cost, (2) time spent by the evaluation staff, (3) time spent by respondents, (4) ease of setting up instruments, (5) difficulty of getting individuals to participate, (6) loss of accuracy due to increased work load, and (7) availability and quality of official statistics.

Imagine an instrument that measures exactly what you want; however, all instruments cost money, and some may be too costly. (Think of sending observers to record clients' behaviors all day, every day.) Some approaches may not be feasible. (Think of supplying a personal computer for daily self-monitoring of some behavior to everyone in a health education program.) Some approaches may produce other problems. (Think of how hostile clients can become if they have to complete 1 hour of paperwork every day for a month.) The key to selecting good measures is to choose a set sufficiently valid and reliable for your study's purposes, yet developed at minimal cost to the project and to the respondents.

An important aspect of economy is collecting no more data than are necessary to achieve the purposes of the particular study. Some investigators developed a 124-page questionnaire requiring 3 hours to complete. This strategy created many problems. The program must bear tremendous costs in time, printing, collating, keypunching, and data processing. Respondents must bear considerable costs in completing the questionnaire. They may become hostile to such a questionnaire and refuse to participate at all, select only questions of personal interest to answer, or actively subvert the data collected. Many may decide not to complete the interview. It is a common finding that investigators collect more data than they can reasonably analyze; the parties incur the costs of collection, but because of report deadlines nothing is ever done with the data. All of these reasons argue for the greatest economy in selecting measures.

The more valid and reliable instruments and methods usually incur more financial and staff costs to the investigator and time costs to the respondents. Sometimes an investigator must simply select the most valid and reliable instrument and method for the amount of money available and accept the resulting errors and problems. In some cases, an evaluation should not be done if resources are not available for instruments and methods that meet minimum criteria for a particular project.

Other criteria or issues in the selection of variables and measures have been identified: the nature and purpose of the study, sequential modifiability of the design, and comparison with other studies (Cox and Snell, 1979); hardness of data (Feinstein, 1977); dross rate; and ability to replicate (Webb et al., 1966).

Nature and Purpose of the Study

A data-collection method must be selected that most clearly meets the nature and purposes of a study, within resources and constraints. An evaluative study can be conducted for a variety of purposes. For a smoking-cessation program (a service production system like that depicted in Figure 6.4), you might conduct an evaluation to assess the output (stopped smoking or not), the acceptance of the output by the environment (social support for continued nonsmoking), the availability of resources in the environment (number of smokers willing to pay for a smoking-cessation program), the quality of the resources, the appropriateness of the structure (is the program well designed), whether the processes are occurring as planned (is the program being conducted according to the design), or whether the processes are related to outputs (are people who attend more sessions more likely to quit). Each topic can be the focus for an evaluation in a particular program. The type of question posed by the evaluator should determine the data-collection method. This criterion for method selection is similar to our strong emphasis on the role of a model in conducting an evaluation, but here we focus on one specific aspect of the evaluation.

Sequential Modifiability of the Design

An important aspect of instrument and method selection is whether a preliminary study can be performed to select and develop measures. As noted earlier, a variety of instruments might be used for any particular variable. If you have the time and resources to conduct a preliminary study, make multiple measures of the same variable in your study. Some thought must go into developing criteria for the selection of the appropriate measures, for example, greater reliability or higher correlations with other variables of interest. If you cannot make a preliminary study, pay greater attention to selecting the instrument and method without the benefit of pretesting. The two primary issues are validity and reliability of the instrument and method for the population you are studying.

Comparisons with Other Studies

In some cases, you may want to compare the results obtained with evaluations done elsewhere or at another time. If so, assess the same variables with the same instruments (questions); otherwise, comparisons cannot be made. If a particular measure has a major flaw, include both the original measure (so comparisons can be made) and an alternative measure, to see if a different pattern is obtained with the new measure.

Hardness of Data

Another important criterion in selecting measures is the hardness of data. There is a feeling among investigators that certain kinds of data are "harder" than others (which are called "soft") and therefore more important to collect. According to Feinstein (1977), the following characteristics are typically associated with data hardness: (1) The data are obtained objectively (e.g., physiological measures) rather than subjectively (e.g., self-reports); (2) the primary data can be preserved for repeated analyses (e.g., a videotape of an encounter, which can be reobserved and checked); (3) the measurement is on a dimensional scale (i.e., a ratio or interval scale).

Feinstein, however, debunks many of these ideas. For example, physiological measures can be highly unreliable. There may be rapid changes in the values of the physiological measure, the variable may not be clearly and precisely related to the phenomenon of concern, or there may be problems of mechanical determination of the physiological values by the laboratory. [In some cases, you may have not collected a sufficient amount of a sample (fluid), or you may have stored it improperly or for too long to perform an accurate test.] Certain variables (e.g., eye contacts) may be very difficult to quantify from a videotape because they are not precisely specified or because they require too much judgment and interpretation on the part of the observer. A ratio or an interval scale does not ensure reliability. Feinstein argues that the criterion of primary concern in hardness is reliability; he also shows how a wide variety of ostensibly soft measures can provide useful and reliable data in clinical trials. His admonition is to collect all variables that are directly relevant to the concerns of a project, regardless of hardness, while paying particular attention to the reliability of data collection.

Dross Rate

The dross rate is the ratio of useless-to-useful information obtained by a particular method for a unit of time. Methods with a high dross rate are obviously inefficient approaches to collecting data. If a program is interested in behavior that does not occur frequently or with some regularity, the amount of useful data obtained per unit of data-collection time can vary widely. For example, an observational study of total eating behavior is inefficient to perform because subjects may snack at many times during the day. Some may have small meals and eat candy bars or potato chips at work or at school. Thus, observers would have to follow subjects for a whole day to be there when eating occurred, but only a small percentage of the full day would be spent on observing eating behavior. A questionnaire is a more efficient approach. In 15 or 20 minutes of directed questioning, an entire day's eating behavior can be assessed. But can subjects accurately remember everything they ate that day or the previous day? The observational approach obtains more dross per unit of data-collection time than does the questionnaire or interview, but it may be a more valid instrument, depending on the issue of concern.

Ability to Replicate

An investigator is able to replicate a study more easily using certain methods than others. For example, a structured questionnaire can be used and reused at multiple times with differing groups. A review of medical records before and after a particular event (e.g., a continuing education course) may not be replicable at a later time period because the medical records will differ due to historical factors.

STEPS TO DEVELOP A MULTI-ITEM SCALE

The primary emphasis in this chapter has been presenting issues in selecting an existing instrument to measure some variable or construct. Given the amount of effort, thought, and time necessary to adequately develop an instrument and the risky nature of such development (i.e., what you develop may not work the way you want), your best bet is to select an existing measure. By doing so, you capitalize on all the resources someone else has brought to bear on the task, usually including considerable expertise in the related content area.

There are times, however, when existing instruments don't measure what you need to have measured. To develop a new multiitem scale, you must go through the following steps. Given the large number of pitfalls and complexities in doing so, start these steps only after you're convinced that no existing scale meets your needs.

Step 1: Select the Conceptual Model

Be sure that you have an agreement with the evaluation committee (policy, management, service, and advocacy domains) about what theory or model provides the foundation for the project. This model will specify the variables to be collected and provide the understanding about how these variables or concepts are supposed to work. Agreeing to the model as the first step will minimize definition and specification conflicts in the future.

Step 2: Become Familiar with the Related Literature

Read as extensively as possible theoretical, basic, and applied research articles related to the model selected or propounded. These articles should give you a clearer idea of what these variables are and how they are supposed to be working. Part of this survey should be a review of copies of questionnaires to see how others have put related ideas into operation. Authors will usually send you copies of their questionnaires, when requested.

Step 3: Obtain Descriptive Information from the Target Population

Theoretical ideas need to be put in language meaningful to a local population. Data must be collected on the many ways in which a theoretical concept can be interpreted in a particular group. This is usually done by means of focus group discussions or in-depth interviews. For example, some evaluators may be interested in the outcome expectancies associated with some behavior, that is, the pros and cons that result from performing a specific behavior. To put into operation a measure of outcome expectancies for a particular population, you must meet with representative people and identify what they believe happens from performing the behavior of interest and whether what happens is good or bad for them. (Don't assume that because you think an outcome is good, they do too.) Most often, many pros and cons are identified. You must then select the most important of these expectancies for inclusion in the instrument. Sometimes it is difficult to translate the theoretical idea into words easily understood by the target population, thereby inhibiting your ability to elicit meaningful concrete examples of the idea. How this translation should be done should be well thought-out in advance. In focus groups, having a backup group leader who is attentive to possible differences in meaning between the primary leader and the group may help.

Step 4: Generate Candidate Items

To encompass the many different aspects of the underlying concept, generate a broad variety of items. Systematically identify aspects of the underlying concept and generate items to encompass each aspect. It is valuable to initially generate at least 20 to 30 items per construct put into operation. The transcripts of the focus groups and/or intensive interviews are a primary source for individual items. The systematic approach to generating items enhances content validity.

Step 5: Evaluate the Items

Several criteria are often used to evaluate the items, including the following:

A statement that is clearly related to the construct being put into operation

Inclusion of only one simple idea per item

No double negatives

Fifth grade reading level (no big words, simple declarative statements)

Half the items stated positively and half the items stated negatively (to avoid yea-saying bias)

Because different people can read different things into the same item, a group should be used to evaluate the items. This group should include people familiar with the theoretical framework (experts) and those familiar with the target population. When major problems are identified, the item should be discarded. (This is why you need to start with a large number of items.) Modifications can be made in items that have only minor problems. This step enhances the face and content validity of the items.

Step 6: Draft an Instrument

A good instrument will have a detailed protocol with several components:

Instructions to the data collector(s) including any procedures for checking or assuring reliability

Instructions to the person completing the items

Items with response options

A manual for converting responses to variables and how to handle missing information or other problems likely to arise

A training program for data collectors

Each component must be carefully constructed. It is at this point that you must anticipate the many types of bias. Consider the criteria for selecting an instrument and generate an instrument that minimizes bias and maximizes validity and reliability.

Step 7: Pretest the Instrument

Although the people generating and evaluating items may believe the items are clear and simple, respondents may not. In an interview format, it is necessary to pretest the complete instrument for

Respondent understanding of the instructions and items.

Possible offensiveness of the items.

Completeness of the group of items.

This pretesting interview is often done by

Administering the full instrument.

Going back to the instructions and each item and asking respondents to interpret in their own words, what each instruction and item meant to them and whether any were offensive (e.g., sexist, racist, ageist).

Asking whether there were related ideas triggered by those items that were not included (i.e., identifying other, possibly better, items).

Items are often deleted and/or modified as a result of this interview to improve them and instructions are often changed.

Step 8: Conduct a Validity–Reliability Study

Data need to be collected on a sample of people representative of the target population. The sample should be a large enough sample to reflect the number of items to be collected and to conduct all the necessary statistical procedures. This study should include the following:

The instrument just developed.

Other instruments that conceptually should be related to the variable in operation

Any checks on particular items (e.g., have an observer check on whether this person did the behavior in a high-likelihood location)

It would be best if at least the newly created instrument were collected on all participants twice in order to estimate test–retest reliability.

The following kinds of tests would ordinarily be conducted with this data:

Internal consistency: Cronbach's alpha on the items in the scale, at both times

Factor analysis: to determine whether all items load on one scale or multiple scales, at both times

Test–retest reliability: correlations between the scales at the two administrations

Construct validity: to determine whether the operationalized variable(s) from the new instrument correlate in the expected directions with variables from the other instruments, or with the checks

Step 9: Review, Revise, and Reassess

This preliminary validity–reliability test may reveal a variety of problems. Based on the findings, the evaluator may want to revise, delete, and add items; revise the instrument; or change the nature of the concept being measured. If any substantial changes are introduced, repeat step 8 because even relatively minor rewordings of items can change the psychometric properties.

Sometimes an evaluator finds an instrument that is close to what is wanted but not exactly right. The temptation is to directly modify the existing instrument and assume it will work as desired. Unfortunately, instruments can function very differently, even after only minor changes in wording. Anytime an instrument is modified or an instrument will be used with a population not previously studied with the instrument, implement all the steps from step 7 onward.

This is a very brief overview of these steps. Evaluators should consult full texts for a more detailed presentation. Useful texts include

Biemer, P. B., R. M. Groves, L. E. Lyberg, N. A. Martinowitz, and S. Sudman. *Measurement Errors in Surveys*. New York: Wiley, 1991.

Bradburn, N. M., and S. Sudman. *Improving Interview Method and Questionnaire Design*. San Francisco: Jossey-Bass, 1980.

DeVellis, R. F. *Scale Development, Theory and Applications*. Newbury Park, Calif.: Sage, 1991.

Nam, C. B., and M. G. Powers. *The Socioeconomic Approach to Status Measurement*. Houston: Cap and Gown, 1983.

Osterlind, S. J. *Constructing Test Items*. Boston: Kluwer, 1989.

Sudman, S., and N. M. Bradburn. *Asking Questions, A Practical Guide to Questionnaire Design*. San Francisco: Jossey-Bass, 1982.

Tryon, W. W. (ed.). *Behavioral Assessment in Behavioral Medicine*. New York: Springer, 1985.

SUMMARY

Health program evaluators should have a conceptual model underlying the evaluative study they are planning. Instruments should be selected to measure the variables in the model. The instruments selected need to be valid and reliable measures of the variables of concern, must have the precision necessary for a particular purpose, be appropriate to the studied population, and must have a protocol that can be thoroughly reviewed. They should not place excessive demands on the participants or the staff. They should be as inexpensive as possible, permit comparisons with important related evaluations, have as small a dross rate as possible, permit the collection of descriptive data, and be replicable. The various threats to the validity of a particular instrument and method should be anticipated. Steps must be taken to counter the threats that are preventable. This is a tall order and requires much effort, but it is not an insurmountable job.

The instruments for measuring the desired variables use many kinds of methods. A broad spectrum of the more commonly used methods are discussed in Chapter 7, in light of the considerations presented here for instrument selection.

7

Data-Collection Methods

"Physiological measures are always more accurate than are social and behavioral measures."

"If I could only get access to that doctor's records, think of all the evaluations I could do."

"Let's just jot down some questions and send them around for people to answer."

"Let's just talk to the next twenty people who come through the door."

"It won't take much time!"

Professional Competencies Emphasized in This Chapter

• Providing mechanisms to assess selected educational methods

• Assisting in specifying indicators of program success

• Helping develop methods for evaluating programs

• Participating in the specification of instruments for data collection

• Training personnel for evaluation, as needed

• Collecting data through appropriate techniques

• Using survey techniques to acquire data

• Evaluating results of the skill development process

Should the health promotion/health education program evaluator use self-reported statements of numbers of cigarettes smoked, observations of actual smoking behavior in certain settings, or physiological indicators of recent smoking behavior, to assess whether a smoking-cessation program worked? Which would be best for a smoking-prevention program in a junior high school? Should you use self-reported frequencies of high-salt food consumption, a 24-hour dietary history obtained by interview, observations of consumption of all foods, or overnight urine sodium tests, to determine dietary sodium restriction among hypertensive patients?

These are the kinds of decisions with which evaluators of health promotion and education programs constantly struggle. Because rights and wrongs are rarely clear-cut, you must become familiar with a broad variety of methods and select the best of good methods or the least bad of unpalatable approaches. In becoming familiar with the strengths and weaknesses of many methods, you should develop skills identified by the Role Delineation Project (U.S. Department of Health and Human Services, 1980a) in four areas, as shown in Table 7.1.

TOTAL QUALITY CONTROL IN DATA COLLECTION

In this chapter, we promote the skills listed in Table 7.1 by taking each method of data collection, identifying its strengths and weaknesses

Table 7.1   Health Promotion and Education Program Evaluator Skills

Assessing and selecting methods	Providing mechanisms to assess selected educational methods Assisting in specifying indicators of program success
Developing methods for a specific evaluation	Helping develop methods for evaluating programs Participating in the specification of instruments for data collection
Training of those employing the instruments	Training personnel for evaluation as needed
Using a variety of methods	Collecting data through appropriate techniques Using survey techniques to acquire data Evaluating results of the skill development process

SOURCE: Adapted from U.S. Department of Health and Human Services (1980a).

(biases), considering the other issues in methods selection, and outlining straightforward steps for developing an instrument and implementing the method. You want the best possible information, that is, the most valid and reliable possible under the circumstances and with available finances. This is called a *total quality control* approach to data collection. There are many facets to collecting quality data. Many problems in data collection were identified in Chapter 6. In total quality control, you must anticipate these possible sources of problems, select the best methods for a particular evaluation, monitor the data-collection quality throughout, and actively work to avoid or minimize the many problems before or as they occur. In this light, you collect the best possible information under the circumstances. No evaluation is perfect, but some are much better than others. An evaluator will become known to colleagues and peers for the care and attention to detail in the methods for collecting information to evaluate programs. The various methods are considered within two categories: obtrusive and unobtrusive methods. First, however, we must emphasize the importance of sampling.

SAMPLING

In Chapter 5, we introduced methods for estimating the sample size needed to make the desired inferences; we also discussed the salience of selection bias. Here we briefly discuss how to obtain that sample. A major assumption in doing any statistical tests of hypotheses or of relationships is that one is doing the test to infer to some population.

That is, one conducts the tests on a sample with the intent to test whether the mean or a relationship in the sample is true of some population. If you are collecting data on the whole population of interest (e.g., the population of all residents of Hephzibah, a small town in eastern Georgia), then there is no need to do statistical tests because anything found about that population would be true of that population. However, whether means in that population or relationships detected in that population are true of some larger population (e.g., the residents of the state of Georgia) could not be determined from studying Hephzibah alone. If one wants to generalize to all children, but only 3-year-old boys are in the sample, then it is difficult to generalize to any girls or to boys other than 3 year olds. The sample of 3-year-old boys (when intending to generalize to all children) is called *biased*, that is, it is not representative of all units to which you want to generalize. Similarly if you want to generalize to all participants in your program but sampled only families with two parents, you couldn't say much about single-parent families.

A sample must be selected with some random component to generalize to a population. There are many types of sampling techniques with random components (e.g., simple random, clustered, stratified) (Kish, 1965; Sudman 1976). The randomness minimizes the likelihood that a systematic source of selection bias will occur among the sample, thereby influencing the degree of representativeness of the population. Simply doing random sampling does not ensure the sample representativeness, but not selecting randomly makes it likely that the sample is not representative. Thus, after a sample has been selected and data collected, you should check to assess the extent to which your sample is representative. Comparing it to variables known about the population (e.g., gender, ethnicity, age from census data) and that can be collected on the sample.

A sample needs to be representative of the population-at-risk to which inferences are to be made. Selecting the next 50 participants in a program (sometimes called quota sampling) may not be representative of all participants. If you could be sure that the entry of any person into a service facility was a completely random event, then quota sampling might be appropriate. Alternatively, the next 50 participants may all be obtained on a Saturday. People who come on Saturday may be different from those who come during the week (e.g., people coming on a Saturday may more likely have full-time jobs). Clients coming in during the week are less likely to have full-time jobs. If employment affects the variables of interest in the evaluation, this could be a serious selection bias in the sample and provide substantially misleading results.

Evaluators are often faced with obtaining data from record systems (e.g., death records, clinic records). A systematic sampling technique is often used in selecting cases from records. In systematic sampling, divide the population (e.g., 20,000 cases) by the sample size needed (e.g., 100), which results in a sampling interval (e.g., 200). If you select very two hundredth record, 100 cases will be systematically obtained. A random component is entered by selecting a random start, that is, randomly selecting a number between 1 and 200 and starting with that case. Thus, if 37 were the randomly selected start, the sample would consist of cases numbered 37, 237, 437, . . . 19,837. A major strength of systematic sampling is ease of implementation. If the sequence of cases is random (e.g., in alphabetical order), then systematic sampling will be an unbiased sampling method. The sequence, however, may not be random (e.g., clinic visits and birth records, which are organized by calendar days), or there may be periodic repeat missing data. In these cases, the interval in sampling (every two hundredth case) may always get a weekday (instead of a representative sample of weekdays and weekend days) or may more likely get cases with missing data. This could bias the sample and render the results uninterpretable. Given the general availability of computers, you should randomly generate sequence numbers when possible, using a computer program to select cases from files, to ensure that no sequencing bias exists in the data.

Developing the sampling procedures for an evaluation is an important step, both to minimize sample bias and to clearly define the population for which measures need to be selected or developed. In developing the sampling procedures, you must specify both the inclusionary characteristics (i.e., characteristics of people to be included; e.g., participants in the program to be evaluated) and exclusionary characteristics (i.e., characteristics of people used to keep them out of the sample; e.g., a disability that impairs their ability to communicate with the evaluator). These inclusionary and exclusionary characteristics define the population to which a certain set of data and findings can be generalized. In developing a sampling procedure, consult any of a variety of texts on sampling (Aday, 1991; Kish, 1965; Sudman, 1976). Consulting a biostatistician may be necessary. With the sample defined, the evaluation can proceed to the consideration of selecting or developing measures.

OBTRUSIVE MEASURES

The term *obtrusive* implies that the person being studied is aware of being measured, assessed, or tested. Methods usually included in the obtrusive category are self-report questionnaires, interviews, and direct observations of behavior. The term *unobtrusive* implies that an individual is not aware of being studied. The methods usually included in the unobtrusive category are record abstractions, physiological measures, and behavior trace methods. Behavior trace methods include such things as measuring the thickness or changes of a shoe sole, to assess how much walking a person has done. Because many of the behavior trace methods require much greater development and validation for general use, they are not further considered in this chapter. Unobtrusive measures are valued because they are supposed to produce less random error and bias because subjects are not aware of being measured. The differences between obtrusive and unobtrusive methods, however, are not always so clear-cut. For example, a skillfully designed questionnaire may ask validly tangential questions that do not tip off program participants about which aspect of their behavior is of concern. Alternatively, if workers in an agency learn that they are continually being evaluated using the agency records they regularly complete, their record-completion behavior may drastically change to protect themselves. Obtrusive and unobtrusive are therefore general categories of methods. Evaluators must be constantly concerned about the obtrusiveness of all measures and what effect this may have on the results.

Obtrusive measures raise validity and reliability questions. Becoming aware of being studied can affect a person's behavior and thought processes. It may influence the person to respond to questions in a way that enables the person to manage and even to tailor the impression made by the responses. For example, the grateful recipient of a program's services may say things to emphasize continued need for the program services and deemphasize things that indicate the services are no longer needed.

Self-Completion Questionnaires

A self-completion (or self-report) questionnaire is an instrument that the respondent can complete by reading the questions and providing answers, without an interviewer or other person taking part. Such a questionnaire can be used with a one person or with a group.

Strengths. The self-completion questionnaire is the most convenient and frequently used method of data collection for program evaluation. It allows data to be collected from many people in a very short period of time. Almost all types of measures can be assessed by self-completion questionnaire. The costs are minimal (interviewers are not needed, printing costs are low). All people are exposed to the same instrument.

Because no interviewer is involved in asking questions, a well-designed questionnaire controls for interviewer effects, that is, differences in responses because of differences in the way in which interviewers ask the question. Moreover, the proportion of unusable data in a self-report questionnaire is low. In contrast, an interviewer may have to listen to irrelevant comments, and an observer may waste time on unproductive observations. In a questionnaire, all the questions are directed at the object of concern. Similarly, the replicability of a questionnaire is high. The same questionnaire can be used in multiple studies.

The self-completion questionnaire is particularly useful when the phenomenon studied is amenable to self-observation, well-defined answers can be elicited in simple straightforward questions, and respondents can read and write. Good references on self-completion questionnaires include Aday (1991), Berdie and Anderson (1974), Bradburn and Sudman (1979), and Barker and Blankenship (1975).

Phenomenon Amenable to Self-Observation. For some phenomena (e.g., attitudes, values, beliefs), self-report may be the only method of data collection. For others (e.g., cognitive processing of information), self-report may be appropriate but not exclusive. And for some (e.g., skill at performing particular tasks), self-report instruments are suspect because the person may not know how the tasks should be done under optimal or typical circumstances. When the object of concern is amenable to self-reflection and self-report, a self-completion questionnaire can be very useful.

Phenomenon Well Defined. When the phenomenon of concern has been studied extensively and much is known about it, a self-report questionnaire can be used. For example, extensive data exist on the many facets of smoking, so an interviewer may not be needed to probe and interrogate subjects to elicit the possible responses. Because the response possibilities are known from other research, a questionnaire can be designed to list all the response possibilities and ask respondents to select which is most descriptive of their own practice. The purpose of the questionnaire in this situation is to document which response possibility is most appropriate for this particular respondent.

Some phenomena are poorly defined (e.g., the reasons why healthy people do not engage in aerobic activity). Not much basic research has been done about these subjects, so the possible responses are not clearly outlined. Data collection about them would benefit from the active questioning of a trained interviewer to identify and document the response possibilities.

Simple, Straightforward Questions. The longer and more complex a question or the more subtle the distinctions a question requires, the more likely it is that a respondent will misinterpret it or have difficulty understanding and answering it. An interviewer may be necessary to explain either a long and complex or a subtle question or to ask further questions to ensure that the respondent understands it. A self-completed self-report questionnaire assumes that the respondent is motivated to read the questions completely, whereas an interviewer can encourage a respondent to attend to longer questions. Self-report questionnaires therefore are most valid and reliable with short, simple, and straightforward questions.

Cognitive Ability of Respondents. Although it may seem obvious, self-report questionnaires assume that respondents can read and write. A self-report questionnaire is inappropriate for the blind, the retarded, nonreaders, and people not familiar with the language. To ensure the greatest applicability, a questionnaire should be developed to be readable at a fifth or sixth grade reading level.

Validity-Enhancing Techniques. At least one technique has been reported that can enhance the validity of self-report questionnaires: the bogus pipeline (Lowe et al., 1986). In this technique, the person collecting the data informs respondents that investigators have other means of collecting accurate information (e.g., conducting a chemical analysis of some body fluid) and informs respondents that a body fluid sample will be collected for such purposes. This is called a bogus pipeline because either no such validating chemical test exists or investigators have no intention of conducting tests on the collected samples. Lowe et al. (1986) report that the bogus pipeline technique obtained a 27% report of use of alcohol among pregnant women, whereas only 14% reported use of alcohol without a bogus pipeline. Similar results have been obtained in the smoking literature, although not all reports have obtained the same results. This raises the question of under what circumstances the technique is effective. Similar methods might be tested in other behaviors (e.g., diet), and other validity-enhancing techniques should be sought. The availability of validity-enhancing techniques significantly enhances the desirability of self-report questionnaires.

Weaknesses. The self-completion questionnaire is susceptible to several biases. Respondents can easily fall into role selection when answering questionnaires because no one is present to observe, clarify, or challenge their role taking. The phenomenon of response sets was originally identified using self-completion questionnaires. Other problems are the following: (1) Telescoping may occur—events that occurred before a time interval of interest are reported as having occurred in the time interval of interest; (2) the questionnaire promotes change; (3) changes may occur in the respondents' understanding of the questionnaire; (4) limits may exist on the phenomena to which a questionnaire can be applied. Beland et al. (1991) demonstrate a consistency in response bias in which questions about attitudes toward a behavior and the behavior itself were included in the same questionnaire; the correlation between attitudes and behavior increased over the case when questions about attitudes and behaviors were used in separate questionnaires.

Although a self-completed questionnaire theoretically controls for possible interviewer effects, the person who distributes the questionnaire often answers questions about it and may give subtle or overt cues to how it should be answered. Another disadvantage is that, although a variety of validating questions can be asked, a questionnaire is limited in the use of descriptive cues. For example, a dietary interviewer may use food models or portion-size pictures to obtain data on the amount of food respondent eats. It would be costly and unwieldy to build portion-size pictures into every question of a dietary self-completion questionnaire.

Steps in Questionnaire Development. A questionnaire obtains information from a respondent through self-reported answers to a series of questions, usually using paper and pencil, although computers can also be used. Good references on questionnaire development include Aday (1991), Berdie and Anderson (1974), Bradburn and Sudman (1979), Schuman and Presser (1977), Kalton et al. (1978), Barker and Blankenship (1975), and Noelle-Neumann (1970). Four general areas in questionnaire development are discussed next: instrument selection, questionnaire development, field testing, and quality control.

Instrument Selection. Do not reinvent the wheel. When an instrument has been shown to be valid and reliable and it directly measures the variables of interest to you, using that instrument makes good sense. Many investigators have developed and applied multiple types of instruments for a variety of purposes. Using developed instruments is valuable for several reasons. First, capitalize on the thoughts of other investigators in the design of an instrument. They have spent time reviewing the literature and considering alternatives for developing an instrument. Using a developed instrument will save you time. Second, other investigators may have spent time assessing and refining the instrument to maximize its validity and reliability. Most investigators go through multiple generations of a questionnaire to increase reliability. Using their instrument will therefore ensure some level of reliability and validity of measurement in your evaluation. Third, using an existing instrument enables you to make comparisons across studies. In most cases the need for or effectiveness of a program is assessed in comparison to other areas, populations, or programs. Assuming similar populations, using measures developed for another study will allow you to make comparisons between evaluations that might not otherwise be possible. Thus, external validity of results are enhanced.

Using developed measures has been encouraged in theoretical and applied research. To facilitate this use, several authors have compiled compendia of measures used in a variety of areas: health behaviors (Reeder et al., 1976), family (Strauss and Brown, 1978), attitudes (Bonjean et al., 1967; Robinson and Shaver, 1973; Shaw and Wright, 1967), and psychodiagnostic testing (Buros, 1972). The Centers for Disease Control (CDC) has published several volumes that document instruments in seven areas of health and behavior research, which should be useful for health promotion program evaluation. (Contact the Center for Health Promotion and Chronic Disease Prevention, CDC, Atlanta, GA 30333, (404) 488-5506.)

Developed instruments, however, should not be used blindly. In a study on the effect of a family intervention to promote behaviors that reduce cardiovascular risks, evaluators used a knowledge test that had been developed for another study. This test—developed in a population of primarily white, middle-class adults—had used item-to-total correlations to assess its internal consistency (Baranowski, Evans, et al., 1980). The knowledge test was then applied to a population of primarily lower-class, black, and Mexican-American adults and children in a different area of the country. Furthermore, the knowledge test dealt with several risk factors not of concern in the second study, and the intervention in the second study showed statistically significant but educationally insignificant differences between experimental and control adults and no significant differences between children. Selecting that knowledge test was an exercise in poor judgment because of the many differences in purposes between the study for which the instrument had been developed and the second study in which it was used. The evaluators in the second study should have intensively reviewed the content for face validity and field-tested the instrument with a sample of the local population, before using it in their program evaluation.

Instrument Development and Field Testing. In some cases, instruments have not been developed for a particular topic, or existing instruments are not appropriate. Even when instruments are available,

Table 7.2   Questionnaire Instrument Development

---

1. Formulate objectives.
2. State objectives in behavioral terms.
3. Review instruments.
4. Review necessary skills.
5. Construct a preliminary draft.
6. Develop data collection–training protocols.
7. Pilot-test the questionnaire.
8. Redesign the questionnaire and protocol.
9. Retest the questionnaire.
10. Make a final redesign.

SOURCE: Windsor, Roseman, et al. (1981).

you usually have to develop some questions specific to your study. Refer to one or more texts (Berdie and Anderson, 1974; Bradburn and Sudman, 1979) and articles (e.g., Barker and Blankenship, 1975) on questionnaire development, to consider and address the essential development issues.

Windsor, Roseman, et al. (1981) propose the following ten steps (summarized in Table 7.2) in questionnaire instrument development (these steps are similar to those in creating multiitem scales, as discussed in Chapter 6):

1. *Formulate objectives.* The first consideration in generating a questionnaire is to ensure that it measures what it was intended to measure (validity). If you have consensually agreed on a model of the structures and processes underlying your program, this often facilitates developing a questionnaire. With the model in hand, you can clearly state specific objectives for the program that the questionnaire must assess.

2. *State objectives in behavioral terms.* The objectives of your evaluation should be stated in behavioral terms—what program participants should be expected to do. Behavioral objectives enhance the likelihood that people will agree on what the objectives are and that appropriate measures can be created.

3. *Review instruments.* If an instrument measuring the phenomenon of concern exists, seriously consider using it. At a minimum, review existing instruments for ideas to be included in a new instrument.

4. *Review necessary skills.* To achieve the desired outcome behaviors, a person must have certain prerequisite knowledge and skills.

Make a complete list of these knowledge and skill items in order to create the questionnaire.

5. *Construct a preliminary version.* Prepare a questionnaire that covers each knowledge, skill, and behavior outcome you wish to measure. Select or write items both so they appear to measure the objective (face validity) and, in cases of a large body of possible items, so they sample evenly from all the things that could be measured (content validity). Write items so that they can be clearly understood. Clarity is often achieved by basing a questionnaire on a fifth grade reading level. This means use of simple sentences (single subjects, verbs, and objects) and the simplest possible words. Although clear time limits for questionnaire completion have not been established, the longer the questionnaire (beyond four pages or so), the more likely it is that a person will refuse to enter the study, provide quick but erroneous answers, or not complete the questionnaire. Pay careful attention to question wording and sequencing (Kalton et al., 1978; Noelle-Neumann, 1970; Schuman and Presser, 1977). Distributing early drafts of a questionnaire to colleagues for review and comment will often identify obvious problems. The coordination committee for the evaluation (see Chapter 2) may also be of value in reviewing early drafts.

In general, use closed-ended instead of open-ended questions. The respondent may not accurately understand an open-ended question, may not want to provide a full answer because it will take too much time, or may give a full and complete answer in his or her view but the program staff finds misleading or uninterpretable. For example, if you are interested in specific foods a person has eaten, an open-ended question might read "What did you eat yesterday?" For some respondents, the answer may take a full page and may not cover all the foods of interest to you. If you are interested in a limited number of foods (e.g., high-salt foods), a reasonable closed-ended alternative would be to list all these foods and ask whether the respondent had eaten any of these foods. This approach is less likely to miss foods of concern because the foods are listed and the list acts as a memory prompt for the program participant. Developing closed-ended questions, however, requires more time and attention to detail than open-ended questions. You must review the literature to ensure that the response categories are mutually exclusive and exhaustive, that is, that they include all the logically or frequently identified alternatives. You must also test the questionnaire to ensure that the alternatives are understandable to the intended program participants. When rating scales are used to obtain responses, the structure of the response scales can be important. Schwarz et al. (1991) demonstrate that respondents differentially interpret and respond to categories labeled −5 to 5 than when they are labeled 0 to 10, although numerically they are equivalent. Baranowski, Tsong, and Brodwick (1990) demonstrate that respondents tend not to use the endpoints of rating scales.

Open-ended questions can be useful in a questionnaire: when you want to learn something about which little is known. In this case, a closed-ended question is posed (usually in a yes–no format), followed by an open-ended question asking for an explanation. For example, the following question provides fascinating results:

Have you decided to breast-feed your baby?
☐ Yes   ☐ No
Why?_____

It elicits a variety of reasons that maintains a high level of internal consistency (Baranowski et al., 1982). Ensuing research, however, used closed-ended questions based on these responses (Baranowski, Tsong, and Brodwick, 1990).

Some investigators recently have employed cognitive psychology techniques to improve the quality of questions (Jobe and Mingay, 1990). These techniques have been applied primarily to questions about behavior, that is, when certain facts might be stored in memory and need to be accurately retrieved. According to this perspective, a good question about behavior will ask for information in a way that is consistent with how people attend to, perceive, store in memory, and retrieve the information (i.e., the major cognitive processes) (Baranowski and Domel, 1993). These investigators used a "talking aloud" procedure early in the development of a questionnaire, in which they asked respondents to report about both the answer to the question and what they were thinking about in formulating their answer to the question. This technique holds much promise and should be considered in the design of questions. Another useful technique from this research is to first ask about a longer time interval for the occurrence of an event, followed by asking about a shorter time interval of interest, in order to overcome the problem of telescoping (Loftus et al., 1990).

The questionnaire should be appealing to respondents. Berdie and Anderson (1974) identify many facets of an appealing questionnaire. Keeping the pages free of clutter and using much empty space make the form visually appealing. Asking several questions that are stimulating or pleasing early in the questionnaire increases the likelihood that respondents will maintain the motivation and attention to complete the instrument. Developing and using clear and simple instructions increase the accuracy of responses to the questionnaire.

Multiitem instruments should be constructed to avoid response sets that can bias the results. You can overcome this problem by keeping the number of questions in which yes is the appropriate response equal to those in which no is appropriate and by including equal numbers of positively and negatively worded items. The response biases may then be detected and corrected. For example, if a person responds yes to all questions, several of which the answers should logically be no, this instrument can be dropped from the analyses.

Finally, develop the questionnaire with the method of data processing and analysis in mind. Because computers are almost always used to process data, the following guidelines are often helpful: group together questions that employ a similar response format (e.g., yes–no vs. a 5-point scale vs. an open-ended response) so that the data-entry clerk can enter the data from the form; or design the form with a column on the right side of the page in which responses from the main body of the questionnaire are coded for data entry. Keep answer spaces to the right-hand side of the page for easy coding or entry. Precode the questionnaire for data entry—that is, assign each response alternative a response value and make sure that each question has an identified and numbered set of columns for coding and data entry. Figure 7.1 illustrates a questionnaire with these characteristics.

6. *Develop data collection–training protocols.* Once the instrument has been developed, protocols for collecting and coding the data must be written. These protocols give the data collectors detailed information on what to say in instructing people to complete a questionnaire, what questions are likely to occur, and how to answer these questions. Writing the protocols at this time will help answer many questions that will arise among staff. These protocols, in turn, provide materials for training the people who will collect the data. Protocols are often revised during and soon after training.

7. *Pilot-test the questionnaire.* Whether the questionnaire is an existing instrument or was developed for your evaluation, it must be pilot-tested as part of a formative evaluation. At a minimum, the purpose of the pilot test is to see whether the intended re-

HEALTH QUESTIONNAIRE			For Computer Use Only
	ID #		_ _ _ _ _
Are you married? (check only one)	Yes ☐	1	
	No ☐	2	(1,06) V2
Do you have any children? (check only one)	Yes ☐	1	
	No ☐	2	(1,07) V3
About how often do you go to a fast food restaurant? (check only one)	Never ☐	1	
	Rarely ☐	2	
	About once a week ☐	3	
	Several times a week ☐	4	(1,08) V4
	About once a day ☐	5	
	Several times a day ☐	6	
Do you like to go to fast food restaurants? (check only one)	Yes ☐	1	
	No ☐	2	(1,09) V5
Why? (please explain) _____			
_____			SKIP
_____			(1,10-1,79)
			Card 1
			(1,80)

Figure 7.1 Example of a Precoded Questionnaire

spondents can complete the set of questions under the specified circumstances.

In the most basic pilot tests, a draft of the questionnaire is given to a sample of people (maybe 10 or 15) representative of the target group of the larger evaluation, under the same circumstances. After each respondent completes the questionnaire, the person distributing the questionnaire interviews the respondent to find out whether any questions were unclear, produced anger or anxiety (e.g., used terms considered racist or sexist), or were too complex. The interviewer also asks detailed questions about the most important aspects of the questionnaire to ensure that the respondents understood what the program staff intended. A more complex pilot test might include several wordings of the same items at different points in the same questionnaire and might compare responses of separate groups of respondents or compare questionnaires completed under various circumstances. In such pilot testing, the program staff will assess the internal consistency of multiitem scales and might look at differences both in responses to the same questions (reliability) and in relationships between questions or other phenomena (validity). Repeating the questionnaire a week later will assess test–retest reliability.

Although it is often valuable to test a questionnaire early in its development with friends and colleagues, a field test should be done with respondents representative of the population to be included in the major evaluation. Careful attention to validity and reliability issues at this stage will avoid many problems in the main part of the evaluation.

8. *Redesign the questionnaire and protocol.* As a result of the pilot test, the questionnaire and protocol are redesigned and rewritten to capitalize on what was learned.

9. *Retest the questionnaire.* The program staff repeats step 7 if the instrument was substantially revised.

10. *Make a final redesign.* The staff repeats step 8.

Although much work has been done to this point, the questionnaire is not yet ready for use in the program evaluation.

Quality Control. Selecting, developing, and field testing a questionnaire are necessary, but not sufficient, to collect valid and reliable data. Error can creep into data collected by a questionnaire. The health promotion and education program evaluation staff should assume that "Murphy's Law" is the law of the land. Therefore, questionnaire quality control checks should be made.

To obtain estimates of reliability, insert methods or procedures into the instrument or protocol for the most important items or instruments. They can be made in several ways: test–retest, internal consistency, or multiple-form reliability (see Chapter 6). At a minimum, an investigator must calculate Cronbach's alpha (or the KR-20, as appropriate) on all multiitem instruments, to obtain an estimate of internal consistency.

Questionnaires are often returned incomplete (e.g., a person turned two pages, instead of one, and missed a whole page of questions) or with obvious inconsistencies (e.g., a person did not answer a set of questions when an earlier response indicated that, according to the logic of the questionnaire, this person should have completed those questions). To control for these sources of error, a staff member should be available at the return of a questionnaire to review it for completeness and obvious inconsistencies. This staff member can approach the respondent immediately (while the information is still fresh in memory) for item completion or clarification.

To recheck incomplete responses, to detect illegal codes to a question, and to detect more detailed inconsistencies, conduct soon a more intensive review of responses. This review is important so that respondents can be contacted while answers are still relatively fresh in their memories and before real changes occur.

Conduct other data-editing and -cleaning procedures after the data have been entered into the computer—for example, after reviewing 10% of the data-entry forms against printouts of the data set. These checks also detect data-entry errors.

Although this appears to be a great amount of work, following these steps will avoid problems in making inferences from questionnaire data. Any error in data will lead either to biases in the results or inability to detect true relationships. We should therefore do everything possible to eliminate or minimize the sources of error over which we have some control.

Agency or Organizational Forms

In many agencies, the best approach to evaluating a particular service is to collect data every time a unit of service is provided. The instrument for collecting such data is most often a *form*. Both Carey (1972) and Staggs (1972) have discussed the specifics of form creation. Carey's comments on the value of a form in business also apply to the health agency setting:

> The form, or document, or report is a management instrument that ties the several parts of the business system, or subsystem, together. It is the cement, or adhesive, of any business. A well designed form confirms, instructs, directs and informs. A quality form ensures that business policies, regulations and directives are accommodated. Just as it is axiomatic that a home run has no value unless the hitter touches all bases, so it is with a

form. Its utility is in direct relationship to the effort made to ensure it will be used effectively. Checks and balances, standards and measures, all contribute to quality and to effective use.

This is a tall order for any form to fill, but forms can be useful in evaluating an agency's services. The strengths and weaknesses discussed in "Self-Completion questionnaires" apply to forms and need not be repeated here.

Steps in Form Development. All the guidelines for creating a questionnaire apply to creating a form. The primary restriction on a form in comparison with a questionnaire is brevity. Whereas a questionnaire should be kept brief (four pages are best), a form should rarely be more than a single page. This is often a challenge for the form developer. The single page must include the instructions as well as the questions; questions must therefore be self-evident, keeping instructions to the absolute minimum.

To be accepted by the staff members who will be filling it out, the form should pose few barriers to completion. Besides being simple, it should request information in a manner that is easiest for the staff to complete. The easiest manner is often the sequence in which the information is obtained by the staff from the task being recorded. If a form follows a client through a health program with multiple staff members completing parts of the form, it is important to keep the information provided by one staff member together on a portion of the form, perhaps separated from other portions by boxes or lines. The sequence of the boxes or lined sections should reflect the sequence in which they are completed in the service delivery process.

Developing incentives for the staff to accurately complete the form can be important. Sometimes it is valuable to use or modify existing forms to collect the desired evaluative information. In this way, you capitalize on whatever incentives exist for completion of the form and avoid the natural resistance to newly developed forms. At times each person in a form-completion chain wants a copy of the form completed to that point. A form can be created using NCR paper (the paper that reproduces impressions on lower sheets without the use of carbon paper) and appropriately pyramided, that is, each person in the chain can detach a color-coded copy to the form as it goes from staff member to staff member, with each successive copy showing and collecting additional information. Showing staff members that the data are used, and how, creates an important incentive. A clerk, who can call the form completer to clarify incomplete, confusing, or otherwise unclear information, should review form data on a frequent periodic basis (every day is best). Providing periodic reports that summarize these form-completion behaviors will promote quality form completion and may even be useful in improving or maintaining high-quality service (Andrasik et al., 1978).

The people who will complete the form and the people who will use the collected information should review a form in several drafts. In one case, evaluators of an emergency medical services system (Bernstine and Baranowski, 1976) had to develop a single-sheet form to serve many purposes: (1) recording clinical information for the use and legal protection of the emergency medical technicians (EMTs) and paramedics providing emergency care, (2) transmitting clinical information for use at the next stage in the patient-care delivery process (e.g., the hospital emergency room), (3) tracking (for the state) the flow of emergency patients' care from preambulance to ambulance care to life-support care at local emergency rooms to sophisticated regional emergency care, and (4) evaluating the quality of medical care at each stage in delivery. The form had to be flexible enough to record the many types of emergency problems from snakebite in remote rural areas to automobile accidents to cardiovascular or cerebrovascular events.

Figure 7.2 shows a draft of this form, which has many of the desirable characteristics discussed. The clinical data are prominent and grouped on the left and bottom of the form. The data on tracking of care appear in the order in which they occur. It is brief and well defined, with all data appearing on a single page. Each section is clearly introduced by a blocked title. The form was developed and refined over a number of meetings with EMTs, various hospital staffs, and state health department employees. At each stage in development, the various groups demanded data in a different format. The state required data in a form that was thorough yet easily computerized because the state had to process hundreds of thousands of these forms each year. This most often meant closed-ended responses to a series of strategic questions. The EMTs and paramedics demanded that major portions of the form be blank lines to record text about the patient. They wanted this open-ended format because they did not want to hunt through checklists on a form to define the patient's status and they believed they could easily, quickly, and accurately interpret clinical notes. The hospital staff members wanted nothing to do with the form because they put no confidence in the procedures, tentative diagnoses, or care provided by EMTs and paramedics (despite their extensive training) and because they did not want the care they themselves provided to be evaluated by the state.

This form was extensively modified in response to the comments of each faction and field-tested in one area of the state. The effort was ultimately a failure because of the conflicts among the various factions using the form (see Chapter 2). The conflict over open-ended versus

WASHINGTON STATE EMSS REPORTING FORM

ATIENT NAME _____ FAMILY PHYSICIAN _____

HOME ADDRESS _____ AGENCY NAME _____

CITY _____ ZIP CODE _____ ATTENDANT'S NAME _____

MED ALERT TAG _____ SEX ____ AGE ____ INFANTS ONLY ____ SIGNATURE _____
(YEARS) (MONTHS)

PRE-AMBULANCE CARE BY
- PRIVATE CITIZEN ☐
- FIRE SERVICE ☐
- PUBLIC SAFETY ☐
- VOLUNTEER EMT ☐

AMBULANCE RESPONSE DATA
- COUNTY CODE
- AMBULANCE CODE
- CASE #
- CALL RECEIVED VIA SINGLE ACCESS PHONE
- DATE: MO. ____ Day ____ Year ____

CLASSIFICATION OF PATIENT PROBLEM   I   II   III
- TRAUMA
- HEAD AND/OR SPINE
- BURNS
- CARDIAC
- PULMONARY
- SHOCK
- NEONATAL-OB
- BEHAVIORAL
- POISONING OR OVERDOSE
- ALCOHOL
- UNCLASSIFIED

INITIAL OBSERVATIONS AND TREATMENT

PULSE	REGULAR	
	IRREGULAR	
PULSE RATE	<60	
	60-120	
	>120	

ECG
EKR
DEFIBRILLATION
DRUGS (SPECIFY BELOW)

STOLIC BP	<110	
	110-140	
	>140	

LEGS ELEVATED
IV FLUIDS (SPECIFY)

RESPIRATION RATE	<15	
	15-25	
	>25	

RESPIRATORY DISTRESS

AIRWAY CLEAR	MANUAL	
	SUCTION	
AIRWAY TUBE	ORAL	
	ESOPHAGEAL	
	TRACHEAL	
	MOUTH	
VENTILATION	BAG	
	RESPIRATOR	
	TUBE	
OXYGEN BY	MASK	
	CANNULA	

CONSCIOUS
MENTAL CONFUSION
UNCONSCIOUS

REPONDS TO	VOICE	
	MOVEMENT	
	PAIN	
	NONE	
PUPILS O or •	RIGHT	
	LEFT	

CONVULSION

BLEEDING	CONTROLLED	
	UNCONTROLLED	
POSSIBLE FX	IMMOBILIZED	
	NOT IMMOBILE	

PRE-AMBULANCE CARE GIVEN
- OBSERVATION ONLY ☐
- EXTRICATION ☐
- CONTROLLED BLEEDING ☐
- SPLINTING ☐
- CPR ☐
- OTHER (SPECIFY) ☐

COMMENTS

BILL TO
- ☐ PATIENT ☐ WELFARE
- ☐ EMPLOYER ☐ BLUE CROSS
- ☐ MEDICARE ☐ PVT. INS.
- ☐ VA ☐ OTHER (SPECIFY)

Name of Insurance Company,
Welfare, Firm, Employer Name,
Other:

POLICY NO

TIMES
- CALL RECEIVED
- VEHICLE DISPATCHED
- ARRIVED LOCATION
- DEPARTED LOCATION
- ARRIVED DESTINATION
- PATIENT TAKEN FROM
- PATIENT TAKEN TO:

WAS HOSPITAL CONTACTED?
- YES ☐ NO ☐
- IF YES: IF NO:
- AT SCENE ☐ NOT NECESSARY ☐
- EN ROUTE ☐ EQUIPMENT UNSATISFACTORY ☐
- HOSPITAL DID NOT ANSWER ☐

WHO GAVE INSTRUCTIONS - RECEIVED FROM
- ☐ PHYSICIAN ☐ NURSE
- ☐ OTHER (SPECIFY)

SIGNATURE OF ED PERSON
COMPLETING THIS FORM:

PATIENT DISPOSITION
- DISCHARGED HOME
- ADMITTED TO HOSPITAL
- TRANSFERRED TO ANOTHER HOSPITAL (SPECIFY)
- REFERRED TO OUTPATIENT CARE

EVALUATION OF PRE-HOSPITAL CARE
- SATISFACTORY ☐ UNSATISFACTORY ☐
- IF UNSATISFACTORY, SPECIFY WHY:

TENTATIVE ED DIAGNOSIS _____

PLAN OF ED TREATMENT: _____

INSTRUCTIONS: CODE THE APPROPRIATE LINE - THEN INDICATE ON ANATOMICAL FIGURE
- • ABRASION-CONTUSION •
- • LACERATION •
- • BURN 1° •
- • 2° OR 3° •
- • CLOSED INJURY •
- • PENETRATING INJURY •
- • BLEEDING •
- • POSSIBLE FRACTURE •
- • AMPUTATION •
- • PAIN •
- • NAUSEA, VOMITING •

Figure 7.2 Example of Agency Reporting Form

closed-ended data was most serious, but the reluctance to be evaluated by the state was a strong undercurrent. This example demonstrates the complexities of form development and the political nature of data collected on forms.

Self-Completion Mail Surveys

When resources are scarce and the target population for the evaluation is dispersed across a broad geographic area, a mail survey is an attractive method for collecting data. The mail survey uses a self-completion questionnaire with the postal system as the vehicle for delivering and retrieving the instrument. Dillman (1978) provides a valuable reference on mail survey research techniques.

Strengths and Weaknesses. Comments about the strengths and weaknesses of the self-completion questionnaire also apply to the mail survey. Given the relatively low cost of mail service, these surveys offer an inexpensive method of obtaining data from areas as large as a city, a state, or even a nation.

The strengths of the mail survey method under some circumstances can be its weaknesses under others. A mail survey assumes that some sampling frame has a particular respondent's accurate address and that mail can be delivered to that address. Problems may exist with both these assumptions. For example, a mail survey of students in a school district revealed that 30% of the addresses were in error. Some were simply out of date; others were nonexistent locations. The latter were probably given by people who wanted their children to attend a preferred school without living in that school district (Nader et al., 1980)

In another study, a mail survey was conducted of all hypertensive patients attending a particular clinic. Roughly 15% of the addresses that were obtained from the patients' medical records were in error. The clinic's financial records, kept separately, had more up-to-date information (Baranowski et al., 1982).

Some people want to maintain anonymity and not have mail deliverable to them. Such people may be illegal aliens, people sought by bill collectors, or people afraid of being sought by criminal elements, publicity seekers, or other undesired contacts. Not being able to deliver mail to such people may bias a mail survey in a particular study. People who move frequently (often those wishing to maintain their anonymity, those staying ahead of creditors, or those in constant search of work) have difficulty receiving mail. Although reachable at one time, they may be unreachable at others (population stability over time). This mobility of the target population may vary by geographic area (population stability over areas).

The greatest recommendation for the mail survey is its low cost as a method for obtaining data from a large geographic area. The dross rate for unreturned or incomplete questionnaires can be high, depending on the nature of the sampling frame. The dross rate on information on the questionnaire is quite low, however.

Steps in Conducting a Mail Survey. If you are contemplating a mail survey, you need to find a sampling frame that contains names, addresses, and, if possible, phone numbers. You must be concerned

Table 7.3 Steps in Conducting a Mail Survey

1. Develop a questionnaire: Use colored paper, make it no longer than four pages, provide an original typed cover letter that is personally addressed, make the response a personal responsibility of the respondent, and set up a tracking system.
2. Send a notification postcard or letter 1 week early.
3. Send out the initial questionnaire: Tape 25¢–50¢ in the upper right-hand corner to encourage response, ensure return postage for undeliverable mail, and provide a return envelope with postage.
4. Send a reminder postcard at 2 weeks.
5. Send a second questionnaire to nonrespondents.
6. Call nonrespondents by phone.

SOURCES: Dillman (1978) and Yammarino et al. (1991).

about the probable accuracy of that information and whether some people who are of interest to the study may not be included or not accurately represented in the sampling frame.

Use the following steps (summarized in Table 7.3) in implementing a mail survey:

1. *Develop a questionnaire.* Follow the ten steps outlined earlier for developing a questionnaire. In addition, print the questionnaire on colorful paper, so respondents can find it when looking in a pile of papers, and make it not more than four pages long (Yammarino et al., 1991). The cover letter should be an original typed letter, personally addressed to each respondent, with the message indicating the personal responsibility of the reader to respond immediately. Work out a tracking system listing the name, address, and telephone number of each respondent in alphabetical order or numerically by identification number, for recording returned questionnaires, updating addresses and phone numbers as new information is obtained, and providing a central data file for conducting follow-ups.

2. *Send a notification postcard or letter.* Higher initial response rates are achieved if a postcard or letter of notification informing respondents of the pending arrival of the questionnaire is sent about 1 week before the initial mailing (Yammarino et al., 1991). It keeps some respondents from initially discarding the questionnaire and entices others to learn more about the questionnaire. With interest piqued, they may look forward to its arrival.

3. *Send out the initial questionnaire.* Send the initial questionnaire to all potential respondents about 1 week after the postcard. Includ-

ing 25¢–50¢ in the upper right-hand corner of the cover letter increases the response rate significantly over providing no financial award and as much as providing a $10 award (Dillman, 1978). Ensure return postage so the post office will return undeliverable questionnaires, thereby enabling other methods to be used to follow up on these potential respondents. A return envelope with return postage substantially increases the response rate (Yammarino et al., 1991).

4. *Send a reminder postcard.* Within a couple of days after the initial mailing, there is a high volume of return of questionnaires. After 3–5 days, the return rate tapers off. Within 2 weeks, 95% or more of the questionnaires that will be returned from the first mailing alone will have been received. Send a reminder postcard to nonrespondents at this 2-week point.

5. *Send out a second questionnaire.* The return pattern from the postcard will follow that of the mailing of the first questionnaire, but the rates will not be as high. Within 2 weeks, 95% or more of the questionnaires responding to the postcard reminder will have been returned. Some people will have discarded or otherwise lost the initial questionnaire; thus, send a second questionnaire to nonrespondents 2 weeks after the postcard.

6. *Call nonrespondents by phone.* Reasons for nonresponse to a second questionnaire may be the respondent never received the questionnaire, refuses to answer, or wants more personal contact or assurance of anonymity. Placing a telephone call can obtain the accurate address of a nonrespondent (to whom a new questionnaire must be sent), may be able to persuade the respondent of the value of participating in the survey, can answer the respondent's questions immediately over the phone, or can administer the questionnaire if needed. In this way, phoning, which is an expensive approach to data collection relative to the mail survey, is used only as the last resort with the fewest number of potential participants, thereby minimizing costs. Telephone interviewing, however, may elicit different information than that from a mail questionnaire because the interviewer can influence the respondent's understanding of the questions or the nature of the respondent's motivation to respond.

Program staff members should expect some percentage of questionnaires to be returned marked "undeliverable." Attempt phone contact with these persons immediately to obtain new addresses for a mailing. On the master list of names, addresses, and telephone numbers, do the following: Monitor the returned questionnaires, revise addresses and enter telephone numbers, and record attempts to reach respondents. Any reasonably organized person can manage the mail and return aspects of a mail survey. Someone, however, must plan for the logistics of doing all these activities and arrange to have staff members available at the likely to be used time.

Following this set of procedures and diligently following up on nonrespondents produce response rates of 70%–95%, with a variety of respondents (Dillman, 1978). An 80% response rate is considered adequate. There appears to be little response bias between those responding and those not with this response level. Conduct analyses with data from the sampling frame (e.g., age, gender, ethnicity, geographic location), to determine differences between respondents and nonrespondents. Differences may bias interpretation of the results of the survey, and any encountered bias therefore needs to be noted.

Self-Completion Diaries and Logs

Investigators have been concerned about two problems in usual methods of obtaining self-report measures: telescoping and memory loss. *Telescoping* means that respondents tend to remember certain events as having occurred more recently than they actually did. *Memory loss* refers to failure to remember the occurrence of a variety of events. Studying the dietary behaviors of children provides an interesting example. Most dietary assessment methods require intensive recall for the past 24-hour period or for as long as 2 weeks. Children, however, demonstrate several limitations in reporting the frequency of their consumption of particular foods: They do not easily remember the foods eaten for a full 24-hour period, have difficulty reporting on frequencies of consumption of particular items across meals and snack times, are often not aware of the names and nutrient content of food products they consume, and are not aware of the methods of food preparation (e.g., salt-shaking habits, use of sauces or condiments, use of margarine vs. butter) followed by their parents, grandparents, or school cooks. Some investigators have used self-report diaries to compensate for these problems. One book (Sudman and Lannom, 1980) and three articles (Laurent et al., 1972; Roghmann and Haggerty, 1972; Verbrugge, 1980) are of particular value on this subject.

Strengths and Weaknesses. Verbrugge (1980) reviewed the available literature on health diaries and came to the following conclusions: (1) Diaries produce higher frequencies for most phenomena than other methods and appear to be particularly better than other self-report methods for reporting low-salience phenomena (e.g., transient, low-impact health problems; symptoms; disability days); (2) telescoping is absent; (3) memory lapse is minimized. In addition, depending on how the diary data were collected, diaries could provide very rich sources of a wide variety of data for intensive analysis.

Verbrugge further reports that two other methodological concerns of investigators did *not* occur: A very high percentage of people contacted agreed to complete diaries, and very few people who agreed to complete a diary failed to complete one during the full recording period. This high completion rate happened without financial or other incentives to complete the forms.

Verbrugge (1980) also reports several problems with diaries. The quality of the data is roughly proportional to the effort expended to collect it. Frequent (e.g., weekly) attempts must be made to collect the diaries. Recontacts must be made with respondents to clarify missing, inconsistent, or otherwise unclear data, not only to verify the responses but also to demonstrate program staff concern about the data quality. These collection efforts are obviously made at a high cost in staff time. Verbrugge estimates these costs as higher per respondent than data collected by interviewers because of the intensive efforts at data collection and because of the need for extensive data coding. Domel et al. (in press, 1993) demonstrate that children can keep reasonably accurate food diaries in school, and the accuracy increased from about 65% against an external observer, when the children were prompted on a weekly basis, to about 85%, when the children were prompted and monitored on a daily basis by research staff.

According to Verbrugge (1980), investigators note two other methodological problems (biases) in diaries: sensitization and conditioning. Investigators note that respondents become more aware of the phenomena simply from monitoring their own behavior, at least initially. This increased sensitivity results in behavior changes (e.g., the person is more likely to seek medical help when the monitored symptoms occur). These investigators also find that the frequency of events decreases anywhere from 5%–25% during the recording period. They report that the respondents increasingly lost interest in the phenomenon (i.e., became bored) over time, which resulted in the lower reported frequencies. All the comments about biases in the self-report questionnaire potentially apply to the diary unless steps are taken to correct them.

The dross rate in diaries varies, depending on how the diary is structured. If the diary calls for open-ended comments, the dross rate may be high. If the diary calls for daily checks on a checklist or frequency counts in a structured format, the dross rate should be low.

One effort at collecting dietary information from children attempted to capitalize on the virtues of the diary method while minimizing the dross (Baranowski et al., 1986). The children were asked to record their daily consumption of specific categories of foods that were high in the nutrients of concern to the project: salt and saturated fats. The categories were food-specific; for example, the high-salt sources category included soy, Worcestershire, steak, and related sauces, and there were three milk categories—whole milk (4% milk fat) and two kinds of low-fat milk (2% milk fat and .5% milk fat). To promote memory of the whole day's intake, the child was asked to remember the frequency of consumption of specific foods within segments of the school day: breakfast, lunch, after-school snack, dinner, after-dinner snack, and bedtime snack. Pictures of the food items were used to prompt memory and make the instrument visually attractive.

Diaries are an attractive, though expensive, approach to data collection when the program staff have reason to believe that telescoping and memory loss may occur if other instruments are used.

Face-to-Face Interviewing

In certain circumstances, there is no substitute for having an interviewer conduct a survey. The literature on survey interviewing methods seems infinite. Several references are useful (Anderson et al., 1979; Bailar and Lanphier, 1978; Bradburn and Sudman, 1979; Cannell et al., 1977; Sudman and Lannom, 1980; Survey Research Center, 1976). This literature is too complex to be conveniently summarized in this brief section; only an overview of the method is presented.

Strengths. Conducted face-to-face, the interpersonal interview is preferable to the self-completion questionnaire when

1. The content area is not well defined.
2. The questions are long, complex, or require subtle distinctions.
3. The respondents have difficulty reading or writing.
4. Personal effort may be needed to contact respondents.
5. Data on other variables (e.g., blood pressure measurements) also need to be collected.

The primary strength of the face-to-face interview is the use of a well-trained interviewer to query the respondent intensively and to detect, clarify, and follow up on perplexing answers or questions. A trained person can obtain answers to questions that are not well defined or for which in-depth answers are needed. Interviewers can be trained to probe interviewees with a variety of questions, attempting to get below-surface responses, that is, flippant or simple answers a respondent may provide. For example, if you are interested in why mothers decide to breast-feed or not, you could ask a simple question —"Why did you decide to breast-feed or bottle-feed your baby?"— and leave several lines for the unstructured response. Alternatively, you might use the power of having an interviewer ask the following series of questions:

> "What do you see as the benefits to your baby of breast-feeding (or bottle-feeding)?"
>
> "What do you see as the benefits to yourself of breast-feeding (or bottle-feeding)?"
>
> "What do you see as the costs to you of bottle-feeding (or breast-feeding)?"
>
> "What do you see as the costs to your baby of bottle-feeding (or breast-feeding)?"
>
> "How important are the costs of breast-feeding to you?"
>
> "How important are the benefits of breast-feeding to you?"
>
> "How important are the costs of bottle-feeding to you?"
>
> "What is the most important reason why you selected your method of infant feeding?"

A respondent finding these questions in a self-response questionnaire would probably answer them with the easiest responses. For example, the answer to the first question might be "Nothing." An interviewer can probe a little deeper, looking for things this mother might like about breast- or bottle-feeding. Thus, for certain situations, the interview is more appropriate than the self-completed questionnaire. However, now that research has documented long lists of possible reasons for breast-feeding (Baranowski, et al., 1990), which have been formulated as multiitem-response scales, the self-report questionnaire may be just as useful for this issue, when used with a literate population.

Interview questions are best formed when the investigator is working from a theoretical framework or a model. For example, the breast-feeding interview was based on an expectancy model that assesses the benefits and costs of two behavioral alternatives (Baranowski, 1992–1993). Questions can be designed to assess the key variables in the model, and the interviewer can be instructed how far to probe respondents to ascertain the data of interest to the program staff.

The interview is appropriate for long and complex questions and those requiring subtle distinctions for the same reasons that it is valuable for poorly defined questions. The appropriateness of an interviewer for respondents who cannot read or write is obvious.

A face-to-face interview is also valuable when extensive effort is necessary to contact a respondent. In some cases, a sample of people is selected from a source (e.g., all previous clients in a smoking-cessation program) that does not maintain their current addresses, or the sample may have addresses not easily reachable by mail (e.g., some people live in inconspicuous lofts, sheds behind other homes, or other quarters not on usual mail routes and without mailboxes). In rural areas, respondents may live in remote houses down dirt roads or accessible only by hiking up trails. Such people may not have a mailbox or telephone or may come to town only a few times a year to pick up their mail. A timely response to a mail questionnaire is highly unlikely. A more mundane example would be the survey that requires a random sampling of households in a particular geographic area. Maps do not usually list all dwellings in an area (the maps that do show dwellings always seem to be several years out of date), indicate which dwellings are abandoned or otherwise not occupied, and note which dwellings are multiple-household units (e.g., apartments or condominiums). Rules can be generated for taking a random sample in such a situation, but a trained interviewer is needed to identify all the sampling units in an area and implement a set of sample selection rules.

The interview provides the most flexible method for the use of descriptive cues. An interviewer can ask a variety of questions and make a variety of judgments about the state of the respondent. With careful attention to detail, an interview can almost always be replicated, which promotes reliability in data collection.

Weaknesses. The face-to-face interview is susceptible to a variety of biases. In an interpersonal situation, respondents are likely to anticipate what the interviewer expects of them and act accordingly (role selection). The probing of particular content areas is likely to focus the attention of the respondent on these issues, which may change the way the respondent thinks about the issues and thereby confound future attempts at measuring this content area (measurement as a change agent). All self-report measures are susceptible to yea-saying and social desirability (response set). Interviewer effects, by definition, may occur in interpersonal interviews. Interviewers become more proficient and more subtle at asking questions, so that later interviews may be different from earlier ones (changes in the research instrument). The interview may not obtain accurate information on highly sensitive issues, for example, sexual or contraceptive behavior (restrictions on content).

Realizing these biases, the health program evaluation staff must take steps to counter or minimize their effects. Interviewers should be trained to ask questions in a warm and nonjudgmental manner and to avoid behaviors that might lead respondents to infer appropriate-versus-inappropriate responses. Questions should be worded in both positive and negative forms to minimize the effects of response sets. Training should be long enough so that interviewers are no longer learning about the meaning of the questions during the course of the interviews. Periodic testing or retraining may be necessary to ensure that the interviewing remains true to the original intent of the study. If obviously unreliable answers will be obtained using an interview format, the data should be collected in other ways.

The dross rate for an interpersonal interview may be high. There are many events in life (other than the topic of the interview) about which respondents would prefer to talk, and respondents may feel uncomfortable addressing the issues posed.

The interpersonal interview is an expensive method of data collection. Because of its costs, it should be used judiciously. Some combination of self-completed questionnaires and interviews may best achieve an investigator's objectives within the available budget. Alternatively, if time permits, a small interview survey may be conducted first to identify all the response alternatives. This complete listing of alternatives can, in turn, be used in a self-completion questionnaire.

Steps in Conducting Face-to-Face Interviews. A good face-to-face interview requires a well-designed interview schedule (list of questions) and a well-trained interviewer. The guidelines and suggestions presented earlier in this chapter for developing questionnaires also apply to developing the interview schedule. Training interviewers requires an equal attention to detail. Table 7.4 outlines the qualities that a good training program provides.

Training should give interviewers enough knowledge of the subject area to enable them to ask intelligent, probing questions. They should not, however, be informed of the study's specific hypotheses; that knowledge might bias the way in which they ask, interpret, or record responses. An answer to any question may be ambiguous, unless clear guidelines or clear categories of response exist for recording the response. For example, to the question "Why do you smoke after eating?" a new smoker might answer, "Well, I'm not too sure. Er . . . well, it gives me a boost right after a meal. I feel like tackling a project after a cigarette, but otherwise I'd feel like taking a nap. But I don't

Table 7.4 Required Qualities of a Good Training Program

1. An understanding of the major ideas that underlie the questionnaire.
2. A guidebook or protocol on probing and on recording responses.
3. Materials for clarifying responses.
4. Procedures for collecting other data.
5. Clear instructions to obtain and contact a sample.
6. Experience in conducting the interview, especially probing.
7. Common experiences in recording or coding self-report information.
8. Sources of information to report or clarify problems.
9. Testing for reliability.

like the taste and all those ashes. I try to puff enough to feel good, but not keep that terrible smoke in my mouth." This is a complex response to an apparently simple question. Some of the comments are positive; some are negative. The basic response to the question is equivocal. A set of rules is needed to guide the interviewer on the depth to probe for clarification and which parts of this response to record.

For some questions, an interviewer needs materials to show the respondent how to answer. Materials might include categories of income printed on a card, so that the respondent can report which category most accurately reflects the family income. A portion-size picture might be used to enable the respondent to estimate how much food he or she consumed.

Sometimes interviewers will collect data other than responses to questions. This might include blood pressure or saliva samples. Clear, detailed guidelines, materials, and thorough training need to be provided. Criteria need to be formulated for screening and possibly rejecting potential interviewers who cannot collect data adequately. For example, potential interviewers with hearing problems will not be able to collect blood pressure readings using a stethoscope. The health program evaluation staff needs to provide the interviewer with area maps or other unit enumeration materials and give the interviewer clear, precise instructions on what constitutes an interview unit and how to select among these units.

Armed with these materials and instructions, interviewers need experience in conducting interviews on a pilot basis. The pilot interviews test the questionnaire and enable the interviewers to develop confidence in implementing the interview and clarifying issues that did not arise in the initial review of materials and procedures. A valuable procedure is to have each interviewer tape-record a test interview and discuss the interview with the evaluator, program staff, and other interviewers. During the review of the tape recordings, all interviewers individually record the taped responses to the questions; they then compare their recordings. Such an experience is particularly valuable because the interviewer gets feedback from the program staff and one another on the appropriateness of his or her recordings, program staff members become aware of a variety of unresolved problems in the interview, and the staff have the opportunity to eliminate, or more intensively train, interviewers who do not obtain or record accurate responses. While interviewers are recording the information from the interviews, the program staff should collect the data and calculate the level of reliability. Such a review session should occur weekly thereafter, to ensure that interviewers are continuing to record in a reliable manner.

If a health program evaluation staff is conducting a community survey, interviewers must be given a phone number to call when they need information or clarification on interview techniques, sample locations, or the many other problems that occur. The program staff must take many steps to promote the reliability of all facets of the interviewing process. Interviewers should be encouraged to maintain logs of problems they encounter, and these should be resolved at the weekly meetings. If physiological measures are being collected, the interviewers' basic data-collection technique needs to be assessed at weekly intervals, and the machine needs to be assessed to ensure that it maintains its calibration.

Interview training may be conducted over a 3- to 5-day period. Table 7.5 presents a common outline for the sequence of training. Before they are sent into the field, interviewers must be furnished with identification. The program staff, in some cases, should announce the impending interviews to the local authorities (e.g., local sheriff or police) and place announcements in the papers so that the populace will expect to be contacted.

Conducting an interview survey is a time-consuming and costly business. We have given an overview of only some of the issues and methods involved. Program staff considering this technique should consult texts on interviewing methods.

Telephone Interviewing

Telephone interviewing is considered an attractive alternative to face-to-face interviewing because the information is cheaper to collect per interview and greater control can be exerted by evaluation staff over the methods of data collection in a central automated center for telephone interviewing. Several telephone survey research centers cur-

Table 7.5   Outline of Training for Face-to-Face Interviewers

Day	Time	Training
1	AM	Presenting the ideas on which the study is based
	PM	Detailed question-by-question review of the instrument, allowing for extensive questioning by interviewers
2	AM	Presenting support materials for obtaining responses Conducting a role-played interview
	PM	Training and testing in obtaining the clinical or physiological measures
3	AM/PM	Conducting and taping two practice interviews (prearranged with people to be interviewed)
4	AM	Reviewing the problems encountered and questions raised Common recording by all interviewers of information from taped interviews and discussions of recordings made
	PM	Continued common recording and discussion of taped interviews Testing of physiological measurement ability
5	AM	Training in procedures for selecting samples
	PM	Last questions Testing physiological measurement skills

rently use computerized centers for such interviews (Groves, 1979). A burgeoning literature has developed on methods of telephone interviewing (Dillman, 1978; Groves and Kahn, 1979; Jordan et al., 1979). Morris and Windsor (1985) demonstrate how useful a telephone survey can be in refining community-based health promotion services provided by a primary-care clinic.

All comments made about face-to-face interviewing apply at some level to telephone interviewing, but telephone interviewing is susceptible to additional biases. A primary concern is population restrictions. Data reveal that over 90% of all households have telephones (Thornberry and Massey, 1978), telephone unavailability is more common among people traditionally considered disadvantaged —for example, those in rural areas, the unemployed, those with lower education and income levels, and the separated and divorced. The telephone company refuses to place telephone cable into many sparsely populated, rural, mountainous areas in Appalachia. Further population-restriction problems arise when trying to reach people with unlisted phone numbers, those who have moved, and those who have changed phones for other reasons since the last public listing of telephone numbers.

To overcome the latter two problems, some investigators propose the method of random digit dialing, which obtains randomly selected phone numbers. The shortcoming of this approach is that it is not usable for contacting some known sampling frame of individuals (e.g., all the former participants in a particular project) or contacting people in specific geographic areas because the first three digits in the telephone number may not be specific to those areas. Jordan et al. (1979) compared a telephone interview survey with a household interview survey conducted on random samples in the Los Angeles area. They report that 6.8% of the units they attempted to contact in the household interviews were ineligible and 36.0% in the telephone interviews were ineligible. Telephone surveys may therefore be a less efficient approach for contacting specific units. Differences may also exist in the populations that can be reached by telephone over a span of time or a geographic area, but these have not been documented.

There may be greater restrictions on content in the telephone than in the face-to-face interview. It is commonly reported that a telephone interview cannot last more than 30 minutes and is best conducted in 20 minutes or less. In contrast, face-to-face interviews are commonly 1 hour or longer. The telephone interviewers in the study by Jordan et al. (1979) report (1) telephone interviews are faster-paced than are face-to-face interviews, (2) pauses of routine length in interpersonal interviews were unbearably long in telephone interviews, and (3) no visual cues were available to the interviewers to gauge when and how long they should probe for responses.

The Jordan team also report comparative analyses of data. In their initial comparison, almost twice as many people refused to answer a question on family income (a highly sensitive question) by telephone than in a face-to-face interview, but few other differences were obtained in demographic variables. This difference in response to family income was lower in comparisons of subsequent telephone and face-to-face interviews, ostensibly because of improved telephone-interviewing techniques. What these techniques were, however, was not reported. Jordan et al. (1979) found no statistically significant differences in means for attitude items or the numbers of responses to open-ended items, but they did find greater yea-saying, more frequent refusal to answer questions, more frequent extreme responses, and greater acquiescence to the perceived desires of the interviewer among telephone interview respondents. Thus, the same mean responses were obtained using the two methods, but greater error was obtained from telephone interviews. Siemiatycki (1979) and Aneshencel et al. (1982) report few differences in means across the methods for collecting the same data and thereby provide greater hope for use of telephone interviews.

Because greater acquiescence is obtained in telephone interviews, the dross rate is probably lower for telephone interviews than for face-to-face interviews; this has not been documented, however. Telephone interviewers can ask for descriptive cues as well as face-to-face interviewers can, so rough parity exists on this issue. The methods are equally replicable. A telephone survey is less expensive than a face-to-face interview, but it cannot be maintained for the same length of time. The relative cost per unit of information remains to be documented.

Direct Observation

Sometimes the accuracy of self-reported behaviors is suspect. In these cases, some investigators turn to direct observation: Weick (1968), Herbert and Attridge (1975), Johnson and Bolstad (1973), Baranowski et al. (1991), and Simons-Morton and Baranowski (1991). Herbert and Attridge reviewed a variety of psychometric and practical concerns in the design of observational instruments. Johnson and Bolstad reviewed a series of methodological studies on observation as the primary method of data collection.

Observational methods are most useful for collecting behavioral and capability data. By definition, behavioral data are amenable to observation. Ability, or skill, data often require a person to perform a task in a controlled circumstance to see whether the person can do it (Windsor, 1981; Windsor, Roseman et al., 1981). For example, a diabetic patient is often asked to perform self-injection to demonstrate that he or she can effectively do it. Direct observation includes a variety of methods. Observational data can be obtained, for example, directly by observers, videotapes, audiotape recorders, and other mechanical and electronic means. In some methods, the observer attempts to be an objective recorder of phenomena; in others, the observer frequently interacts with the subjects and may, in fact, participate with the subjects in various key social events (Emerson, 1981). Observational studies may be concerned simply with identifying the frequency of certain phenomena or, at a more complex level, with the relationships between events. There are many other ways to segment observational research literature. The rest of this section relates primarily to cases in which the observations are done by trained observers attempting to be objective recorders of the frequency of predefined phenomena.

Direct observation is one of the most expensive approaches to obtaining behavioral data. One or more observers must be present for extended periods of time to document the behavior of concern; extensive observation records must be maintained; multiple coders must search the observation records and code the phenomena of concern, or expensive lap-top computers must be used in the field to record

Table 7.6   Components Necessary for the Direct Observation
Method

1. *Observation instrument* that reflects the theory, model, or other purposes
   of the study: forms or observation-recording spaces in a computer and
   definitions of observation-recording categories or symbols
2. *Protocol* that outlines all rules relating to the issues of observational data
   collection
3. *Observers* trained to use the instrument and protocol
4. Procedures to assess *interobserver reliability*
5. *Protocol for coding data*
6. *Coders* trained to use coding protocol
7. Procedures to assess *intercoder reliability*

the observations. Using the self-report method, a single investigator
can use a self-report questionnaire with multiple respondents and in
1 hour obtain data from each respondent covering an hour, a day, a
week, a year, or even a lifetime of experiences. In contrast, a single
observer in 1 hour can obtain data on only 1 hour in the life of one
person or an interacting group of people. Observation therefore can
be cost-effective when used with small samples to validate data obtained using other methods (Simons-Morton and Baranowski, 1991).
These other methods can then be used with larger samples.

Steps in Conducting Direct Observation. Consult Herbert and Attridge (1975) on creation of an observational form. They identify 23
rules for consideration in the design and implementation of the form
and a system of data collection. At a minimum, the method of direct
observation of behavior requires all the items listed in Table 7.6.

The observation instrument includes the format for recording
(which could be spaces on a sheet of paper or on the screen of a small
computer), the definitions of terms, and the protocol for converting
observed phenomena to observation categories. The instrument could
use a checklist format displaying the possible observational items
within categories for easy reference and should include a sufficient
number of boxes to check the occurrence of the item at timed intervals. Figure 7.3 is an example of a checklist-type form for recording
observations of a child's physical activities. Alternatively, the instrument could rely on observer memory and simply provide spaces for
recording symbols remembered by the observer to represent specific
observation categories.

Pay careful attention to defining the items for observation. The
activity categories in Figure 7.3 define the aerobic activities, which

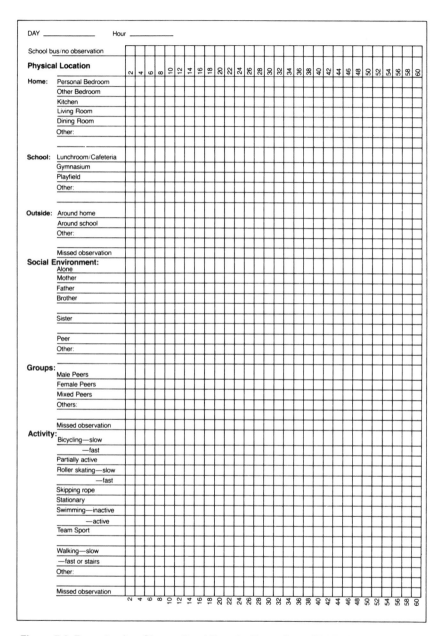

Figure 7.3 Example of an Observational Form for Recording a Child's Aerobic Activity

can lead to cardiovascular benefit, usually performed by children in the South (where the research was done). (Notice cross-country skiing, a common activity in the North, was not included.) Consensus must exist among the observers and other research staff on the meaning of terms. Distinctions among the proposed items must be amenable to observation, requiring as little judgment as possible on the part of the observer. For example, the distinction between partial activity and full aerobic activity requires judgment. With periodic reliability testing, agreement can be increased by extensive practice and consensus among observers. Observers must also agree on which aspects of the environment correspond to the categories in the instrument. For example, if observations are conducted in home, which room is the living room, and which is the playroom? Where does the kitchen end and the dining room begin? Is the new person who entered the room a cousin, a niece, or an aunt?

The protocol must specify whether the observer should record (1) the predominant activity during a specific time interval (dominant activity recording), (2) all activities during a specific time interval (complete activity recording), or (3) those activities performed at an instant of observation (time-sampling method). The dominant recording method characterizes long-duration activities occurring in an interval but may miss important short-duration activities. The complete recording method obtains all short- and long-duration activities but loses any sense of which activities predominate in an interval and may overly burden an observer. The time-sampling method is the easiest to implement but misses information on what happened between instantaneous observations. There are no automatically right and wrong choices of method. Select the one that obtains the most useful data for the purpose at hand. In the study in which Figure 7.3 was used, the second option, recording all events, was selected because the investigators were concerned with longer-duration bouts of continuous activity (Puhl et al., 1990)—that is, any occurrences of no activity negated a continuous bout of activity, thereby negating its being aerobic.

The protocol must specify procedures for contacting, training, and/or interviewing the persons to be observed; times at which all activities are to be conducted; sequences of activities within observation sessions; and procedures for preventing or ameliorating anticipated problems. The protocol should include the definitions of items and examples of the cases that are difficult to distinguish. It should clarify whether single or multiple checks or entries are disallowed, allowed, encouraged, or required within time intervals of categories of observational items. Procedures for recording field notes should be stated.

Table 7.7 Outline of Training for Observers

Day	Time	Training
1	AM	Reviewing the conceptual framework underlying the research Discussing the observational form and protocol, item-by-item
	PM	Jointly observing a movie or videotape depicting the expected observation scene Assessing reliability of the joint observation reports
2	AM	Observing the phenomenon of concern under realistic conditions
	PM	Discussing the problems encountered Revising the form or protocol, as necessary
3	AM	Simultaneously observing the phenomenon of concern by two or three observers
	PM	Assessing interobserver reliability Discussing problems of reliability Revising the form or protocol, as necessary
4 and on	AM/PM	Repeating of day 3 as necessary to achieve the desired reliability

The protocol should also specify periodic times for joint observations to obtain interobserver reliability. Several references are useful in discussing interobserver reliability: Tinsley and Weiss (1975), Bartko and Carpenter (1976), Green (1981), House et al. (1981), and Windsor (1981).

Observer training is a primary method of promoting the reliability of direct observational data. Training might proceed according to the outline in Table 7.7.

If not done by computer, people who code information from the observation instruments also may not agree on coding specifics, due to differences in interpretation or understanding of the coding task, temporary distractions, or errors in memory or perception. A protocol is needed for coding data from the observation instrument into meaningful variables. Many of the same issues covered in the observational protocol must be covered in the coding protocol. People doing the coding need to be trained in performing their task, although the training may not have to be as long because the task is more clearly defined and the data are not lost once the coding is done. Coding of the same form by two coders must be built into the daily tasks of the coders to obtain periodic estimates of intercoder reliability.

Johnson and Bolstad (1973) identify five key problems in observation methods: (1) Reliability estimates may not be made on the same coding and time units; (2) the days on which reliability is assessed may not be representative of other days on which observations are conducted; (3) the instrument may decay due to the passage of time; (4) the observers may respond in some unknown way to having reliability assessed; and (5) the people being observed may respond in some unknown way to being observed. Methods for counteracting these problems have been developed.

First, constant monitoring of the reliability of observational data is necessary. Data must be collected in a manner that facilitates comparing the data collected by two people on the same event. Obviously, both observers must use the same event-coding system. Another problem is the possibility that two observers will report the same frequency of events when each is reporting different occurrences. The observational form should use the same time unit for recording events to avoid this. How long the time unit needs to be will vary with the phenomenon observed. The Johnson and Bolstad (1973) study required 3- to 5-second intervals. Other studies have used 1 second, 1 minute, 2 minutes, and 5 minutes, depending on the type of behavior observed and the purpose of data collection. For the form in Figure 7.3, observers used 2-minute intervals because this was short enough to obtain relatively discrete information yet long enough not to fatigue the observers during a full day of observation.

Second, because human behavior is variable, some days may have many occurrences of a particular event, but a long time may transpire before the event of interest occurs again. For example, some people rarely engage in aerobic activity, and an event of aerobic activity may not occur on the day on which interobserver reliability is estimated. Thus, reliability must be estimated at multiple points in a project. In addition, artificial simulations of infrequent events should be created for observational tests (e.g., in a movie or videotape), to estimate the interrater reliability.

Third, Johnson and Bolstad (1973) report a study in which the interrater reliability of two observers remained reasonably high during the course of the study, but correlations of their observations with those of a third party became progressively lower. This phenomenon indicated that over time the two observers created their own mutually agreed-to approach to categorizing events, which progressively diverged from the aim and methods of the original coding scheme followed by the third party. This has been called *observer drift*. The authors redressed this problem by having more than two observers and conducting interobserver reliability checks on different pairs of observers over the course of the project and by periodically checking observers against a known standard videotape.

Fourth, the behavior of observers can be as responsive to environmental factors as that of the people being observed. Johnson and

Bolstad (1973) report that the reliability of observers significantly declined right after training, but the decline varied depending on which reliability-monitoring system was employed. Cases in which reliability was assessed by having a second observer conduct observations on selected and announced days (the spot-check method) had the overall largest slide in reliability, except on days when the spot checks occurred. To promote maximum reliability, Johnson and Bolstad recommend the following components of training for a reliability monitoring system:

1. Have all the observers read and study the observation protocol.
2. Have the observers complete programmed instruction materials on precoded interactions.
3. Conduct daily, intensive-training programs on precoded scripts enacted on videotape or by actors.
4. Provide field training with an experienced observer, followed by reliability testing.
5. Randomly assess interobserver reliability in the field.

Finally, Johnson and Bolstad (1973) note that people being observed are affected in major and minor ways by the observational process. The literature, however, is not clear about which behaviors are most likely to be affected, in what ways, or for how long. Investigators must be watchful of the reactivity of observational methods. There is reason to believe that the less obtrusive (or obvious) the observer is, the less effect the observer will have on the behavior in question. After some period of time, the effects of the presence of an observer appear to wear off or decrease. Investigators should therefore work to minimize the obtrusiveness of the observer and allow long enough observation periods to reduce the effects of the observer's presence.

Observational techniques have been particularly useful in assessing the extent to which self-report methods have provided valid data (Simons-Morton and Baranowski, 1991) and in assessing whether usual training provided to patients in clinics resulted in their having the skills necessary to perform the desired health maintaining behaviors (Manzella et al., 1989; Windsor, 1981; Windsor, Roseman, et al., 1981).

Focus Group Interviews

There has been a growing interest in using more qualitative methods in conducting evaluation (Patton, 1990; Steckler et al., 1992). The more quantitative methods (such as those presented to this point) are based on testing causal models of programs and behaviors, whereas the more subjective methods attempt to record subjective perceptions and understandings (Patton, 1990). Many evaluators are attempting to find ways to integrate qualitative and quantitative methods (Steckler et al., 1992). The utility of the focus group has been briefly discussed in Chapters 3 and 4.

One commonly used qualitative technique is the focus group interview method (Basch, 1987; Krueger, 1988; Sussman et al., 1991). In this method, an investigator convenes a group of usually 8 to 12 people representative of the population of interest and, using a detailed protocol of sequenced questions and probes, asks a series of questions and follows leads presented by the participants.

Focus groups allow an investigator to get more detailed information than is possible from other methods because the protocol is designed to ask open-ended in-depth questions, the interviewer can deviate from the protocol to follow up on points that arise in discussion, and multiple respondents are present who can stimulate one anothers' thoughts on the topic of discussion. The focus group method has been used

To qualitatively evaluate programs.

To develop questions for use in a questionnaire, when the investigator is entering an area about which little is known.

To review results from quantitative questionnaires to help interpret the results and give case examples.

To develop general ideas on methods for intervention to achieve a particular behavior change.

To develop or refine specific procedures for components of an intervention.

To develop ideas for use in media productions.

To evaluate early drafts of media productions.

The focus group method is particularly useful in generating a range of alternatives for consideration for inclusion in a questionnaire, in an intervention, or for whatever it is being used.

Weaknesses. There has been little quantitative evaluation of the focus group method (Sussman et al., 1991). The major advocates of focus groups (e.g., Krueger, 1988) recognize that one person can dominate the focus group, making it difficult to obtain the opinions and perceptions of all group members. Thus, a focus group must be considered a sample of one (instead of a sample of the number of members of the group). Reliability of estimation is a particular problem for focus group research. In the section on sample size estimation, we discussed that one or a small number of cases will not be enough to represent a population; in the section on sample selection, we discussed that a sample must be selected using some randomization procedure in order to be representative of a population. These same concepts apply to focus groups. If you need (by calculation) to conduct 100 interviews to estimate a quantity or relationship in a particular sample to generalize the findings to a larger population, then, in the worst-case situation, you may have to conduct 100 focus groups to obtain similar information. If an average of 10 people are involved per group, this is a sample of 1000 people. How many focus groups are necessary to reliably estimate different kinds of phenomena has not been investigated. Evaluators using focus groups, however, need to be concerned about this issue and must not assume that they have unbiased information after conducting 4 or 5 focus groups.

Because questions are not asked consistently across focus groups, the responses may reflect answers to substantially different questions. Sometimes the same questions are not even asked from group to group because the interviewer is following new important leads. Thus, tabulation of responses from focus groups cannot be accepted as estimates of prevalence and must be interpreted with caution.

The information from focus groups may be misleading. One focus group interview reveals that children like vegetables primarily under certain circumstances: when served raw with dips or when served with sauces as prepared in their homes (Baranowski, Domel, et al., 1993). However, data collected from the same children at a subsequent time on their preferences for fruits and vegetables reveal that the methods of preparation had little to do with preference—children like or do not like broccoli no matter how it is prepared (Domel, Baranowski, et al., in press). It is not clear whether children are not reliable reporters of preference information, the sample of focus groups was not large enough, or some group dynamic might account for these inconsistent results.

The skill of the interviewer in conducting focus groups in general and in dealing with a particular audience can be critical. For example, a professional highly experienced in conducting marketing-type focus groups with educated adult female consumers may not be able to elicit information on fruit and vegetable consumption with fifth grade students from a lower-income minority population.

In a quantitative experimental evaluation, Sussman et al. (1991) report that 31 focus groups with high school students reveal no more ideas for recruiting teenagers into a smoking-cessation clinic than does an open-ended prequestionnaire. The students became more convinced of the value of their original suggestions (a group polarization effect) and also were more willing to participate in such sessions, as a result of having participated in the focus groups. These results may be specific to high school students and/or the issue of recruitment to smoking-cessation clinics. It suggests that focus groups should be used as part of the intervention to commit students to participation in the ensuing intervention and not to elicit information.

Because of the limitations in focus group methods, data obtained from focus groups should be considered as suggestive, identifying a variety of possible answers to a research question, rather than as definitive data.

Steps in Conducting Focus Group Interviews. Focus groups appear to be most successful when the research team has a well-formulated idea of what it wants to learn, a detailed protocol for conducting the focus groups, and a realistic appreciation of what to expect from focus groups (i.e., the generation of possible alternatives for consideration). Table 7.8 lists the steps in developing and conducting focus group interviews.

Focus group interviews are a sophisticated technique requiring much planning and substantial resources. Because of the many potential biases in any group discussion, attention must be paid to overcoming these limitations and to conducting a sufficient number of focus group interviews to ensure that reliable information is obtained.

Table 7.8 Steps in Developing and Conducting Focus Group Interviews

1. Formulate a specific set of questions to be answered.
2. Formulate a detailed protocol to conduct the groups; these include media used to generate discussion, early self-completed questionnaire to generate initial thoughts on the topic, an explicit set of questions to be asked in sequence, and specific probes for each question to get at the underlying conceptual question.
3. Find and train an experienced focus group interviewer or provide training to someone facile in dealing with a particular group.
4. Find a friendly location in which participants can be comfortable, conversations recorded using audiotape or videotape, and refreshments provided.
5. Provide an incentive for coming and reminders of time and location.
6. Identify potential participants representative of the population of interest.
7. Conduct focus groups until no new information is elicited by additional groups.
8. Abstract information from the discussions in a valid and reliable manner.

Hopefully, more research such as that conducted by Sussman et al. (1991) will be conducted to clearly specify all the strengths and limits of the focus group method.

UNOBTRUSIVE MEASURES

Although interviewing, self-report, observation and focus group methods are very flexible and can tap a variety of data, they are also subject to many of the biases identified by Webb et al. (1966). The Webb team argued that, because every method of data collection is subject to one or more (often many) sources of bias, an investigator should use multiple methods. Select methods that are subject to different sources of error. If the same results are obtained despite differing sources of bias, investigators can be more confident that the sources of bias by themselves do not account for the results. This has been called *triangulation.* For example, if a school health education program promoting dietary change shows that participants reported eating fewer low-fat foods after completing the program, critics could object that the subjects in the study were only reporting what the investigators wanted to hear. If observational data also show that the subjects no longer enter a particular corner store that was frequently used and if physiological tests show a weight loss for these subjects, then skeptics would be harder pressed to question the evaluation conclusions.

There are several methods of collecting unobtrusive data. Under certain circumstances, each method is subject to the biases identified in Chapter 6. For example, if people completing medical records become aware that someone has started using these records to evaluate their performance, they may complete the forms in a self-protective and self-justifying way, thereby making the records a biased source of information. Similarly, hospital accounting records that contain total family income are probably biased downward on this variable because a lower report of income will often mean a lower or no charge for care. The unbiased character of any unobtrusive method is maintained only as long as people are not aware they are being studied and there is no other incentive for them to provide biased information. Several unobtrusive methods used in health research are reviewed next.

Abstraction of Existing Records: Medical and Clinical

Some investigators consider the medical record a readily available and accessible source of rich data at little cost. Imagine the millions of medical records across the country with millions of laboratory and physiological tests on a vast variety of health problems: a veritable gold mine but filled, perhaps, with fools' gold. There are very limited occasions when a medical record abstraction is appropriate and valuable. These occasions can be identified after listing the biases in record abstraction.

Strengths and Weaknesses. Entries are made in one or more medical records every time a patient receives care from a physician or other health care provider. This is an enormous quantity of data. If the health care provider or institution can be persuaded to share these records, the body of data becomes available for evaluative purposes. The primary cost is incurred by hiring staff to enter and abstract the desired data from all the data available.

There are, however, many limitations. Not every person receives medical care for a particular problem. Although some of the major barriers to care have been overcome in the United States and western Europe, study after study indicates that the poor and ethnic minority groups are less likely to receive care for a health problem than others. Differences in care are lower for painful acute problems (e.g., otitis media) and greater for less painful, more chronic conditions (e.g., hypertension). Thus, population restrictions for results of studies made of only those receiving care may be more or less severe depending on the topic of the study.

Because the evaluation team has little or no control over how much information gets recorded or over the quality of that recorded information, an enormous set of problems can arise. For example, in regard to restrictions on content, Ferber (1968) abstracted variables primarily related to medical care (information likely to be in the record) and avoided abstracting data related to health education or health promotion (which were much less likely to be in the record). He reports easy access to accurate information on a limited number of demographic variables (e.g., age, sex, hospital accommodation, marital status, and employment status but not occupation) and difficulties in abstracting every other type of information. Windsor, Roseman, et al. (1981), in conducting a retrospective medical record review of 996 diabetic patients, found that only 40% had a baseline assessment and only 6% a discharge behavioral assessment.

Feinstein (1970) explains the unreliability of medical record information by examining the three major purposes of maintaining a medical record: patient management, science, and legal concerns. In regard to patient management, Feinstein notes that physicians more frequently relied on their personal memory of a case than on the record. Thus, much clinically useful information is not recorded, and what gets recorded varies with the characteristics of the patient. Physicians also tend to record only "scientific" information, leaving "softer" (but clinically relevant) data out of the record. Physicians typically do not record, or do not consistently record, variables that are pertinent to someone else's study. The same variable may be recorded in several places in the medical record, and because medical records are not diligently updated, conflicting information on the same variable may appear in different locations in the record.

The way in which scientific facts are clinically obtained in medical practice does not reflect the compulsion and concern for replicability given to data collected for scientific research. In this light, even if the scientific data were systematically recorded, they would be of questionable accuracy for research. Few physicians maintain records for scientific reasons, and so replication is not important to them. Medical records, however, do provide evidence in cases of malpractice. If a physician is concerned about malpractice, the information in the medical record may be biased in the direction of protecting the physician from malpractice awards. How this affects any particular variable depends on the variable, the perceived probability that this item is related to malpractice litigation, and the direction of distortions necessary to protect the physician.

The stability of the content of medical records varies over time and across diseases and medical conditions. For example, the International Classification of Diseases (ICD) is a set of codes for major categories of causes of death and disability. Hospitals use several ICD codes in the planning of health services. Different hospitals use different ICD codes, creating variations in data among locations. Moreover, the ICD codes are periodically updated to reflect the latest medical knowledge. Data collected before and after code changes are therefore not directly comparable because the diagnostic criteria for making a particular judgment may have changed. Newly revised ICD codes may be employed earlier in one geographic area and later in others. These differences may preclude comparisons across geographic areas in a particular year or for several years or within an area across time periods. Related issues arise. As medical science advances, new diagnoses are made possible. Diagnoses that were impossible before this research become common. Increasing frequency of a new diagnosis may not reflect an increasing incidence but simply a new interpretation of a long-term problem. Fads also occur in the popularity of diagnoses. Certain diagnoses that are poorly defined and little used at one time become popular at others. Cases that are not clearly defined are more likely to be coded using the more popular disease categories. Any patient may have multiple medical problems; which medical diagnosis gets recorded? For example, was the major cause of this person's death the heart attack or the 20-year history of insulin-dependent diabetes mellitus? Informal convention on priority in the coding of multiple medical diagnoses will differ by time and geographic area, making comparisons difficult.

Another potentially major bias in using medical records for data abstraction is the guinea pig effect. If medical records are used over an extended period of time, physicians and others become aware of this use of the records and may attempt to change their recording behavior to protect themselves from criticism. This change in recording may bias the validity of a longitudinal evaluation based on medical record abstraction.

The dross rate in medical record data is high. Great quantities of information must be sifted to find the few variables of interest. Familiarity with the record and training can assist the abstracter in locating information efficiently. As more information is desired from the medical record, abstracters become less likely to adhere to the abstraction rules, and more inconsistencies become obvious. Only a limited number of variables can be obtained from medical records to describe the selected sample. Effectively done, record abstractions can be replicated.

Steps in Abstracting Medical Records. A medical record abstraction can be useful when demographic data and simple, commonly recorded medical data are desired and when attempts to control for reliability are made. One study that attempted to abstract relevant information on hypertensive patients in a family medicine clinic illustrates the steps required in conducting abstractions of medical records. Figure 7.4 presents a page from this study's abstraction form. Six different drafts of the form were developed. The first three were revised to reflect the purposes of the study more clearly as these purposes became more clearly defined through staff discussion. Reliability analyses were conducted on the next two drafts by having sets of two out of three abstracters jointly abstract 20 records. Reliability indices were calculated on the 20 jointly abstracted records for each variable, for each pair of abstracters. All cases in which differing values were obtained were intensively reviewed against the medical record, and rules were generated to refine the search or the recording process.

On the second set of reliability abstractions, rules for abstraction were further refined, and variables for which a reliability of abstraction of 0.75 or higher was not achieved were dropped from the study. The sixth draft was used for the final abstractions. Search and coding rules were printed on the abstraction form to make their use convenient. A limited set of demographic, commonly recorded, and more serious variables was finally obtained from the medical records. Less

```
10.  Date of last visit to clinic for      ☐☐       ☐☐        ☐☐
     any reason
     SOURCE: SOAP sheets.                   Month     Day        Year
                                          V22(2,53-54) V23(2,55-56) V24(2,57-58)


11.  Blood pressure most recently
     recorded (right justify)(prefer        ☐☐☐  /  ☐☐☐   mm Hg
     recording second sitting blood
     pressure.  If this is not avail-     v25(2,59-61)   v26(2,62-64)
     able, record lowest blood pressure
     of session.) Source: Blue SOAP sheets
     (Objective) or shingles

12.  Pulse rate (most recently recorded                ☐☐☐  beats/minute
     value if recorded in last six months)              V27(2,65-67)
     (right justify)

Priority among sources: 1. blue SOAP sheets (Objective)
                           or shingles
                        2. CV flow sheet

13.  Patient's weight (most recently recorded)
     (right justify)                                   ☐☐☐  lbs.
     Priority among sources: 1. blue SOAP sheets
                                or shingles            V28(2,68-70)
                             2. CV flow sheet

14.  Patient's height (right justify)

     Priority among sources: 1. physical exam sheet    ☐☐  inches
                             2. blue SOAP sheet or
                                shingles               V29(2,71-72)
                             3. dietary consult

15.  Most recent values on physiologic measures
        BUN (most recent value)
        To get most recent value,                      ☐☐☐  mg/100 ml
        all sources must be searched:
        1. Single value blood chemistry form           V30(2,73-75)
        2. 660 form
        3. 1260 form
        4. a report of laboratory values in
           blue SOAP sheets (Objective)
        5. hospital discharge summary
        6. CV flow sheets
        7. Old records
        (If multiple values are obtained for one day, take value in
        order of the above priority listing)
```

Figure 7.4 Sample Page from a Medical Record Abstraction Form

than half the variables originally desired were included in the final form. Particular attention was given to the development of rules for abstraction because Boyd et al. (1979) show that explicit criteria for abstractions can more than double the interabstracter reliability values.

Abstraction of Existing Records: Financial and Accounting

Financial records are also considered an attractive source of data because of their ready accessibility and availability. Accountants and others have spent many hours developing reliable systems for recording the income and outflow of money to and from organizations. All of the comments made about medical records potentially apply to financial or accounting records. There is one major difference, however. Data in financial or accounting systems tend to be more up-to-date and more reliable because of financial incentive. If a company or organization does not maintain accurate, up-to-date financial records, it cannot collect the money necessary to maintain itself. This is especially true for organizations dependent on fees for services (e.g., clinics); it is less true for organizations receiving grants, bequests, or contributions (e.g., voluntary health agencies). Despite the incentives for accurate records in agencies that rely on fees, a wide disparity still exists in the quality of financial records these agencies keep. (See Appendix C for data needed in cost studies.)

Other limitations exist in abstracting these records. Financial record systems rarely have extensive nonfinancial data. Names and addresses may be systematically recorded, but the rest of the information is often financial. This is a benefit if the primary concern of an evaluation is financial, for example, a cost–benefit or cost-effectiveness study; otherwise, it is a hindrance. Even when finances are the data of choice, abstracters may need special expertise to understand how the financial data are categorized, to locate the desired information, and to check and abstract the most appropriate data. Organizations may be reluctant to permit access to their financial records. Finally, if financial records from more than one organization are of interest, completely different coding systems may be (and often are) used by organizations using differing accounting systems because the recorded information is defined in a completely different manner. Thus, investigators must be careful in using financial records.

Clinical, or Physiological, Measures

Clinical, or physiological, measures are used in a variety of health education and promotion studies. In some cases, the physiological measure is the primary outcome measure—for example, blood pressure determinations as measures of effectiveness of programs to control high blood pressure. In other cases, physiological variables act as checks on the validity of self-reported measures—for example, serum thiocyanate level to validate smoking cessation. McNagny and Parker (1992), who report that 72% of men with a positive urinary assay of benzoylecgonine (a metabolite of cocaine) denied use of illegal drugs in the previous 3 days, highlight the importance of obtaining physiological validation of self-report information. In some studies, physiological variables reflect the subject's health status or disease risk, which may be affected by habitual behaviors. Examples include serum cholesterol, which may be affected by diet and exercise and is predictive of atherosclerosis, or a submaximal stress test, which measures physical fitness and should be affected by aerobic activity. The great attraction of physiological measures is that they are not obtrusive in the many senses that behavioral measures are: It is not obvious to subjects that they are being observed, and the measures are reactive only to the extent that they encourage people to perform the desired behaviors when they are aware of the values.

Despite the aura of complete objectivity of these "hard data" measures, they are subject to as many but different sources of error as the "soft data." For example, physiological indicators are often subject to daily, weekly, and other cycles in values. Recent studies of blood pressure, using continuous or frequent monitoring instruments, show marked variations between waking and sleeping hours, between mornings and evenings, between conversation times and times alone. Blood pressure readings taken in an office or clinic are roughly 10 mm Hg higher than those taken in the home. Blood pressures rise and fall in response to the person's emotional or arousal state. Thus, systematic bias may occur in a study from simply taking a blood pressure measurement at different times in the day or in different settings. Due to minute-to-minute variability, resting blood pressure readings should be taken three or four times over successive minutes to obtain reliable estimates of resting blood pressure, and diastolic blood pressure readings obtained by auscultation may not reflect true diastolic pressures as assessed by intra-arterial sensors (Moss and Adams, 1963).

Although physiological measures seem simple and straightforward to make, extensive detailed protocols have been developed for obtaining them, including (1) extended training procedures (for even well-credentialed individuals); (2) specification of the environmental conditions in which the measure is taken (e.g., blood pressure readings for a research project are typically taken in a well-lit room, with the sphygmomanometer at eye level, and with low environmental noise); (3) specification of the state of the subject (e.g., an individual who has fasted for 12 hours before a blood sample for serum cholesterol analysis is taken); (4) procedures for handling the specimen (if one was taken); (5) identification of the specific machine and how it should be run, periodically tested, and corrected; and (6) procedures for ongoing quality control of all elements of the data-collection process. A primary difference between physiological measures and the behavioral and self-report measures is that the many sources of error in physiological measures are often known and more amenable to control if highly structured procedures are compulsively employed.

Human and other errors can occur at every stage in the taking of physiological measurements. Medication compliance provides an interesting example. Biron (1975) notes that having enough medication flowing in a person's circulatory system to be effective in fighting a disease (a therapeutic plasma concentration) requires prescription of an adequate amount of medication for the size of the person's body or other personal characteristics, consumption of all the medication prescribed (patient compliance), and action by the body to make the medication available in the bloodstream as expected (bioavailability). Biron argues that most physicians do not know enough about pharmacotherapy to prescribe amounts that promote therapeutic bioavailability; there are severe problems in compliance, for many reasons; and there is high variability from person to person in how the body absorbs, metabolizes, and stores the same medication (Alvares et al., 1979). With regard to bioavailability, Biron (1975) also points out that a pharmaceutical company can make the same product within a relatively wide band of variation, some of which promote bioavailability of the product while others retard it. These are all potential sources of error prior to taking a blood sample to test for bioavailability of the drug. Plasma concentrations at less than a therapeutic level may therefore be due to factors other than patient compliance.

An important source of error that has come to light from doing multicenter studies is interlaboratory variability (Laboratory Standardization Panel, 1990; McShane et al., 1991). That is, even among high-quality laboratories where procedures are intensively followed, substantially different values can be obtained for the same samples. The most common procedure for handling this source of error variability is for a central quality control center to prepare several compounds with known, systematically controlled levels of the chemical of interest and to send samples of the compound to the participating laboratories. Based on the values obtained at each laboratory in comparison with the known values for each controlled compound, an adjustment value can be given to calibrate values obtained by the machine and procedures at each laboratory. This calibration must be done periodically to control for laboratory drift (similar to observer drift).

A variety of other errors can occur. The needle for taking a blood sample from a child may be too narrow, destroying many red blood cells and contaminating the serum sample. The blood sample may not be collected in an inappropriate test tube, leading to coagulation and destroying the sample for a particular analysis. The centrifuge for separating red blood cells from serum may not be functioning properly. These and a host of other errors should disabuse program evaluation staff of blind faith in the value of physiological measures. Furthermore, certain procedures for obtaining a physiological measure (e.g., obtaining a blood sample or making an X-ray film) pose health risks for the individual (e.g., infections arising from an improper blood-collecting technique or cancer arising from X-ray exposure) or sometimes to the staff (e.g., accumulated X-ray exposure or exposure to AIDS-containing body fluid samples). Health program evaluation staff must consider the issue of whether the importance of obtaining the physiological measure overrides the risk(s) to the individual and the staff.

Steps in Using Physiological Methods. The listing of the problems in implementing a physiological measure should not discourage program staff from selecting such a measure when it is appropriate. First, consult medical and other personnel (e.g., a clinical pharmacist) on the appropriateness of a particular measure to answer the question at hand. The measure should clearly validate some behavioral measure, be the primary outcome of concern, or be a health or risk indicator of primary concern.

Second, select (or develop) a protocol to monitor *all* phases of physiological data collection and processing. Almost all physiological measures that an evaluator may want to use have been used in other studies. The protocol that best meets the needs of the evaluative study should be employed.

Third, continually monitor data collection and processing for reliability to ensure that the same high-quality data are obtained throughout the project. Most protocols detail a set of quality control procedures. It should be clear from this discussion that collecting physiological variables can be a very expensive proposition, even aside from the substantial laboratory costs for actually conducting the tests.

TOTAL QUALITY CONTROL OF DATA COLLECTION

Cummings (1992) identifies four principles of quality control in food production. Paraphrased for evaluation data collection, these principles include the following:

1. The quality of data collected is higher with more consistency in the development and implementation of procedures for collecting it.

2. Continuously monitoring data collection provides the supervisor with an understanding of the process of data collection, points and times of failure, and opportunities for improving it.

3. Reliable methods function well, even in trying circumstances; use the most reliable methods appropriate to a study's purposes.

4. Provide evaluation data whose average quality is equal to that expected by those authorizing the evaluation.

Table 7.9 Steps in Total Quality Control of Data Collection

1. Select the instrument most appropriate to the particular need and targeted population; under only rare circumstances, create your own instrument.
2. Pretest the instrument with a subsample of the target population; for self-report data, test for understanding of items, difficulty of recall-report, offensiveness of items, and other sources of difficulty (e.g., interviewer embarrassment).
3. Select data collectors with prerequisite skills.
4. Train data collectors in specific procedures to some preset level of reliability; use modeling, role playing, "fish bowl," double interviewing, and reliability testing with feedback throughout training.
5. If a new instrument has been developed or an old instrument has been modified; identify a representative sample of the target population; collect data under circumstances as if in major study; recollect same data within 1–4 weeks (to assess test–retest reliability); collect other variables with which the target variables should be related (to assess construct validity); estimate reliability and validity from collected data; if reliability and validity are unacceptable (e.g., less than .8 reliability), revise the instrument and reconduct the reliability and validity study; and if reliability and validity are acceptably high, find a way to abbreviate data collection to reduce participant burden, yet collect acceptable quality data.
6. If using a validated instrument, devise an environment for optimal data collection and continuously monitor consistency (e.g., on a 10% subsample), including assessing interobserver or test–retest reliability, checking consistency daily, and retraining data collectors if reliability falls below a preset level.
7. Assess coding or transcription reliability.
8. Once data are fully collected, estimate reliability and validity of the data collected and include them in the report.

Consistent with these quality control guidelines, Table 7.9 gives the general procedures for total quality control of evaluation data collection.

The ideal health promotion and education program evaluator will have a certain level of compulsion in following consistent, thorough procedures for the design, development, and preliminary testing of instruments and in attaining consistency among data collectors. Data-collection procedures must be continuously monitored using appropriate reliability checks to ensure that levels of consistency are maintained throughout data collection. All data-collection efforts encounter trying circumstances. The more reliable methods are more likely to withstand the difficulties and produce higher-quality data. People authorizing an evaluation are usually expecting high quality from the data collection; thus, high-quality methods should be used to collect that data. If high-quality data are not expected, then perhaps the evaluation shouldn't be done.

SUMMARY

The issues in selecting and developing methods are complex. Each method is susceptible to various threats to reliability and validity. Although many of these threats can be overcome, they are overcome at a cost. The job of the evaluator is to select and develop the most reliable and valid methods and instruments appropriate to the issues at hand, within the funding and other resources available.

A common distinction is made between obtrusive and unobtrusive measurement techniques. Unobtrusive measures are often desired because reactive bias is less likely to appear in these data. Under certain circumstances, however, even the measures that seem most unobtrusive can become obtrusive. Furthermore, unobtrusive measures are not always appropriate for collecting the type of information needed in a particular evaluation. The evaluator must be sensitive to bias issues in every evaluation conducted and must select and employ the most appropriate measurement methods.

Many skills are involved at each stage in selecting and developing methods and instruments. The novice evaluator should not become intimidated or discouraged. Despite the collective skills and intelligence of teams of evaluators, anticipated and unanticipated problems occur in the best of evaluative studies. No evaluative (or other) study has been perfect. Novice evaluators should, instead, have a realistic respect for the problems likely to be encountered, build their skills to the maximum possible, and involve consultants knowledgeable in the particular type of evaluation contemplated. The best way to learn these skills is to participate in the selection and development of methods under the supervision of others already skilled in these tasks. To build their skills, aspiring evaluators should seek professionals conducting program evaluations and volunteer or otherwise participate in these activities.

8

Simple Methods to Analyze Program Data

"The results are significant, but how do we explain that?"

"First they ask me for an evaluation; now they tell me to skip the details."

"It has taken me six months to evaluate this project, and they simply do what they want!"

"Detailed evaluations often rise in emotional appeal as they decline in intellectual clarity."

Professional Competencies Emphasized in This Chapter

• Specifying types of data

• Presenting data

• Describing and comprehending descriptive statistics

• Differentiating among selected types of distributions

• Selecting analytic methods

• Applying analytic methods

One of the world's greatest statisticians, Sir Ronald Alymer Fisher, hated mathematical nitpicking. What made Fisher so great was his intuition and insight into problems. For many health evaluators, *statistics* is a word suitable for use only at night with a full moon on Halloween—it's scary! In this chapter, we focus on statistics as a tool of intuition and insight for persons involved in health education and promotion programs, not for mathematical nitpicking. This is a difficult task. Mathematics is the one area of scholastic performance in which people are comfortable admitting failure. Health workers are not afraid to say, "I haven't had math since algebra, and I failed that." Unfortunately, admission or submission to failure at the outset will prevent the absorption of these valuable tools.

Those who suffer from learned helplessness should not read this chapter. What will follow may surprise you as you read. Learning about statistics is similar to evaluating a nutrition program in rural Mexico—you must understand the language before you can get at the concepts. The notation and jargon get easier and are an insufficient reason to skip this chapter. But do not lose the forest for the trees. The concepts are the meat; the jargon and notation are the mathematical nitpicking. The chapter has been written with the assumption that you have taken an elementary statistics course. This is not a necessity for the earlier portions of the chapter, but it is an asset in the more detailed treatment of statistical methods in the latter portions.

This chapter covers a large amount of information used in dealing with the analysis of program data. It is not intended to be a statistical text on these topics. Numerous texts exist; repeating them would require far more than a single chapter. Our basic notion is to give you access to various statistical texts, so that these techniques can be understood and applied with the full complement of discussion provided in the array of books available.

The important concepts in evaluation are the *appropriate classification of the design* and the *type of study* used. The use of statistical tools is a means, not an end. The importance of statistics as a tool cannot be overemphasized, but the achievement of statistical significance does not imply, in and of itself, that an intervention has been successful. You must ask a series of additional questions to support statistical techniques for a full analysis of the data. Keep in mind that the simple techniques for analyses are (1) understanding of the problem and (2) careful and unbiased assessment of the results obtained.

THE EVALUATOR AS A CONSUMER

The title of this chapter promotes the notion that you as an evaluator can apply simple methods to program data and obtain sufficient information to shed an objective light on the value of a health education and promotion program. To do this, you must first become a competent consumer of other evaluations. Experience is an excellent teacher. The more you are involved in evaluations and face the difficult decisions, fatal flaws, competing demands, and critical problems identified in other evaluations, the more efficiently you can perform as a creator and provider of results.

To be a competent consumer, you should become aware of the key issues in presenting information in evaluation reports. (Appendix A gives you guidance about how to prepare an evaluation report.) Some evaluations consist of nothing more than verbal testimonials on the efficacy of a program. We will not consider such statements of faith in this chapter. Although potentially meaningful and of some value, they cannot generally be used in an objective manner. The purpose of an evaluation and of statistical methods for analyzing program data is to assist the decision-making process. Analysis should be done in an unbiased manner, void of the interpersonal issues that come into play after the information is presented. Virtually every tool that is useful in making this kind of objective decision can be summarized in some numerical form. The tool may be nothing more than a simple count of qualitative findings.

TYPES OF DATA

Given the numerical representation of data, several key questions must be asked. The first is, What do these data represent? It is important to recognize which numerical class the data fall into because analytic methods are often restricted to one class of information. There are generally three classes of data representation.

Nominal, or *naming*, *data* refer to arbitrarily labeled characteristics such as male-female, black-white, infant-child-adolescent-adult, or numbers on a football jersey.

Numerical data consist of two subclasses—discrete and continuous data. *Discrete data* can be placed on an integer scale, such as the numbers 1, 2, 3. Often these data relate to counts or frequencies. *Continuous data* are numerical measures that can be measured to infinitely fine degrees, provided greater measurement capabilities exist. For example, weight is a continuous measure; you can measure it not only in kilograms or grams but also in milligrams or even finer increments (nanogram—parts per million), if such measurements are deemed appropriate and technically feasible.

The third class is *ordinal data*, a combination of nominal and numerical data. Ordinal data give arbitrarily labeled information, such as low, medium, or high. Corresponding to this labeling is an underlying numerical scale. Thus, if investigators talk about low-risk, medium-risk, and high-risk individuals with regard to serum cholesterol levels, they assume that the low-risk individuals have, by definition, lower cholesterol levels in actual, measured numerical values than medium- or high-risk persons. Nominal and ordinal data are both subsets of a class called *categorical data.*

ACCURACY AND PRECISION

As noted in Chapters 6 and 7, once you have identified the type of data, you must examine the degree of accuracy and precision with which the measurements have been made. *Accuracy* is the measurement of explicitly what is present, and *precision* is the ability to obtain the same results each time the same object is measured. Accurate measurements need not be precise, and precise measurements need not be accurate. Accuracy is analogous to validity, and precision is the same as reliability. The additional jargon has arisen from the fact that research involving health educators is often multidisciplinary. It is common to have the terms *accuracy* and *precision* used interchangeably with *validity* and *reliability*. However, the latter terms are used almost exclusively when discussing behavioral instruments; the former are often found in the laboratory.

When a measurement is accurate but not precise, the evaluator's confidence dwindles. When a measurement is precise but not accurate, the evaluator attempts to identify the extent of inaccuracy and adjust for it. If you were surveying a population and asked people their weight, generally they underestimate it. Although people are fairly precise, the extent of their consistent underestimate would be the inaccuracy.

The term *bias* is used to describe a measure of inaccuracy. A very precise measurement can be biased. When the bias is known, this presents no problem. One of the major problems in evaluation is unrecognized bias. To detect such bias, it is imperative to have a clear, explicit explanation of how the data were measured. As noted in Chapters 6 and 7, a danger of bias may exist in the instruments, in their application, or in the recording or transfer of data. It might result from the biases of the interviewers or the biased responses of those being interviewed. Investigators must ask how these individuals were recruited and the data acquired. Questions must be asked perpetually to uncover and assess the underlying information.

Some settings in health promotion and education may not lend themselves to random selection of program participants. When your program participants are volunteers, you cannot ignore the population segments you are not measuring. As noted in Chapter 5 (causation), you must think about and anticipate how measurement of the group excluded from your analyses would alter the data and findings you observed.

You must also ask, are there any logical structures present in the data that bias or limit application of the results? For example, are the responses independent of one another? Are the measurements taken on the same individual before and after an intervention or on two unrelated, independent samples? If you interview all persons in the same household, does the fact that they live together make their responses more alike? You must also ask questions about these more subtle distinctions. If you are providing a family intervention, the unit of analysis is actually the family, not the individual. You must then be cautious in analyzing data by individuals because the response within a family is likely to be related—a person is more likely to respond the way another family member does than the way a person from a different family does. This violates an important assumption of the statistical procedures used to analyze individual data. In essence, if these questions are neglected, you may end up with statistical analyses that look like textbook examples but are misleading.

READING TABLES

As a consumer of evaluations, you need to know how to get the most out of tables, graphs, and figures. Also, with the availability of computer graphics, be careful in what you are viewing.

A table usually consists of rows and columns of numbers or other items. Graphs and charts are pictorial representations of numbers. Graphs usually use lines to connect points on X and Y axes or bars showing frequencies. Charts usually display data in circles (pie charts) or by size and shape. The distinctions are not universal and usually are unimportant. Developing the ability to extract information from tables, graphs, and charts is essential to good evaluators. Similarly, they must be capable of organizing information properly in tables, graphs, and figures. The key to tabular presentation of data is a properly constructed, adequately labeled table that can be read and understood without consulting the accompanying text.

Table 8.1, for example, tells a reasonably complete story. The title states that the body of the table will contain counts—the number of new users of cervical cancer screening clinics by year for five Alabama counties. The footnote explains that in Wilcox County in 1977 the clinic was not in operation; therefore, no data could be obtained for that cell of the table. The asterisk conveys more than would a zero. The use of a zero would be acceptable and accurate coupled with an asterisk to explain why. At the top of the table, the column headings under "Year of Initial Visit" identify the year in which the new users first came to the screening clinics. The left-hand (or stub) column lists five counties in Alabama. Knowing these facts, readers can identify any number in the table. The number 90, for example, represents the number of new users of the screening program in Sumter County in 1979. The number 96 represents the number of new users in Marengo County in either 1978 or 1980. The total on the row or column is called the *margin*. Margins provide summaries and are often used to provide information on overall trends. The table is the basis of the spreadsheet programs widely used on personal computers. These

Table 8.1 Number of New Users of Cervical Cancer Screening Clinics by Year for Five Alabama Counties

	Year of Initial Visit				
County	1977	1978	1979	1980	Total
Hale	63	60	135	94	352
Marengo	250	96	140	96	582
Perry	61	66	41	42	210
Sumter	79	51	90	87	307
Wilcox	*	44	33	54	131
Total	453	317	439	373	1582

*Clinic not in operation.

programs offer a general approach to creating, manipulating, and displaying data.

All too often, individuals read the text of a document and ignore the information provided in the tables. Ignoring the tables is unwise. Tables, graphs, and charts are normally provided to highlight the important points presented. Thus, you should be able to gain as much from them or more than from the verbiage put forth by the authors. In addition, your interpretive ability will enable you to reach a conclusion about the information presented in tables and graphs without the bias of the author's opinion. This does not mean that you should not read the articles, but scan the tables and figures first. Then, when the author presents a point, you are armed with the author's data to decide whether his or her interpretation seems reasonable or is merely a "beauty in the eye of the beholder" statement.

RULES FOR CONSTRUCTING TABLES, GRAPHS, AND CHARTS

There are several general rules to follow in the construction of tables, graphs, and charts. For tables:

1. Divide the data into categories.

2. Label the axes carefully and include footnotes if necessary.

3. Provide an accurate and descriptive title.

4. Include totals of rows and columns.

5. Do not clutter the display with too much data.

6. Try several displays to see which conveys your best primary message.

Regardless of the type of data (nominal, numerical, or ordinal), establishing categories can be a confusing task. Consider the data in Table 8.2 on blood pressure measurements of 20 people. Looking at the 20 diastolic blood pressure readings in this table does not immediately convey a message to you. If 2000 people were screened, the display of individual data would be prohibitive. An alternative is to group the data into summary categories.

The majority of categorizing problems come from numerical data. When presenting numerical data in tabular form, you need to group the data into numerical categories called *classes*. A class is a grouping of common characteristics. You want to create neither too many classes nor too few. Having too many classes makes the tabular presentation not very different from looking at the *raw* (uncategorized) data themselves; having too few classes does not provide enough dif-

Table 8.2 Diastolic Blood Pressure

Person No.	Diastolic Blood Pressure (mm Hg)
1	62
2	93
3	73
4	60
5	70
6	78
7	70
8	94
9	66
10	107
11	97
12	88
13	70
14	64
15	63
16	72
17	61
18	70
19	80
20	76

ference to detect the pattern of responses in the raw data. Table 8.3 summarizes the raw data on blood pressure readings into four classes: the number of persons with diastolic blood pressure between 50–64 mm Hg, 65–79 mm Hg, 80–94 mm Hg, and 95–109 mm Hg. From this table, you can better understand a pattern in the data. The greatest number of observations, 9 out of 20, is in the class 65–79 mm Hg. About equal numbers fell in the 50–64 mm Hg and 80–94 mm Hg classes, and two were over 95 mm Hg. Many desktop computer software programs will enable the creation of these tables, but the choice of intervals should be based as much as possible on a rational basis. In this example, the intervals were chosen to correspond to hypertensive levels (>95 mm Hg), borderline levels (80–94 mm Hg), normal levels (65–79 mm Hg), and low blood pressure (<65 mm Hg).

Tables often show what is called the *relative frequency*. This is nothing more than the percentage or proportion of all the observations in the table in a specific class. For example, in Table 8.3, 45.0% (9 out of 20) were in the 65–79 mm Hg class. In general, we want at

Table 8.3 Diastolic Blood Pressure Groups of 20 Subjects Screened

Diastolic Blood Pressure Group (mm Hg)	Frequency	Relative Frequency
50–64	5	25.0
65–79	9	45.0
80–94	4	20.0
95–109	2	10.0
Total	20	100.0

least 5 cases per class and a maximum of approximately 10 classes. There can be as many as 20 classes for some continuous data and as few as 2 or 3 for certain nominal responses. The actual number of categories may also depend on the number of observations and the categories used in published literature. Categorical responses generally follow the nomenclature associated with the nominal or ordinal data.

A second criterion is that the limits for each class should agree with the precision of measurement of the raw data. Thus, if weight is measured to the nearest tenth of a kilogram, the class limits should not be in terms of the nearest hundredth kilogram. Intervals should be chosen that are of equal width. This facilitates comparison, is not misleading to the reader, and makes other calculations and computations easier. It is important that class intervals not overlap; classes must be mutually exclusive. Thus, age intervals of 25–35 and 35–45 are not mutually exclusive, for an individual who is 35 years old would not clearly reside in one interval or the other. Open-ended intervals should be avoided, although in many publications they occur very naturally. A common example is the class of persons 65 years of age or older. This creates difficulties in summarizing the data and inhibits maximum use of the results from the table.

Tables should be clearly labeled. The title should describe the body of the table and the characteristics in the table. Totals should be noted in tables. If proportions or percentages are shown, the denominator should be clearly identified in either the column headings or the title. When there is possible uncertainty about the units of measurement, the units should be clearly identified in the body of the table. Extremely complicated or complex tables should be avoided, even though they tend to save space in an article or report. Tables should be simple and clear enough so they do not require excessive time to read.

Graphic techniques for displaying data, such as charts, are com-

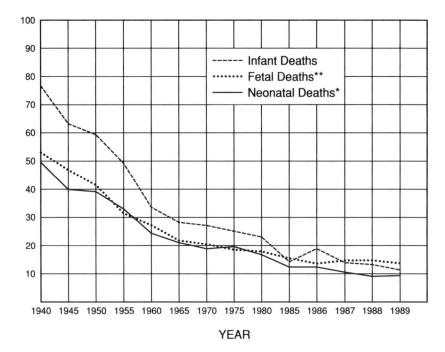

YEAR

*Rate per 1000 Live Births
**Ratio per 1000 Live Births

Figure 8.1 Trends in Fetal, Infant, and Neonatal Mortality, Jefferson County, 1940–1990
SOURCE: Jefferson County Department of Health, Bureau of Health Statistics and Vital Records, *1989 Annual Report* (Birmingham, Ala.: Jefferson County Department of Health, 1990), Figure 5.

monly used and follow many of the same rules of thumb as tables. *Histograms*, commonly called *bar graphs*, are reasonably straightforward and, like nearly all the techniques discussed in this chapter, can be found in any elementary textbook on statistics or computer program. *Line graphs, frequency polygons,* and the like are pictorial ways to present data. Such pictures must be proportional in size to the actual numbers they represent, so that the data are not distorted by appearance and do not cause misinterpretations of the results. In creating graphs and charts, it is exceedingly important to label the scales, space the scales appropriately (often equally), and make the intervals on the axes consistent.

All evaluators, at one time or another, need to read or create tables, graphs, and charts. The importance of characterizing them correctly should be clear from this brief discussion. Consider Figure 8.1. This line graph of infant, fetal, and neonatal deaths has several deficiencies, although it is well labeled in terms of a title, a legend, and appropriate footnotes. The unlabeled Y axis is not clearly delineated via the legend but could appear on the axis as "Per 1000 Live

Births." The X axis, the year, gives an improper pictorial representation. Looking at it casually, you might draw the conclusion that little reduction of mortality has come from the efforts put forth by the health department and others in recent years. Administrators might use this graph to argue that additional money should not be spent on fetal and infant death. They might maintain the status quo because the pattern has bottomed out. This is a misinterpretation. Looking closely at the X axis, you would see that the spacing of 5-year intervals between 1940 and 1985 is the same as the spacing of 1-year intervals between 1985 and 1990. An accurately drawn figure would show the 1990 data in the spot where the 1986 data appear. Completing the curve on that scale demonstrates a continued downward trend not inconsistent with the prior data. The mislabeled plot of 1986–1990 demonstrates the variability in the yearly rates and gives the appearance of a change in the rate of decline, but this is a visual change rather than a mathematical one. This type of problem is frequently encountered when using readily available computer graphics software.

DESCRIPTIVE STATISTICS

Many of the methods we describe in this chapter we assume are familiar to you. We will highlight them without elaborate discussion and provide a laundry list of tools to use in various circumstances. Our goal is to try to motivate you to use more of the tools in specific circumstances, not to provide a detailed understanding of these statistical tools. For readers lacking an understanding of the tools provided, we recommend any elementary statistics book. The material outlined in this chapter combines two semester courses in statistics.

Summary Counts

Program data have attributes that can be summarized in several ways. Frequency data constitute one of the most common summaries found in program analyses. Many interventions are designed to bring people into programs, keep them in the programs, and encourage them to take certain actions. Each purpose lends itself to measurement of the number of individuals who take a particular action. This counting, often called *pigeon counting*, is a descriptive statistic that represents the volume in a program. Although numbers of people attending represent achievements, it is as important to count nonusers. Count data frequently appear that attest to the success of a program without giving any notion of the eligible population pool. Lack of descriptive information about the available population gives an inadequate summary for count data. Methods for count data are described later in the chapter. Analytic methods to assess differences among various sub-groups of count data for certain program decisions are discussed below. However, major issues with count data are whether the counts are adequate and whether they meet the purposes of the evaluation.

Summary Location (Central Tendency) Measures

Continuous data commonly measured as part of community health programs include items such as age, weight, height, blood pressure, income, improvement in cognitive score, a behavioral questionnaire score, etc. Two useful summary indicators in describing such information are a measure of summary location (central tendency) and a measure of spread or variation. The concept of a summary location measure is the familiar representation of numerous situations by a single experience, a sort of average of what happened. Measures of location, often called *averages,* are the mean, the median, and the mode.

Mean. The *mean* is the arithmetic average for a series of observations. It is the sum of the observations divided by the sample size.

$$\text{Important Formula: Mean}$$

$$\bar{x} = \frac{\sum\limits_{i=1}^{n} x_i}{n}$$

This formula uses several important notations. The bar(–) above the x is used almost uniformly to represent a sample mean. The Σ is a standard symbol to represent the addition of a series of numbers. The numbers are represented by the subscripted letters x_i, and the notation $i = 1$ indicates that x_1 corresponds to the first number, x_2 to the second, and so on. The letter chosen is arbitrary; it could be y_i, z_i, or any other letter of your choosing. Thus,

$$\sum_{i=1}^{3} x_i = x_1 + x_2 + x_3$$

If we had 200 numbers, then

$$\sum_{i=1}^{200} x_i = x_1 + x_2 + \cdots + x_{200}$$

The notation $+ \cdots +$ means to continue adding in sequence until x_{200}.

Consider the diastolic blood pressures shown in Table 8.2. The mean of these blood pressures is

$$\bar{x} = \frac{\sum\limits_{i=1}^{20} x_i}{20} = \frac{62 + 93 + 73 + 60 + \cdots + 76}{20} = \frac{1514}{20} = 75.70$$

This implies that the average diastolic blood pressure value is 75.70 mm Hg. This mean value may or may not be equal to the true value; you rarely will measure everyone to determine it exactly. Usually there is only a subset, a sample, from which you estimate the mean. A statistical convention is to use Greek alphabet letters for true values and Latin alphabet letters for estimates, that is, μ and $\bar{x}$ for the true mean and sample mean, respectively.

The arithmetic mean is the point where, if the data were placed on a number line, you could pick up that number line and have it balance. It is the equivalent of a fulcrum for a teeter-totter. The observations are the weights of the individuals sitting on this teeter-totter, and the fulcrum is the mean. The arithmetic mean has a number of very powerful mathematical properties that make it a very common and important measure of central tendency.

For evaluators to talk about the average blood pressure in a community before and after an intervention is an important, reasonable, commonsense descriptor. The mean, however, can suffer certain deficiencies as measure of central tendency. Its major disadvantage is that it is seriously affected by extreme values. For example, suppose you are describing the average income of the individuals who attended a particular meeting. Five individuals were present whose incomes were $34,000, $25,000, $28,000, $30,000, and $74,000. Using the mean as the measure of central tendency, the average income was $38,000. However, only one of the five individuals had an income greater than $38,000. This mean gives an impression of a wealthier group than on the whole was present. The single aberrant income, $74,000, has distorted the representation of this group by the mean.

Median. A measure less sensitive to extreme observations is often used as a competitor or in conjunction with the arithmetic average. It is known as the *median* and is defined as the middlemost observation (50th percentile). The median is the observation above which half of the observations occur and below which half of the observations occur. It is not as mathematically powerful as the arithmetic average, although there is increasing interest in it among theoretical statisticians, facilitating increased understanding of the median's properties. As a measure of central tendency, the median is unaffected by extremes. Consider the income example: the mean was $38,000, but the median is $30,000. The median is often used for data such as income or serum cholesterol and glucose levels, where there is *skewness*—a stretching out of the observed results in one direction compared to the other. The mean and median are the same in certain situations, but when skewness is present, they are different. This fact can be useful because a comparison of arithmetic average to the median can identify skewness, which might be important in interpretation and evaluation.

Mode. The last measure of central tendency is called the *mode*, the value that occurs most frequently. Sometimes it is important in evaluation to cite the most commonly occurring point. The mode is rarely encountered as a descriptive measure in the scientific literature and almost never is used in statistical procedures, but it does occur in evaluation research. The mode may be used to point out the peak times at a clinic or the most important day of the week in a program or clinic operation. It is frequently used where ordinal or time-dependent data are found.

Measures of Variation

The mean and the median are by themselves or together not sufficient. They do summarize masses of data into a single number that can be presented as a representative value for an entire group. However, as a single figure, they do not provide enough information for all situations. Consider the following sets of numbers: 10, 20, 30, 40, 50 and 28, 29, 30, 31, 32. Both sets of numbers have the same median, 30, and mean, 30. If these were income figures (in thousands of dollars) for two groups and the evaluation report cited the average income of $30,000 for each group, investigators might erroneously surmise on that basis that the two groups were the same. The five people whose incomes range from $10,000 to $50,000 are likely to be far more diverse in background, education, interests, employment, social standing, and the like, than the other group of five, which is economically more homogeneous. Although the means and the medians are the same, the actual data on the two groups clearly convey some sense of difference. To accommodate this apparent failure of the location summary statistics, various measures of spread or variation are often used.

Range. The first and the simplest measure of variation is the *range*, which is defined as the highest value minus the lowest value. Thus, the range for the two income groups would have been $40,000 for the first and $4000 for the second. Reporting the descriptive statistic of a mean income of $30,000, with a range of $40,000, and a mean income of $30,000, with a range of $4000, provides clear summary information. The summary represents the differences that appear in the numbers and does so in the simplified form of two statistics.

Although many individuals think that the range consists of the lowest and highest observations (e.g., the range is from 10 to 50 or 28 to 32), technically this is not correct. The range by definition is a measure of spread, the difference between highest and lowest observations. The main drawback to the range is that it is heavily influenced by the extreme values. It has the further drawback of ignoring all the information in the sample except for two observations, whether there are 1000 or 10 individuals in the sample. This lack of utilization of the data bothered statisticians, and they searched for a measure that could be used to represent a population and utilize all of the data.

Variance and Standard Deviation. The first choice of a measure to replace the range might seem to be the average deviation from the mean. This represents, on average, how far people were from the central value. Following this logic, you would compute the difference between each observation and the overall mean. Then you would add these differences and divide by the number of observations to arrive at an average deviation from the mean. This is a reasonable measure, but it has one drawback: Because the mean is the point at which all the numerical values of the observations balance, it is also the point at which all positive and negative deviations balance, and adding the deviations together must result in zero.

To get around this problem of the average deviation being zero, statisticians use various approaches. If all deviations are measured in *positive* units and then averaged, this summary measure describes an average deviation. Such a measure ignores whether the deviation is above or below the mean, and it is called the *mean deviation*. The mean deviation has its limitations—it takes the absolute value of the deviation, ignoring the sign of the difference. The mathematical problems associated with that approach are numerous.

Another simple solution has been found. You can take the square of the difference between an observation and the mean, add these squared deviations from the mean, and divide the sum of the squares by the sample size. This quantity is an estimate of what is known as the population *variance*. Variance is an esoteric term that means nothing more than the average squared deviation from the mean. Certain mathematical properties are present in this statistic that make it attractive to mathematicians and statisticians.

What becomes confusing to most individuals when using this as a summary statistic is the denominator, which is a little more complicated than simply sample size. Statisticians found that dividing by the sample size produced a variance slightly smaller than they expected. Discussion of this phenomenon can be found in any statistics book. The solution is simple. The common quantity used to estimate the variance is the sum of the squares divided by the sample size minus one.

Important Formula: Sample Variance

$$S^2 = \frac{\sum\limits_{i=1}^{n}(x_i - \bar{x})^2}{(n - 1)}$$

Again, consider the blood pressure example of Table 8.2. Following the formula exactly, we would obtain

$$S^2 = \frac{\sum\limits_{i=1}^{20}(x_i - \bar{x})^2}{(20 - 1)} = \frac{\sum\limits_{i=1}^{20}(x_i - 75.70)^2}{19}$$

Remember that $\bar{x}$ was found to be 75.70. Then, continuing to insert the values from the table into the equation,

$$S^2 = \frac{(62 - 75.70)^2 + (93 - 75.70)^2 + \cdots + (76 - 75.70)^2}{19}$$

$$= \frac{(-13.70)^2 + (17.30)^2 + \cdots + (0.30)^2}{19}$$

$$= \frac{187.69 + 299.29 + \cdots + 0.09}{19} = \frac{3436.20}{19} = 180.85$$

Although this formula is correct, it is cumbersome. It requires computing the mean first and then the variance. This is not efficient. Computers and calculators can generate the mean and variance from a single entry of each data item. Using elementary algebra, the formula for S^2 can be rewritten as shown below.

Important Formula: Computing Formula for Sample Variance

$$S^2 = \frac{n\Sigma x_i^2 - (\Sigma x_i)^2}{n(n-1)}$$

This requires only adding the numbers and adding the numbers squared, yielding the exact same result as the previous formula but in one pass through the data.

A conceptual problem in utilizing the variance is that, for presentation and interpretation purposes, explaining the variance to an audience is a difficult task. For the previous income examples, the variance of the five persons with incomes of $10,000 through $50,000 is $250,000,000. This figure is not only overwhelming but also incomprehensible in terms of meaning. For the second group, the variance is $2,500,000. The difficulty arises because variance is computed in units squared, and most people are not trained to think in terms of squared units. Thus, a simple solution, if the units are squared, is to take the square root of the quantity. This gives a number that is in the same unit as the raw information. Taking the square root provides an estimate of the average deviation from the mean obtained from the average squared deviation from the mean. This measure is known as the *standard deviation*. The standard deviation for the income example is $15,811.39 for the first group and $1581.14 for the second. This measure of variation is now represented in the units of dollars and is interpretable directly in relation to the raw data.

A common way to present results is to give the mean plus or minus the standard deviation. For example, to report the income example, you might show that the average income of the first group was $30,000 ± $15,811.39 and of the second was $30,000 ± $1581.14. A rule of thumb for the number of decimal places is that the mean and standard deviation usually carry one decimal place more than the raw data. This is generally done. If you are reporting on blood pressure, you would talk about a mean of, say, 80.5 mm Hg because the measurements of blood pressure are in full integers. Income means and deviations are usually given in customary figures, however. A standard deviation of $1581.1 is not used; one more decimal place, $1581.14, would be used to match the customary unit, dollars and cents.

Standard Error of the Mean. The literature often reports another statistic, the *standard error of the mean* (SEM or SE). This is a measure related to the standard deviation and the sample size.

Important Formula: Standard Error of the Mean

$$\text{SE} = \frac{S}{\sqrt{n}} = \frac{\sqrt{\sum_{i=1}^{n}(x_i - \bar{x})^2/(n-1)}}{\sqrt{n}} = \frac{\sqrt{\sum_{i=1}^{n}(x_i - \bar{x})^2}}{n(n-1)}$$

Important Formula: Computing Formula for Standard Error

$$\text{SE} = \frac{\sqrt{n\sum_{i=1}^{n}x_i^2 - (\sum_{i=1}^{n}x)^2}}{n^2(n-1)}$$

When reading the literature, you must be careful to note whether the author has presented the mean plus or minus the standard error or the mean plus or minus the standard deviation. Vastly different meanings and conclusions can be drawn depending on which of these quantities was used. Certain rules of thumb apply to the mean plus or minus the standard deviation. It is known for some common situations that the mean ± 1 standard deviation generally encompasses 66⅔% of the observations, the mean ± 2 standard deviations roughly encompasses 95% of the observations, and the mean ± 3 standard deviations encompasses virtually 100% of the observations from most unimodal and symmetric distributions. This approach provides not only a summary measure of location and the overall variability of the population but also where and how far the sample of values extends.

You must be clear, in an evaluation, that the sources of variation can be identified. Some sources of variation relate directly to the outcome. Any one observation will have some deviation from its mean. This is a natural sampling phenomenon. Other sources of variation can be measurement effects, testing effects, and even temporal effects. The various sources of variation provide interesting information and insights into the evaluation process. When you gain experience in perceiving means, variances, and standard deviations, your understanding of the extent and potential sources of variability can give you keen insight into programmatic considerations that can be useful in evaluations.

DISTRIBUTIONS

A *distribution* is a series of counts or measurements. The numbers in a distribution are called *variates.* Frequently, the term *distribution* is used to imply a set of measurements, such as the distribution of weights, blood pressures, cholesterol levels, or educational levels. Often the manner of presenting data as a distribution is in an ordered fashion, such as the frequency of measurements of various blood pressures. At other times, the term *distribution* is used as a theoretical concept: what the data would look like ideally if an underlying mathematical model were true. The mathematical representations permit computations of probabilities, average values, and variances. In any mathematical distribution, the sum of all the probabilities equals 1.

Binomial Distribution

In program evaluations, individuals are commonly characterized as successful or unsuccessful. Persons may attend, comply with their medical regimen, or not comply. When evaluators look at the total group, they often are interested in characterizing the number of successes and failures. A simplified mathematical model of this is called the *binomial distribution*.

The binomial distribution characterizes situations in which a number (n) of independent attempts or trials are conducted with only two possible outcomes. The outcomes are arbitrarily called *success* and *failure*. For example, suppose you invite five people at random to a health education training program, and the probability (the relative frequency of occurrence) that a person will attend the meeting is .60, the same for all persons. You can compute, in advance, the chance that all five persons will attend. Using the assumption that each person is independent (i.e., no peer pressure to avoid or come), the chance of all of them attending is the product of the individual chances:

$$\text{Probability—all will attend} = (.60)(.60)(.60)(.60)(.60)$$
$$= .078$$

This means—if you were to invite groups of five over and over again—less than 8 out of 100 times would all five show up.

What is the probability there will be four attenders and one nonattender? In this situation, you must figure out the probability of four successes and one failure, taking into account that any one of the five could be the nonattender. The probability of attending is .60. The probability of not attending is the sum of all the probabilities (1.0) minus the probability of attending (.60), or .40 (1.0 − .60 = .40). Thus,

$$\text{Probability that four will attend and one will not} = \text{the number of}$$
$$\text{different sets of four attenders and one nonattender} \times$$
$$(.60)(.60)(.60)(.60)(.40)$$

That is, there are four successes each with a probability of .60 and one failure with a probability of .40. You must then figure out the number of different combinations of four attenders and one nonattender that there can be. Because choosing any one person leaves four remaining, you might see that there are five combinations. This logic seems easy, since the counting seems obvious. If the number of attempts or trials gets large, however, it is often easier to use a formula to compute the results. A general formula for figuring out the number of combinations of successes (x) and failures $(n - x)$ from n attempts is shown below.

Important Formula: Number of Combinations

$$_nC_x = \frac{n!}{(n - x)!x!}$$

The symbol ! stands for *factorial*. Factorial simply means continued multiplication of integers descending until the integer 1 is reached:

$$n(n - 1)(n - 2) \ldots 1$$

Mathematicians define 0! to be equal to 1.

Consider, for example, the number of combinations of three successes out of five trials. By formula, this would be

$$_5C_3 = \frac{5!}{(5 - 3)!3!}$$

$$= \frac{5 \cdot 4 \cdot 3 \cdot 2 \cdot 1}{(2 \cdot 1)(3 \cdot 2 \cdot 1)}$$

$$= 10$$

To see this more clearly, label the five persons A, B, C, D, and E. The combinations of three successes and two failures are as follows:

	Successes	Failures
1	ABC	DE
2	ABD	CE
3	ABE	CD
4	ACD	BE
5	ACE	BD
6	ADE	BC
7	BDE	AC
8	BCD	AE
9	BCE	AD
10	CDE	AB

If each of the five persons has the same probability of success, say, .60 (probability of attending), then the probability of a single combination of three successes and two failures is as follows:

$$(.60)(.60)(.60)(.40)(.40) = (.60)^3(.40)^2$$

To find the total probability of three successes and two failures, you must count all the correct combinations and add the probabilities together. This is the same as multiplying the probability of a single correct combination by the number of combinations:

$$\begin{aligned} \text{Probability (3 attenders)} &= {}_5C_3(.60)^3(.40)^2 \\ &= 10(.60)^3(.40)^2 \\ &= .346 \end{aligned}$$

Note that the sum of the exponents (3 and 2) is the same as n (5). Another way of writing this would be

$$(.60)^3(.40)^{5-3}$$

That is, if there are three successes, the rest will be failures. In general, if the probability (the relative frequency of occurrence) of success is p, the same for all persons, you can compute in advance the probability that exactly x of the n persons will be successes, using the following formula.

Important Formula: Binomial Distribution

$$P(x \text{ successes}) = ({}_nC_x)p^x(1 - p)^{n-x}$$

If the probability of failure $(1 - p)$ is represented instead by the letter q, the formula is

$$P_x = P(x \text{ successes}) = ({}_nC_x)p^x q^{n-x}$$

Often the problem is not simply to find out the probability of exactly x successes but rather the probability of x or more successes. This is easy with the binomial formula because you simply add the successive probabilities:

$$P_x + P_{x+1} + P_{x+2}, \ldots, P_n$$

For example, the probability of three or more invited persons attending would be the sum of the probabilities of three or four or five persons attending:

$$\sum_{x=3}^{5} {}_5C_x p^x q^{5-x}$$

$$= [{}_5C_3(.60)^3(.40)^2] + [{}_5C_4(.60)^4(.40)^1] + [{}_5C_5(.60)^5(.40)^0]$$

$$= .3456 + .2592 + .0778 = .6826$$

The chance of observing a particular event (or any event less likely than that one), such as x or more successes out of n trials, is called a p-*value*. The p-value has this meaning regardless of the theoretical model. Sometimes it is stated as a *two-sided* p-value. For example, in a binomial distribution, a two-sided p-value would mean the chance of fewer than some number of successes or greater than some number of successes.

The use of the binomial is frequently encountered in health education research. Success and/or failure labels can be given to many outcomes such as a person attends a patient education session (success) or fails to attend (failure) and a woman obtains prenatal care (success) or she does not (failure). Further, the arbitrary calling of events success or failure can be used. For example, to examine whether the appeal of a program was equal for women and men, one might define being female as a success and male as a failure and use this tool to see what is the chance of having a certain number of women attend a program if it were equally of interest to men and women. The substitution of these arbitrary levels makes this a powerful tool to use for the analyst.

When we discussed descriptive statistics, we said a mean was not sufficient. Often a probability is not sufficient. In evaluating a program, you might want to know the average number of attenders. This figure can be obtained because mathematical distributions have these descriptive statistics. The mean or average number of successes from a binomial distribution is the number of attempts (n) times the probability of obtaining a success (p), or np. This is intuitive to most people. If the average quit rate is 25% in a smoking-cessation program and the intervention is applied to 100 people, how many would probably quit? Most people would answer 25. The other descriptive statistic discussed was the variance. The variance is not as intuitive, but it is easy to compute. The variance of a binomial distribution is the number of attempts times the probability of success times the probability of failure (npq). So, if the probability of cessation were .25, the mean would be $n(.25)$ and the variance $n(.25)(.75)$. For an n of 100, the mean would be 25 and the variance 18.75.

Poisson Distribution

When using the binomial distribution, if the number of trials (n) is very large and the probability of success (p) is very small, the binomial distribution becomes difficult to compute. Consider an evaluation of a breast self-examination (BSE) program to detect early cancers. The relatively low incidence of breast cancer may involve tedious computations using the binomial distribution. Suppose the probability of finding a cancer using BSE is 1 in 1000, or .001. If 2000 women are screened, what is the probability that three or fewer cases of cancer will be detected? Using the binomial distribution, this would be the sum of the probabilities of detecting 0, 1, 2, and 3 cases:

Probability (0 cases) $= 2000_0^C(.001)^0(.999)^{2000} = .135$

Probability (1 case) $= 2000_1^C(.001)^1(.999)^{1999} = .271$

Probability (2 cases) $= 2000_2^C(.001)^2(.999)^{1998} = .271$

Probability (3 cases) $= 2000_3^C(.001)^3(.999)^{1997} = .181$

Computing $(.999)^{2000}$ and so on can be tedious even with modern calculators. The overall probability of detecting three or fewer cases is .858. If we were doing this for the state of Alabama, the number of trials would exceed 3 million, but even the exact n is not known.

Mathematicians have found that a formula can be derived that does not depend explicitly on the actual number of trials. This form or distribution assumes that the number is so large that a mathematical constant can be used to summarize the series of multiplications. This is known as the *Poisson distribution*. It is the distribution that results from increasing the number of trials and assuming that the probability of success becomes small. The expression used to calculate the probability of x successes is shown below.

Important Formula: Poisson Distribution

$$P(x \text{ successes}) = \frac{e^{-\lambda}\lambda^x}{x!}$$

where $\lambda = np$, the mean number of successes
e = a mathematical constant, 2.71828
x = the desired number of successes

Consider the BSE screening example. Using this formula, the probability of detecting 0, 1, 2, and 3 cases is a function of λ (or *np*). In this example,

$$n = 2000$$

$$p = .001$$

Thus,

$$\lambda = 2000(.001) = 2$$

In many instances, you do not know *n* or *p* exactly. However, you might have tumor registry data that shows for a particular time period an average 2 to 2.5 cases are detected. These "numerator" data can be used as your estimate of λ. They are very valuable in many community programs where denominator data (the potential target populations) are not explicitly known. Using λ = 2, you can now find the probabilities for the same duration of time.

$$\text{Probability (0 cases)} = \frac{e^{-\lambda}\lambda^x}{x!}$$

$$= \frac{e^{-2}2^0}{0!}$$

$$= \frac{(.135)(1)}{1}$$

$$= .135$$

$$\text{Probability (1 case)} = \frac{e^{-2}2^1}{1!}$$

$$= \frac{(.135)(2)}{1}$$

$$= .271$$

$$\text{Probability (2 cases)} = \frac{e^{-2}2^2}{2!}$$

$$= \frac{(.135)(4)}{2}$$

$$= .271$$

$$\text{Probability (3 cases)} = \frac{e^{-2}2^3}{3!}$$

$$= \frac{(.135)(8)}{6}$$

$$= .180$$

Thus, the probability of three or fewer cases is the sum of these probabilities (.135 + .271 + .271 + .180), or .857. This is close to the actual binomial computation of .858. The small difference between the two probabilities is from the Poisson assumption of an infinite population; although 2000 is a large population, it is not infinite.

Consider another example. Suppose the average number of encephalitis cases in a large community has been two per year. With the cutback in federal funds, spraying for mosquitoes has been substantially reduced. The director of the health department is concerned and wants you to institute a public health education program aimed at citizen control and awareness. Six months later, she returns to say that your program was obviously not effective because there were twice as many cases as on average in the past. Using the Poisson distribution, you can compute the probability (p-value) of four or more cases occurring if the mean (λ) were truly two. This would be the sum over all the population of four, five, six, and so on, cases. Mathematically, you would use summation notation and write

$$P(4 \text{ or more cases}) = \sum_{x=4}^{n} \frac{e^{-2}2^x}{x!}$$

However, remember that n is very large, and this would be quite a bit of computation. If you obtain the probability of fewer than four cases arising, 1 minus that probability must be the probability of four or more cases arising. (This "trick" of finding the complementary event is widely used in statistics.)

$$P(4 \text{ or more}) = 1 - P \text{ (fewer than 4)} = 1 - \left(\sum_{x=0}^{3} \frac{e^{-2}2^x}{x!} \right)$$

$$P(x = 0) = \frac{e^{-2}2^0}{0!} = .135$$

$$P(x = 1) = \frac{e^{-2}2^1}{1!} = .271$$

$$P(x = 2) = \frac{e^{-2}2^2}{2!} = .271$$

$$P(x = 3) = \frac{e^{-2}2^3}{3!} = .180$$

$$P(\text{fewer than } 4) = .135 + .271 + .271 + .180$$
$$= .857$$

$$P(4 \text{ or more}) = 1 - .857 = .143$$

Given this probability, or p-value, you can assess the director's statement. After these calculations, you mention to the director that, although you do share some concern about the effectiveness of your program, if the average number of cases had not changed, you would expect four or more cases to arise about 14 times out of 100. Although four cases is a higher incidence than you wish, it can occur somewhat frequently by chance variation alone rather than simply because of a program failure. Because spraying was stopped, it is unclear what level the number of cases might have attained without the public health education program, and there is no statistically significant increase in cases. One might conclude the program was not a failure.

The Poisson distribution has further properties that make it very useful in program evaluation. With the binomial distribution, not only the mean but also the variance depended on n and p. The Poisson distribution has the very useful property that the mean and the variance are the same. That is, the mean equals λ and so does the variance. This can be illustrated with an example. As we noted, the Poisson is the result of a binomial when n is very large and p is very small. Suppose n is 1,000,000 and p is .0001, then the binomial mean and variance are

$$\text{Mean} = np = 1,000,000 \ (.0001) = 100$$
$$\text{Variance} = npq = 1,000,000 \ (.0001)(.9999) = 99.99$$

If n were increased to 10,000,000, the mean would be 1000 and the binomial variance 999.9. Increasing n would eventually make the mean and variance equal for all practical purposes. This is a very valuable asset because it gives an estimate of the mean and variance for program planning from numerator data alone.

Normal Distribution

The normal distribution, or Gaussian distribution, is so commonly used that its complexity (as seen in the following formula) has long been overcome by the utility of the curve. You have encountered this curve in discussions of IQs or grading on a curve or many other instances of the familiar bell-shaped curve. One reason for wide usage of the normal distribution is a remarkable mathematical theorem called the *central limit theorem*, which states that, for most situations in the real world, if you take a random sample of observations, compute the sample mean, and repeat the process over and over, the distribution of the means of the samples will be a normal distribution irrespective of the shape of the distribution of the original observations. The variance would be the standard error of the mean discussed briefly above.

The density function of the normal distribution is

$$f(x) = [1/(\sigma\sqrt{2\pi})]e^{-(x-\mu)^2/(2\sigma^2)}$$

where e = the exponential constant 2.71828
x = the random variable of interest
σ = the standard deviation
μ = the mean

The way probabilities are generated is by integrating (a calculus concept) the area under particular portions of the curve. This would require tedious computations and a knowledge of calculus except for a simple relationship with what is called a *z score*. A *z* score is nothing more than the number of standard deviation units above or below the mean. Any normal distribution can be transformed into a standard normal distribution, which is the distribution of *z* scores. This standardizing is accomplished by subtracting the mean and then dividing by the standard deviation.

Important Formula: *z* Score

$$z = \frac{x - \mu}{\sigma}$$

This standard normal deviate *z* can be compared to a universal table based on standard deviation units from the mean irrespective of the underlying data.

Tuberculosis (TB) has become an increasing problem due to drug-resistant strains that are evolving. People exposed to these strains need special counseling. To identify these people, a general TB skin test is often used. This test provides a raised area that is measured to determine if a person needs further detailed screening for the multiple drug-resistant strains. The size of reaction (induration) is used to evaluate a patient. Of course, this means that some patients will be falsely evaluated because they were not exposed but rather had an unusual reaction to the test. Others fully exposed will not show a large enough reaction.

Suppose you know that the mean induration of a TB skin test is 1 centimeter (cm) in a healthy population, with a standard deviation of 0.5 cm. The z score associated with an induration of 2 cm is

$$z = \frac{2 - 1}{0.5} = \frac{1}{0.5} = 2$$

The value of z, 2, can be compared to a standard normal table to obtain the probability of any observations 2 standard deviations or more above the mean. The table shows this probability as .02275. Thus, if the critical value of 2-cm induration is used to identify people for further follow-up, we would expect 2.275% to be false positives, given that induration in a healthy population is normally distributed with a mean of 1 cm and a standard deviation of 0.5.

The normal distribution has certain values commonly used.

z = 0.845 → corresponds to the 80th percentile

z = 1.645 → corresponds to the 95th percentile

z = 1.96 → corresponds to the 97.5th percentile

z = 2.328 → corresponds to the 99th percentile

90% of all observations yield z scores between −1.645 and 1.645

95% of all observations yield z scores between −1.96 and 1.96

99% of all observations yield z scores between −2.576 and 2.576

These values are frequently used to judge the significance of differences in evaluation research and are found by computing z scores and comparing them to standard normal tables. Examples of this process are illustrated in the section on Student's *t* distribution later in this chapter.

Normal Approximate to the Binomial Distribution

The normal distribution is used as an approximation to other distributions. It is frequently used in evaluation research to approximate a binomial or Poisson distribution to further save on computations. When the sample size or number of successes is large, computation of the factorials needed in the Poisson and binomial distributions becomes rather tedious. To avoid this problem, evaluators use the normal distribution. They are allowed to use it because of the central limit theorem. When computing the probability of x successes out of n trials with a probability of success p, convert this to a z score, or so-called normal approximation to the binomial, by subtracting the mean np and dividing by the standard deviation $\sqrt{npq}$. Thus, a normal approximation to the number of x or more successes can be found by finding

$$z = \frac{x - np}{\sqrt{npq}}$$

For example, if you wish to know the probability that 100 or more people will participate in a program aimed at lowering infant mortality out of 150 invited, use the probability of their participation p and compute a z score. You believe that, based on past experience, 40% of those invited will participate. Thus, $p = .40$. To find out the chance that 100 people will attend out of 150, compute

$$z \geq \frac{(100) - (150)(.40)}{\sqrt{(150)(.40)(.60)}} = \frac{10}{\sqrt{36}} = \frac{10}{6} = 1.67$$

$$\geq 1.67$$

Using a standard normal table, you find the corresponding probability of 100 or more successes, which is .047.

Similarly, you can approximate a Poisson with a normal distribution. You standardize the variables in the same manner. First, subtract the mean and divide by the appropriate standard deviation. For a Poisson distribution, the mean and variance are λ. Thus,

$$z = \frac{x - \lambda}{\sqrt{\lambda}}$$

Suppose, as the evaluator for your state health department, you are told there have been 280 encephalitis cases in the last 12 months, when the past data show an average of 250. The question is whether an educational intervention aimed at getting the public to spray for mosquitoes is needed. If there is an indication of an epidemic, such a program would be worthwhile. However, the effort and expense are not trivial. Before you claim that an epidemic exists, you would like to know the probability of 280 or more cases arising when the usual experience is 250. For this you compute a z score based on a Poisson distribution approximated by a normal distribution. Since λ is 250,

$$z = \frac{(280 - 250)}{\sqrt{250}} = \frac{30}{15.81} = 1.91$$

The probability, using the standard tables, is .029, or 29 times out of 1000. This means that, if the average is really 250, only 29 times out of 1000 would you expect 280 or more cases to arise. From this, you conclude that a problem exists and are more confident in recommending a public health education program.

Student's *t* Distribution

The normal distribution works well for numerous situations especially when the sample size is large. Many evaluations involve only small samples. However, it is then unreasonable to assume that σ, the true standard deviation, is known. This is an assumption of the normal distribution above. When n is large, the differences in the probability associated with the z squares are not great, but for a small n, differences arise when σ is unknown or estimated from the data. What is commonly done is to use s, the sample estimate of σ in the computation of the z score. When this is done, a true z score is not obtained; rather, a closely related score called *Student's* t *score* or simply t *score* is obtained. The *t* score comes from a distribution of scores just as the z score relates to the normal distribution. The *t* distribution is virtually indistinguishable from the normal distribution when the sample size is over 100. The *t* distribution has been tabulated, but it requires another parameter (population value or fixed constant) besides the mean (μ) and the variance (σ^2), which are the only parameters that are necessary for the normal distribution. The *t* distribution depends on n, the sample size, whereas the normal does not. This is because the reliability of the estimate of the variance improves as the sample size increases. This dependence is described in terms of $n - 1$, referred to as *degrees of freedom* (d.f.). The smaller the value of $n - 1$, the greater the variability in the *t* distribution. The use of the *t* score is nearly identical to the z score, the only difference being in the table used to obtain the probabilities after that score is computed.

When you want to know if a mean is different from some hypothesized value, you can use a table based on z scores or *t* scores. The process of comparing these values found in the table to some a priori level of probability is called a test. The test derived from the *t* distribution is the well-known t *test*, a statistical test used to compare a single value to a hypothesized value.

Important Formula: t Score for a Sample Mean

$$t = \frac{\bar{x} - \mu}{s/\sqrt{n}}$$

where $\bar{x}$ = the sample mean
μ = the hypothesized true mean
s = the estimated standard deviation, $\displaystyle\sum_{i=1}^{n} \frac{(x_i - \bar{x})^2}{(n-1)}$
n = the sample size
$s/\sqrt{n}$ = the sample standard error (of the mean)

To test whether it is likely to have arisen from a distribution with the hypothesized means, this t score is compared to the tabled value of the theoretical t distribution with the parameter of $(n - 1)$ d.f. A value of t less than the lower critical value or above the upper critical value would be an indication that the result obtained occurs so infrequently by chance variation alone that you can reject the supposition that the sample was drawn from a normal distribution with mean μ.

Suppose you are trying to reach young black males with a blood pressure screening program in hopes of reducing the high morbidity and mortality rates associated with untreated high blood pressure among black males. You design a mass-media campaign to increase utilization of the community adult health clinics. From past data, you find that the average age of black males screened has consistently been around 40 years old. Your new messages are designed to reach the under-40 group. After 3 months of operation, you ask, Is it working? One simple measure is to test whether the average age is lower. Although only a formative evaluation, it would provide a simple and quick indicator of success. If more young black men came in to be screened, the average age would have declined. The numbers are collected, and the results are that the mean age of black males screened in the three months of the program was 38.1 years, with a standard deviation of 12.5 years. The total number of black males screened was 72. Is this evidence of success, or could it have happened by chance?

The average age is lower, indicating the direction you anticipated. However, you do not know how likely the result is from chance. If the true average age were 40, 50% of the time you would observe a random sample less than 40 years of age and 50% of the time a random sample over 40 years of age. Thus, you might say you had a 50/50 chance of supporting your program's effectiveness even if no change occurred. This is due to sampling fluctuations. However, you can assess the *statistical significance* of this result using the t test. Here, the t score is

$$t = \frac{\bar{x} - \mu}{s/\sqrt{n}}$$

$$= \frac{38.1 - 40}{12.5/\sqrt{72}}$$

$$= \frac{-1.9}{1.47} = -1.29$$

Remember, you are seeing if the mean age observed differs from 40 years, which is assumed to be a fixed quantity. The negative sign indicates the observed mean is less than that hypothesized. This result is compared to the lower end of the t distribution (implicitly, because the actual table values are identical for the positive and negative sides and all tables are given in positive values only). You look at the table value with $n - 1$ d.f.—that is, 71 d.f.—and you find that the probability of observing a sample mean of 38.1 years *if* there had been no change in the true mean of 40 is about 1 out of 10. This gives you some encouragement that the program is working. You need more analyses to pinpoint the success. A p-value of 10% or less is all right for a formative evaluation (pilot data) but would be met with skepticism in a full-scale program impact evaluation.

The t test can be used for other testing than the sample's mean. Frequently evaluators use this test to compare two means as follows.

Important Formula: t Test for Two Groups

$$t = \frac{(\bar{x}_1 - \bar{x}_2) - (\mu_1 - \mu_2)}{\sqrt{(s_1^2/n_1) + (s_2^2/n_2)}}$$

where $\bar{x}_1$ and $\bar{x}_2$ = the means of samples 1 and 2, respectively
μ_1 and μ_2 = the respective hypothesized true means
(if you are testing for equality of these,
$\mu_1 - \mu_2 = 0$)
s_1^2 and s_2^2 = the respective sample variances
n_1 and n_2 = the respective sample sizes

This test statistic has approximately $n_1 + n_2 - 2$ d.f.

Consider a study of the efficacy of an intervention to improve pill taking among hypertensive patients. Before implementing the intervention in all of the community health centers, you carry out a formative evaluation. In this pilot study, you randomly allocate 25 newly

Table 8.4 Compliance Index Based on Pill Counts Related to Medical Therapy 3 Months Postintervention

Intervention Group (n = 13)	Control Group (n = 12)
90	92
88	84
96	99
72	75
71	68
92	76
81	85
63	67
84	85
87	91
91	73
90	76
81	
$\Sigma x_{i1} = 1086$	$\Sigma x_{i2} = 971$
$\Sigma x_{i1}^2 = 91846$	$\Sigma x_{i2}^2 = 79671$
$x_1 = 83.5$	$x_2 = 80.9$
$s_1^2 = 93.6$	$s_2^2 = 100.1$

identified hypertensive patients either to a three-arm intervention including diaries, education, and home blood pressure monitoring (*E* group) or to no intervention beyond medical care, *C* group. Three months later, you measure compliance through pill counts of each individual. The data in Table 8.4 are obtained. If you are attempting to see whether the pilot data support your intervention's efficacy, the hypothesis you are testing is that there is no difference between the two groups' average compliance index. Thus, if you can show that the observed difference is unlikely to be a chance occurrence—that is, if it has a small *p*-value—the effectiveness is shown and called *significant*. From Table 8.4, you learn that the mean compliance index for the *E* group after 3 months is 83.5, and for the *C* group it is 80.9. Although the difference is in the direction of your supposition, the *t* test is needed to tell you the statistical significance (i.e., how likely this difference is due to chance vs. the alternative of a true difference). Only this knowledge tells you the real-world importance of the numerical difference. The *t* test can be computed. Because you are assuming no difference and testing the likelihood that your observed difference is due to chance alone, the hypothesized true difference is zero, $\mu_1 - \mu_2 = 0$. The sample variances 93.6 and 100.1 are computed and shown in Table 8.4.

$$t = \frac{(\bar{x}_1 - \bar{x}_2) - (\mu_1 - \mu_2)}{\sqrt{(s_1^2/n_1) + (s_2^2/n_2)}}$$

$$= \frac{(83.5 - 80.9) - (0)}{\sqrt{(93.6/13) + (100.1/12)}}$$

$$= \frac{2.6}{\sqrt{15.5}} = .66$$

This quantity, $t = .66$, is then compared to tables of Student's t distribution with $n_1 + n_2 - 2$ (in this case, $12 + 13 - 2 = 23$) d.f. The tables show that the probability of this result occurring by chance alone is greater than one out of four ($p > .25$). This suggests that the result is somewhat likely to occur by chance. Even though it is in the direction of your beliefs, there is not sufficient statistical evidence to say that the E group differs from the C group.

Whether one would conclude that the program should be abandoned is not just a statistical issue. A pilot study such as this is still supportive and can be used to refine a larger undertaking. As discussed in Chapter 5 (sample size), such a small sample (13 and 12 in each group) is not likely to have shown any but very large effects. Thus, the support is weak, and you need to consider the broader context of the program. If firm data were needed, a much larger sample ($E = 50$ vs. $C = 50$) should have been used in your formative evaluation.

The t test for two groups assumes independent samples. Often, pairing of outcomes occurs, such as pretest and posttest outcomes on the same person. This pairing violates the independence assumption; for example, pulses taken on the same person by two methods are more likely to agree than a pulse taken on one person by one method and on another person by the other method. This lack of independence has impact on the variance, usually by decreasing the value. Using the formulas in independent samples, you miss important differences. To get around this problem, evaluators use a so-called *paired t test*.

Important Formula: Paired t Test

$$t = \frac{\bar{d} - \delta}{\sqrt{s_d^2/n}}$$

where $\bar{d}$ = the average difference of the n pairs of data
δ = the hypothesized true average difference, often assumed to be zero
s_d = the standard deviation of the differences over the pairs
n = the number of pairs

This statistic is now in the same form as a single sample t test. It makes inferences about the sample of differences between the n pairs. This is compared to a theoretical t distribution with $n - 1$ d.f.

Suppose you implement a cancer prevention program. The first group attending the program is to be evaluated using a pretest and posttest of knowledge, attitudes, and beliefs about cancer screening, diagnosis, and treatment. You obtain a valid and reliable instrument to use in testing the participants. The scores are those shown in Table 8.5. The average pretest score is 64.7, compared with the average posttest score of 69.5. The average difference is 4.8 units higher. Note that the average difference is the difference between the averages. This is always true; what changes are the variance and standard deviation. The standard deviations on the pretest and posttest scores are both larger than the standard deviation of the differences. This is indicative of the benefit of pairing. To test whether your intervention has been successful in raising the scores, you carry out a paired t test

Table 8.5 Pretest and Posttest Scores for Knowledge, Attitudes, and Beliefs about Cancer Screening, Diagnosis, and Treatment

Partici-pant	Pretest	Posttest	Change (difference)
1	53	64	11
2	38	50	12
3	87	94	7
4	72	74	2
5	56	68	12
6	74	78	4
7	62	68	6
8	66	66	0
9	70	70	0
10	48	52	4
11	82	78	−4
12	68	72	4
	$x_{pre} = 64.7$	$x_{post} = 69.5$	$\bar{d} = 4.8$
	$s^2_{pre} = 198.8$	$s^2_{post} = 136.9$	$s^2_d = 26.0$

on the 12 pairs (note that δ is assumed to be zero—i.e., on average, zero improvement in the scores):

$$t = \frac{\bar{d} - \delta}{\sqrt{s_d^2/n}}$$

$$= \frac{4.8 - 0}{\sqrt{26/12}} = \frac{4.8}{1.47} = 3.26$$

The value 3.26 is compared with tables of the Student's t distribution with $n - 1$ (or 11) d.f. The tables show that the result obtained would occur by chance less than 1 time in 100, indicating that it is unlikely to be a chance result. The result is considered statistically significant, demonstrating the effectiveness of the education program in changing knowledge, attitudes, and beliefs. Note that if you had used an unpaired or usual t test, the t value would be .91, a nonsignificant result!

Chi-Square Distribution

The *chi-square distribution* is used in testing hypotheses that a sample of data arises from a completely specified distribution. This might test whether a sample could have arisen from a normal distribution. However, another use is in testing for associations through specification of probability rules.

Use of the chi-square distribution is straightforward. The following six steps summarize the process:

1. Arbitrarily set intervals covering the range of data for one or more variables.
2. Count the number of observations in each interval or class.
3. Calculate the probability for each interval based on the hypothesized distribution.
4. Calculate the expected number in each interval by multiplying the probability times the total sample size.
5. Calculate the chi-square statistic.
6. Calculate the significance level or p-value by comparing the results to the upper area of the chi-square distribution.

Evaluators are likely to use the chi-square to test whether characteristics could be considered to behave independently of one another in a probability sense. The alternative is that the two characteristics behave dependently—the frequency of one characteristic's occurrence is altered on the basis of the other characteristic's occurrence. More detail of this theory can be found in most elementary statistics books; here it can be summarized as follows: If two characteristics that can occur together behave independently, the probability of both occurring, that is, P(AB), is equal to the probability of one occurring, P(A), times the probability of the other occurring, P(B). For example, the probability of drawing the jack of hearts from a deck of 52 cards is 1/52 because there is only one jack of hearts. However, because suits and numbers can be considered independent characteristics (i.e., there is the same number in each suit), we can apply the basic probability rule. A jack occurs 4 times out of 52 and a heart 13 times out of 52. Thus,

$$P(AB) = P(A) \cdot P(B)$$

$$P \text{ (jack of hearts)} = P \text{ (jack)} \cdot P \text{ (heart)}$$

$$= (4/52)(13/52) = 52/(52 \cdot 52) = 1/52$$

Probability statements such as this are the basis for the chi-square test for association.

The general formula for a chi-square statistic for a table with r rows and c columns is shown below.

Important Formula: Chi-Square Statistic

$$\chi^2 = \sum_{i=1}^{r} \sum_{j=1}^{c} \frac{(O_{ij} - E_{ij})^2}{E_{ij}}$$

where E_{ij} = the expected frequency in the cell of row i and column j; this expected frequency is usually obtained from the assumption that the element of the cell arises from the independent application of the row probability times the column probability

O_{ij} = the observed frequency in the cell of row i and column j

The statistic has $(r - 1)(c - 1)$ d.f. The larger the discrepancy between the observed and expected frequencies, the less likely the independence assumption would be. However, if you obtain a frequency of 20 and you expected 10, the difference is 10; if you obtain 200 and you expected 190, the difference is again 10. Intuitively, 200 seems closer to 190 than 20 does to 10. To accommodate this notion, the squared deviation is divided by the number expected. Thus, $(20 - 10)^2/10$ yields a contribution to the chi-square statistic of $100/10 = 10$, whereas $(200 - 190)^2/190 = 100/190 = .526$.

A computing formula for the chi-square eliminates the need to calculate each expected frequency and still yields the overall summary statistic.

Important Formula: Computing Formula for Chi-Square

$$\chi^2 = N\left(\sum_{i=1}^{r} \sum_{j=1}^{c} O_{ij}^2/O_{i.}O_{.j}\right) - N$$

where N = the total number in the table
O_{ij} = the frequency of the cell in row i and column j

$O_{i.} = \sum_{i=1}^{c} O_{ij}$, the row total of row i

$O_{.j} = \sum_{i=1}^{r} O_{ij}$ the column total of column j

r = the number of rows
c = the number of columns

The degree of freedom is the parameter of the chi-square distribution that enables comparison of the computed statistic (also called the *test statistic*) to the percentiles of a theoretical chi-square frequency curve. When the chi-square value exceeds the critical value (that percentile above which you would reject the hypothesis of independence), the result is said to demonstrate a significant association.

Suppose the staff of a blood pressure screening program is concerned about the effects of referrals on the kinds of persons utilizing the resource. Since women tend to be seen more frequently than men by physicians, the staff is concerned that differences by gender may occur in whether patients follow referral guidelines. Records are kept of all referrals, and, 6 weeks after the initial referral, patients who have not returned a card documenting a physician's visit are called. The caller elicits information on what happened and then classifies the patient's status as refused, referral pending, or successfully referred. The number of persons completing 6 weeks of follow-up is 130. The results are categorized by gender as shown in Table 8.6. To assess whether men are different from women in following the referrals, a chi-square statistic can be computed. This chi-square would test the independence of gender and referral class, in a probability sense. A significant chi-square would indicate that the row variable, gender, is not independent of the column variable, referral class, im-

Table 8.6 Referral Status of Potential Hypertensives by Gender Six Weeks after Referral

	Referral Status			
	---	---	---	---
Gender	Refused	Referral Pending	Successfully Referred	Total
Male	10	38	28	76
Female	4	16	34	54
Total	14	54	62	130

plying the gender difference. Applying the computing formula (this is what is most often used in computer programs and hand-held calculators) to this example,

$$\chi^2 = N(\sum_i \sum_j O_{ij}^2 / O_i.O_{.j}) - N$$

$$= 130[(10^2/76 \cdot 14) + 38^2/76 \cdot 54) + (28^2/76 \cdot 62) + (4^2/54 \cdot 14)$$

$$+ (16^2/54 \cdot 54) + (34^2/54 \cdot 62)] - 130$$

$$= 130(1.06646) - 130$$

$$= 138.64 - 130$$

$$= 8.64$$

This statistic of 8.64 is compared to table values of the chi-square distribution with $(r - 1)(c - 1)$ d.f., in this case $(2 - 1)(3 - 1) = 2$. The probability of observing a chi-square value of 8.54 or greater under the model of statistical independence is less than .013. This low probability of the results in the table if gender and referral status were independent indicates an association between gender and referral. This statistic does not tell which gender group follows the referral guidelines better; the program staff must return to the actual data to find the direction of the difference. The proportion of men successfully referred is 36.8% (28 out of 76) compared with 63.0% (34 out of 54) for women. Thus, the staff can conclude that women have a statistically significant difference over men in achieving referral.

F Distribution

The F statistic arises from the ratio of two chi-square statistics. Its most common uses in evaluation research are in two methods called *regression analysis* and *analysis of variance*. The F distribution, a frequency distribution of F statistics, requires two parameters, the degrees of freedom associated with the estimated variance of the numerator of the statistic and the degrees of freedom associated with the denominator variance. Commonly, the test or statistic involves the ratio of an estimate of variance between groups (called the *mean square among groups*, or *MS between*) and the variance within groups (also called the *MS within* or *mean-square error*). The variation *among* measures the differences among the various groups or categories under study, and the variation *within* is a measure of random error, a euphemism for all those factors that are uncontrolled and/or unobserved. Frequently, this statistic takes the following form:

$$F = \frac{MS\ among}{MS\ within}, \qquad \text{with } (k - 1) \text{ and } (n - k) \text{ d.f.}$$

where k = the number of groups
n = the sample size

From a regression analysis, it takes the following form:

$$F = \frac{MS\ regression}{MS\ residual}, \qquad \text{with } k \text{ and } (n - k - 1) \text{ d.f.}$$

where the regression is a linear regression equation, which acts like the differences among groups in the analysis of variance.

The F distribution requires more background to motivate the understanding of its use, but such a discussion is beyond the intent of this chapter. Simply, when the variances are equal, the ratio should be 1.0. The F test provides a statement regarding the probability of the observed statistic occurring by chance. How likely is it that the observed ratio is this large compared to 1.0 merely by chance? The value of 1.0 indicates that the variation within groups equals the variation among groups. In other words, there is no difference over chance between the levels of the independent variables. In regression analysis, if the F statistic is significant, you can conclude that using these independent variables will help you predict or estimate the response or dependent variable. For example, age is important in predicting blood pressure. The variation in blood pressure within a group of 30-year-old persons is smaller than the variation between persons 30 to 60 years old.

Similarly, in analysis of variance, if the F statistic exceeds 1.0, this indicates that the deviation within a treatment group is less than the deviation between two treatments. For example, if you measure diastolic blood pressure in patients of low, medium, and high socio-economic status, a significant F statistic would indicate that average blood pressure differed by socioeconomic status.

ANALYTIC METHODS AND APPROACHES

When deciding on appropriate analytic tools for an evaluation, the first major operational decision is choosing a design and, by virtue of that choice, a specific analysis. Will the study involve a single group, two groups, or multiple groups? Although this may seem like an obvious and simplistic categorization of studies, it becomes critical in the interpretation and understanding provided by the evaluation.

Single-Group Designs

The simplest form of single-group design is a prevalence survey. These studies ascertain the characteristics of a population—attitudes, beliefs, physical characteristics, and so on—at a single point in time. Prevalence surveys may be formally designed cross-sectional surveys, telephone surveys, household interview surveys, convenience samples, clinical samples, and so on. The prevalence survey (needs assessment) is an important method to evaluators because it can be the basis for a program intervention. Too often information from cross-sectional surveys is not used in understanding a problem. Testimonials and experiences of others are used for the needs assessment of a particular program, especially for nationwide problems. This can lead to the development of under- or overutilized programs because the planners failed to understand the local setting.

A variety of analyses can be applied in a cross-sectional design. Many of these were described in the sections on display techniques and descriptive statistics. Often, however, it is necessary to go beyond the descriptive statistics in a design and ascertain relationships of various characteristics within the cross-sectional survey. There are two primary, simple methods for doing this.

Chi-Square Test of Association. The first method is use of a chi-square statistic to assess whether two characteristics behave independently of each other or are related. For example, in a smoking-cessation program, the evaluation has focused on identifying the types of individuals who successfully complete the program. Suppose success is defined as cessation 1 month following the intervention. Table 8.7 shows hypothetical data for 625 individuals enrolled in the program. After 1 month, 290 were classed as successful and 335 as unsuccessful in their attempts to quit smoking. Of the 625, 158 were single, 226

Table 8.7 Smoking-Cessation Results by Marital Status

	Marital Status					
Cessation Result	Single	Married	Separated	Divorced	Widowed	Total
Successful	68	89	19	101	13	290
Unsuccessful	90	137	16	79	13	335
Total	158	226	352	180	26	625

χ^2 = 13.03 with 4 degrees of freedom
p = 0.011

married, and so on. Overall, 46% (290/625) stopped smoking. The question arises, Is marital status independent of the ability to quit smoking as represented by the population of this smoking-cessation program? In a statistical sense, the program evaluators want to know whether the probability of quitting is different for people who are single, married, separated, widowed, or divorced. Is the program more successful in some marital groups than others?

Although the chi-square test will not tell which category appears to be different, the evaluators can compute the chi-square statistic for an overall test of any association. When this is done for these data, the chi-square value of 13.03 is obtained with $(r - 1)(c - 1)$ d.f., r being the number of rows (2), and c being the number of columns (5). Thus, the value of the computed statistic, 13.03, is compared to a chi-square statistic with 4 d.f. Looking this up in a table, the evaluators find that the p-value is .011. That is, 98.9% of all computed chi-square statistics with 4 d.f. would obtain values below 13.03, if the null hypothesis were true. Because the chance of finding a chi-square statistic as high as 13.03 occurs only 1.1% of the time (100% − 98.9%), this suggests a lack of independence between marital status and success in quitting smoking (i.e., they are associated).

Although this illustrates the utility of the chi-square test of association in a single-group situation, it does not indicate the existence of a *causative* relationship between these characteristics. Evaluators must then ask themselves, What is this overall test of significance measuring? Since smoking-cessation programs do not obtain a random sample of participants, the meaning of this statistical test must be considered in a dual context. First, what possible selection biases could be operating to bring in people of different marital categories? Which of these might be associated with their motivation to quit? The chi-square statistic could be measuring a lack of independence induced by the selection of people who come into the program, their motivations for coming, and their ability to quit, rather than the effects of the program. Once the concerns of the first question are satisfied, a second question can be asked, Is there something in the message or the program being implemented that works selectively? For example, divorced persons seem to have better success rates than the other categories, and separated individuals might also have better success rates. If the program gives heavy emphasis to family support for quitting smoking, this finding might indicate program deficiencies rather than strengths. Of course, far more analyses are necessary to establish the link between the finding and its importance, but the chi-square statistic provides an initial indicator of areas worthy of subsequent analyses.

Correlation Coefficients. A second common method of analysis to assess relationships in single-group studies is a correlation coefficient. The Pearson product moment correlation coefficient is usually used. This coefficient is used only for variables considered to be continuous, such as age, IQ, and other measured responses. Computation of the correlation coefficient is straightforward. It measures the tendency for two variables to deviate from the respective sample means in a related way. That is, the correlation coefficient measures the tendency to get similar differences between pairs of scores on two characteristics of interest. Suppose you have the data in Table 8.8 on measures of the pulse as taken by an observer and by an automated device at the same time in a blood pressure intervention study. You are confronted with the decision whether to use the automated device. Use of the observer requires personnel time and training, among

Table 8.8   Diastolic Blood Pressures by Human Observer and Automated Device

Participant	Pulse by Observer	Pulse by Automated Device
1	80	82
2	65	77
3	51	58
4	67	66
5	72	75
6	68	81
7	64	72
8	91	99
9	71	72
Average	69.9	75.8

$r = 0.905$

other things. The automated device provides a permanent record and minimizes the use of personnel.

For this particular decision, you are confronted with nine pairs of observations. Each pulse was taken once by a trained observer and simultaneously by the automated device. The correlation, or what may be referred to as the *reliability coefficient*, can be computed using the following formula.

Important Formula: Correlation Coefficient

$$r = \sum_{i=1}^{n} \frac{(x_i - \bar{x})(y_i - \bar{y})}{\sqrt{\Sigma(x_i - \bar{x})^2 \Sigma(y_i - \bar{y})^2}}$$

$$= \frac{n\Sigma x_i y_i - (\Sigma x_i)(\Sigma y_i)}{\sqrt{[n\Sigma x_i^2 - (\Sigma x_i)^2][n\Sigma y_i^2 - (\Sigma y_i)^2]}}$$

where x_i = the value of one characteristic or measurement on person i

   y_i = the value of the other characteristic on person i

Applying this formula to the data in Table 8.8, you obtain a value of $r = 0.905$. What does this value mean? A correlation coefficient can obtain a value from -1.0 to 1.0. The negative values indicate that, as one characteristic increases, the other decreases. A value of ± 1 indicates perfect correlation—knowledge of one variable implies the other. However, a more readily interpretable statistic is provided by squaring r, obtaining a quantity known as the *coefficient of determination* (r^2 or R^2). This quantity is a key statistic when derived from a *regression analysis.* It tells how much of the variation in one variable is determined or explained by the other variable. In the pulse example, $R^2 = 0.819$, meaning that over 80% of the variability of one observation (pulse by observer) can be explained by the other (pulse by automated device). This correlation coefficient would be found highly significant on standard tests of significance. There is certainly more agreement between these two measures than would be expected by chance alone. However, the existence of statistical significance between the characteristics should not be overinterpreted without careful scrutiny. Although the correlation is very high, comparison of the data shows that the average mean pulse is nearly six beats lower when taken by observer than when taken by the automated device. A paired t test on the differences between readings shows that the average difference is 5.89 beats, with a standard deviation of 4.91 beats, yielding a statistically significant difference between the observer and the automated device. The basic implication is that the

Table 8.9   Number of New Users of the Cervical Cancer Screening
Clinics by Quarter for Hale and Marengo Counties, Alabama

Year	1978				1979				1980			
Quarter	1	2	3	4	1	2	3	4	1	2	3	4
Hale	13	20	12	15	14	89	12	20	15	50	18	11
Marengo	22	36	23	15	32	45	34	29	27	29	40	32

automated device yields higher readings than those obtained by the observer ($t = 3.60$ with 8 d.f.). This information is important for making the decision to use such a device routinely or not. Your responsibility is then to try to ascertain which is the more accurate response. The correlation coefficient can be used to measure the reliability or reproducibility (i.e., the precision) of an estimate. The discrepancy between the two responses, if it tends to remain relatively constant, is a measure of bias. In this example, it is not clear which measurement is more accurate. You need to review the literature to help make your choice.

Analysis of Pretest, Posttest Data. Another design often used in a single-group situation is the multiple pretest, posttest design or single time-series design (TSD). Chapter 5 described the cancer screening study in Hale County, Alabama. Table 8.9 shows the number of new users of cervical cancer screening clinics by quarter for Hale and Marengo counties, a more refined categorization of some of the information in Table 8.1. These data might be seen as summarizing program impact in a single time series design. (See Case Study 1 in Chapter 5.)

Consider the data for Hale County in the year 1979. The intervention periods for this study occurred in the second quarter of 1979 and the second quarter of 1980. Substantial and favorable impact during the two intervention quarters is suggested by the array of data. When the data available for analysis are simply frequency data, options are limited, and formal tests of significance are often avoided because of the assumptions. Percentages are used as descriptive statistics, and increases in the percentage of utilization are often used to summarize change. If you can assume that (1) counts arise from a large population, (2) the number of individuals availing themselves of a clinic screening follows a Poisson distribution, and (3) the periods are independent of one another, the Poisson distribution can be used in a simple pretest, posttest design.

Assume that the baseline period or the baseline and postintervention average is the mean value of some Poisson distribution. Given this parameter, you can ask, What is the probability of observing the number of new cases during the 1979 intervention period given this mean from a pretest period based on a Poisson distribution (as described in the section on distributions)? This test, although quick, ignores the fact that the pretest period is not the true parameter value; a test that takes into account the inherent variability in both the pretest and intervention periods would be more desirable. Although this test requires several assumptions, using a normal approximation to the Poisson, an approximate test can be used. Here you approximate the difference between two Poisson distributions and ask whether the underlying means are the same. To do this, use as the means of each sample (x_1 and x_2) the actual number of new users in quarter 1 and quarter 2 in 1979. The variances of a Poisson are equal to the mean, so we use the sum of x_1 and x_2 as the denominator representing the variance of the difference:

$$z = \frac{(x_2 - x_1)}{\sqrt{(x_2 + x_1)}} = \frac{89 - 14}{\sqrt{89 + 14}} = 7.39$$

The probability of a z score greater than or equal to 7.39 is vanishingly small ($p < .0001$). Thus, utilizing this pretest, posttest design, you could reject the hypothesis that these two frequencies have arisen from the same underlying Poisson distribution.

This, of course, is a weak demonstration of impact because it incorporates all reasons for these numbers to be different, but it may improve on the eyeball method. The use of a single TSD with one group has many limitations, as seen in the discussion of threats to validity in Chapter 5. Analogous tests may be conducted using paired *t* tests for a pretest, posttest design and testing the hypothesis that the difference is zero, as was done above.

Analysis of Time-Series Data. The idea of a time series is neither new nor necessarily complicated but generally requires discussions beyond the scope of this text. In its simplest form, a time series is a collection of numerical observations arranged in the order in which they occurred. Formal analysis of time series goes back at least as far as the Romans, who made sufficiently accurate observations to construct the cycle of approximately 365¼ days in the Julian calendar. Data that contain only one periodic component are relatively easy to handle. More complicated series are often characterized by methods not appropriate for this chapter; furthermore, those tools are often useful not in the assessment of impact but rather in the search for periodicities, or other confounding factors that have impact on many intervention programs (i.e., studying behavior of women, taking into account hormone fluctuations).

In using time-series data to evaluate community programs, four types of time issues are of concern (Windsor and Cutter, 1981):

1. The trend in the data (generally increasing or decreasing)
2. Cyclical fluctuations (multiple-year or multiple-month ups and downs)
3. Seasonal variations (annual ups and downs)
4. Intervention effects (increases or decreases after a program)

These issues are critical to the assessment of program impact. Generally, the term *cycle* is used for short- or long-duration changes or repetitive changes, and *seasonal variation* is used for changes that occur with climate changes. Trend is an important and potentially misleading component. Suppose your program resulted in the utilization results shown in Figure 8.2. Average pretreatment use was 70 people [(80 + 60 + 70)/3] per period (leftmost triangle). In the intervention period shown at the arrow, there were 110 new users, a 57% increase in utilization over the pretreatment average. This increase could convince you that the program had a substantive effect. Even the increase in the posttreatment period, an average 110 users [(90 + 100 + 140)/3] (rightmost triangle), might be claimed as a long-term benefit or sustained effect of the intervention. However, you must be honest—even in your wildest dreams, did you really think the program could produce such a sustained impact? You must ask whether other forces were at work.

The simplest assessment of a trend is to plot the data on a properly constructed graph as shown in Figure 8.2. Eyeballing this figure gives the impression of an upward trend, represented by the dashed line. The comparison of before, during, and after the intervention periods (averages of 70 vs. 110 new users) is called the *method of semiaverages* because it divides the time series into two parts and a line can be fitted to the two averages. The method of semiaverages is useful in identifying a trend when no intervention effect is present, but it does not clarify a situation where an intervention effect has occurred because of this method's sensitivity to outliers. A second method, less susceptible to the impact of a single intervention period, is the *method of moving averages*. This computes the mean of a fixed number of successive observations and examines these averages or "smoothed" results. The term *smoothed* is used to indicate that the averaging process reduces some of the random fluctuations expected in real data. The moving averages for three-period increments of the data in Figure 8.2 are 70 = [(80 + 60 + 70)/3]; 80 = [(60 + 70 + 110)/3]; 90 = [(70 + 110 + 90)/3]; and so on.

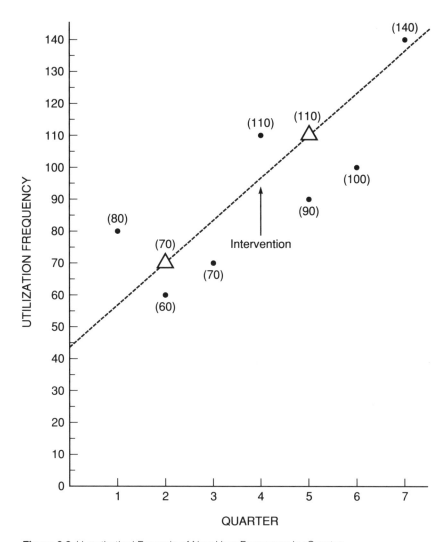

Figure 8.2 Hypothetical Example of New User Frequency by Quarter

SOURCE: R. A. Windsor and G. Cutter, "Methodological Issues in Using Time Series Designs and Analysis: Evaluating the Behavioral Impact of Health Communication Programs," in *Progress in Clinical and Biological Research*, vol. 83: *Issues in Screening and Communications*, ed. C. Mettlin and G. Murphy, 517–535 (New York: Alan R. Liss, 1981).

When these three-period moving averages are plotted on a graph, they fall on a straight line, demonstrating the upward trend in utilization and raising the question of how one intervention shown at the arrow could produce this effect. The moving average method is a technique that reduces cyclical variations—regular up and down changes of results (oscillatory movements). Although the series presented in Figure 8.2 is too short to determine a cycle explicitly, the pattern of a peak, two lower values, and a peak is repeated twice with the terminal peak of 140; yet this movement is smoothed by the moving average process. Such cycles are important and may be confused with seasonal variations.

The methods used to isolate patterns and variations are the same as those for identifying oscillatory movements.

Even when the suggestion of trend is graphically present, the significance of it is often an important issue in assessing the program.

Linear Regression. Several methods are useful in assessing a trend, but one of the most common is *linear regression analysis.* Simple linear regression is a model that states that the average response or dependent variable y has a straight line relationship to the independent variable x.

Important Formula: Simple Linear Regression Model

$$y = \beta_0 + \beta_1 x$$

where β_0 = the intercept of the line
       β_1 = the slope of the line

The calculation of the line is usually accomplished by a procedure known as *least squares.* That is, the coefficients β_0 and β_1 are estimated in such a way as to minimize the square of the differences between the actual observations and the expected observations. The equations for β_0 and β_1 are derived from the n pairs of observations (x_i, y_i) by the following formulas (commonly used in calculators and computer program packages).

Important Formula: Coefficients for Simple Linear Regression

$$\hat{\beta}_1 = \frac{n\Sigma x_i y_i - (\Sigma x_i)(\Sigma y_i)}{n\Sigma x_i^2 - (\Sigma x_i)^2}$$

$$\hat{\beta}_0 = \bar{y} - \hat{\beta}_1 \bar{x}$$

where $\bar{y}$ and $\bar{x}$ are the respective means of the x's and y's. The slope β_1 is equal to zero when there is no linear relationship between x and y. The slope is equivalent to assessing the correlation coefficient r.

The square of the correlation coefficient r^2 tells us the proportion of variance in y explained by x. When there is no relationship, $r = 0$, $r^2 = 0$, and no variance is explained. The slope in this situation is zero. The same value is predicted for the dependent variable y no matter what the value of the independent variable.

Both r and β_1 can be tested—that is, the probability of the result can be found, using a t test. Thus, to test the hypothesis that $\beta_1 = 0$, you would compute

$$t = \frac{\hat{\beta}_1 - \beta_1}{\text{SE } \hat{\beta}_1} = \frac{\hat{\beta}_1 - 0}{\text{SE } \hat{\beta}_1}$$

This is compared to a t distribution with $n - 2$ d.f. In analyzing trend data, evaluators often use time (t_i) as the independent x variable, and y remains the response. Consider the example from Figure 8.2. The least-squares equation that characterizes these data is

$$\hat{\beta}_0 = 52.9$$

$$\hat{\beta}_1 = 10.0$$

$$y_i = 52.9 + 10.0t_i$$

That is, average usage is 52.9 people plus 10 additional people for each time period (quarter) of observation.

The R^2 value is 0.64 for the unsmoothed data. The regression is significant, indicating the existence of a trend. You must ask whether the trend is overriding the intervention or whether there is an intervention effect over and above the trend. In this situation, with the strong trend evident and an apparent seasonal pattern, the success of the intervention could be questioned, especially if the likelihood of a sustained impact is small.

Outliers or Successful Interventions. Given an understanding of the series, the question remains how to measure and assess an impact. When no trend, cycle, or seasonal variation exists, impact can be assessed by comparing the intervention period results to the before and after periods as was done in the earlier example when a trend existed. A statistical appraisal can be made using a method for the detection of outliers in data sets. Although many criteria have been proposed and used, a simple test (Grubbs, 1969) can be used to assess whether the value appears to have arisen by more than chance variation; if so, this indicates a program impact. This statistic G is easily computed by the following formula:

$$G = \frac{\text{Intervention observation } - \text{ Mean of all observations}}{\text{Standard deviation } \sqrt{n - 1}}$$

This parallels a t test except for the adjustment in the denominator. Where the standard deviation of all observations is used, the resultant value G can be compared to available special tables, provided the data can be assumed to be normally distributed. Another test is to compute a z score by comparing the intervention observation to the mean and dividing by the standard deviation. If this value is larger than 3.2, the result is considered significant.

A similar analysis can be carried out when a significant trend exists, as in the example in Figure 8.2. In this situation, the expected value from the trend line is used in the Grubbs formula and compared to the standard error (S) of the regression line:

$$G = \frac{y_i - \hat{y}_i}{S_{\text{regression}} \sqrt{n - 2}}$$

Application of this technique to the example in Figure 8.2 yields no statistically significant deviation from the trend line, indicating there is no intervention effect.

Example of Applied Analysis. To give a more complete example, we applied the methods to the Hale County study of cervical cancer screening described in Chapter 5 and briefly above. The data are presented in Table 8.10. We will consider only the total users for the moment. The intervention periods occurred at the second quarters of 1979, 1980, and 1981. A brief scanning of the data shows large peaks for those quarters. This is, of course, consistent with the hypothesized effect of the broadcast messages and screening efforts and could be taken as a strong indication of success of the cancer screening program (CSP). However, as pointed out, evaluators should not be content with a statement of program impact based merely on observing the data.

These data offer, on closer inspection, additional information that can be used in evaluating the program. For example, in the first five quarters prior to the first intervention period, average utilization was 50.8 total users per quarter. This can be compared to an average in excess of 70 users for the three quarters prior to the last intervention—that is, quarters 3 and 4 of 1980 and quarter 1 of 1981. This

Table 8.10 Frequency of New and Repeat Cancer Screening
Program Users by Quarter, 1978–1981

Year	Quarter	New Users	Repeat Users	Total Users
1978	1	13	28	41
	2	20	34	54
	3	12	21	33
	4	14	51	65
1979	1	14	47	61
	2	89	87	176
	3	12	43	55
	4	20	58	78
1980	1	16	54	70
	2	50	96	146
	3	18	51	69
	4	11	62	73
1981	1	19	60	79
	2	40	141	181

SOURCE: Windsor and Cutter (1982).

suggests an increasing trend and can be evaluated using the techniques described earlier.

To investigate the effect of the trend with attempts to eliminate some of the variability caused by the impact of the intervention, we chose to use a 1-year moving average. This 1-year moving average, in effect, dampens the impact of the intervention periods, which occurred annually. Table 8.11 shows the results of the 1-year moving averages from quarter 4 of 1978 through quarter 2 of 1981. In the column under "Total Users," the smoothed average shows a striking increasing trend by quarter. Simple linear regression analysis of the total number of users on the sequence number of the 11 quarters shows the rate of increase in total users estimated at 3.9 additional users per quarter, which is significantly different from a zero slope. From this, we see that there is a trend in the data collected. At this juncture, we need to ask how plausible it is that the trend is a result of program intervention.

Because this is a cervical cancer screening program, as a patient enters the system, she is encouraged to follow the screening guidelines, which suggest that new users have repeat physicals annually for 3 years. This implies that the intervention should not only increase the total number of users during the intervention quarter but also cause increases in subsequent years as a by-product of entry into the system. To address the question of impact, the 1-year moving averages were computed for new users and repeat users. These averages

Table 8.11   One-Year Moving Averages by Quarter

Year	Quarter	New Users	Repeat Users	Total Users
1978	4	14.75	33.50	48.25
1979	1	15.00	38.25	53.25
	2	32.25	51.50	83.75
	3	32.25	57.00	89.25
	4	33.75	58.75	92.50
1980	1	34.25	60.50	94.75
	2	24.50	62.75	87.25
	3	26.00	64.75	90.75
	4	23.75	65.75	89.50
1981	1	24.50	67.25	91.75
	2	22.00	78.50	100.50
		$R^2 = 0.01$	$R^2 = 0.88$	$R^2 = 0.59$
		$\beta_0 = 24.25$	$\beta_0 = 36.05$	$\beta_0 = 60.38$
		$\beta_1 = 0.25$	$\beta_1 = 3.67$	$\beta_1 = 3.91$
		Not significant	$p < 0.01$	$p < 0.01$

are also shown in Table 8.11 and clearly reveal a strong linear increase in the number of repeat users by quarter. The new users, on the other hand, do not exhibit any trend by quarter; hence, the temporal trend in the total users group is clearly a carryover effect of the repeat screening process and not simply increased utilization across the board over time. This breaking up of the trend enables us to identify findings consistent with the goals of the screening program, both at the utilization level on a cross-sectional basis and in terms of bringing people into the screening system. *Thus, it provides new evidence that the intervention in fact succeeded.* With the knowledge of the trends in the data and the trends appropriate to the intervention, the next stage of the analysis is to assess the data on the impact of the intervention effect itself.

Applying the z score test described above for the existence of an outlier within the data shows that the second quarters of 1979, 1980, and 1981 are all significant, with *p*-values less than 0.05, even without taking into account the trend (i.e., using the standard deviation of all quarters). Testing the significance of these values relative to the standard deviation of the regression line shows all values to be significant at the 0.01 level. Similar tests applied to the new and repeat users also show significant increases during each intervention quarter. Further, graphic analysis, as exhibited in Figures 8.3 and 8.4, shows the in-

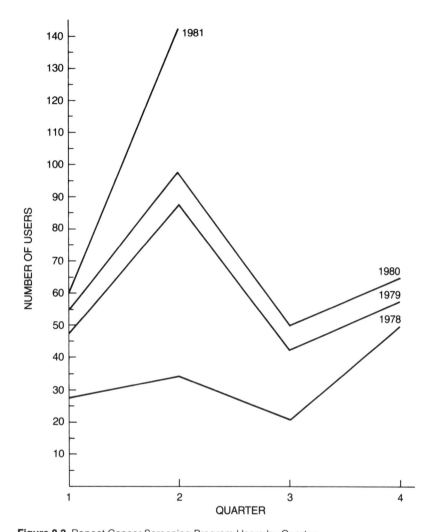

Figure 8.3 Repeat Cancer Screening Program Users by Quarter

SOURCE: R. A. Windsor and G. Cutter, "Quasi-Experimental Designs for Evaluating Cancer Control Programs in Rural Settings," in *Advances in Cancer Control Research and Development*, Proceedings of the Third Conference on Cancer Control, ed. C. Mettlin and G. Murphy, 517–555 (New York: Alan R. Liss, 1982).

crease in both repeat and new users. *The increasing peaks during the second quarters and the parallelism of the curves for repeat CSP users clearly demonstrate the increased utilization brought about by the communications effort.*

The increased number of new users during the second quarters is shown in Figure 8.4 decreasing in 1979, 1980, and 1981. This provides exceedingly useful information to the screening program. It il-

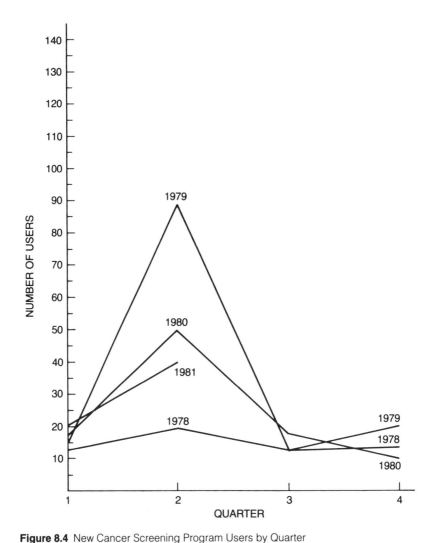

Figure 8.4 New Cancer Screening Program Users by Quarter

SOURCE: R. A. Windsor and G. Cutter, "Quasi-Experimental Designs for Evaluating Cancer Control Programs in Rural Settings," in *Advances in Cancer Control Research and Development*, Proceedings of the Third Conference on Cancer Control, ed. C. Mettlin and G. Murphy, 517–555 (New York: Alan R. Liss, 1982).

lustrates a law of diminishing returns as well as the possibility that the intervention was not applied with as much vigor in later years as in the first year. Thus, the program planners must question how long such an initiative should be continued and for what return. A second issue that is noticeable in the 1978 curve, the baseline period, is a slight increase during the second quarter. This raises the question of whether the effect is partly seasonal. Upon further investigation, we learned that the second quarter coincided with National Cancer Screening Month, and the publicity attending that effort had a consistent effect over time, although of small magnitude.

We have attempted to show with this analysis that, through the collection of rather simple data elements and the application of some fairly simple and straightforward techniques, analysis of time-series data enables us to demonstrate the impact of a community intervention effort, understand which components of the program have been affected by the intervention, and learn what return can be expected in the future on investment of this effort (Windsor and Cutter, 1982).

Two-Group Designs

As noted in Chapter 5, two-group designs occur in two basic ways: by randomization or nonrandom selection. The process of randomization implies that the two groups can be considered equal or comparable. That is, through the randomization process, investigators attempt to ensure that the two groups to be compared have similar characteristics. A nonrandomized design may be a case control study, a nonequivalent control group, or two samples matched on certain characteristics.

In studies or evaluation proposals, the randomized, equivalent control group is a very powerful tool. These two-group studies assign persons randomly to a treatment or a nontreatment group. The statistical tools that are then applied look at either (1) posttreatment measurements, (2) changes from baseline, or (3) number and/or percentage improved, cured, or controlled.

For the first type of analyses, standardized z scores or t scores are computed for the differences between the changes. Table 8.12 shows data on 20 hypertensive individuals randomized to two groups (10 to treatment and 10 to control) before the administration of an educational program designed to improve pill-taking behavior. Random pill counts were used as the dependent measure, and a compliance index of pills taken to pills prescribed was computed. The values before and after treatment are displayed in Table 8.12. The changes in the indices for each patient are shown in the right-hand set of columns. The evaluators by leaving all aspects of comparability to randomization may fail to consider the initial before-treatment measurements and simply analyze the after-treatment compliance indices. This yields a mean compliance index of 99.9 in the treatment group and 94.0 in the control group. Using the approach of two independent samples and applying the t test to the difference between these means, under the hypothesis that there is no difference between treatment and con-

Table 8.12   Compliance Indices Before and After Intervention to Improve Pill-Taking Behavior

	Before		After		Changes	
	Treatment	Control	Treatment	Control	Treatment	Control
Compliance	86	85	110	95	24	10
Index	80	84	102	91	22	7
	86	82	94	101	8	19
	86	83	98	103	12	20
	85	86	100	92	15	6
	84	82	98	94	14	12
	82	82	104	91	22	9
	84	80	102	93	18	13
	88	84	96	89	8	5
	80	78	95	91	15	13
Mean	84.1	82.6	99.9	94.0	15.8	11.4
Standard deviation	2.685	2.366	4.818	4.570	5.67	5.10
t-score	1.33 with 18 degrees of freedom		2.81 with 18 degrees of freedom		0.55 with 18 degrees of freedom	

trol, yields a t statistic of 2.81 with 18 d.f., which is significant at the 1% level, a treatment benefit.

This form of analysis might be used by an evaluator, but actually it is not the most powerful analysis given the design of this study. Because it is always recommended to take measurements of compliance prior to treatment, those data can be used. The before-treatment data show a tendency for the treatment group to have slightly higher compliance indices than the control group—a mean of 84.1 compared with 82.6. The difference in means, when tested with a t statistic, yields a t statistic equal to 1.33 with 18 d.f., which is not statistically significant. However, in observing the difference between these two treatment groups, even given randomization, an evaluator might be advised to assess the difference in the change scores of the treatment and control groups. (Technically, an approach using what is called *regression gain scores* is preferred, but that will be noted here only in passing. The technique analyzes the residuals by group of a regression of after-treatment results on before-treatment levels, plus the treatment group variables.) Doing this assessment in the third set of columns yields a mean increase in the compliance index of 15.8 for the treatment group compared with an increase of 11.4 for the control group. Applying a *t* test to these changes results in a *t* statistic of 0.55 with 18 d.f., which demonstrates no significant difference in increased compliance between the treatment and control groups. It should be pointed out that this example is not included to show the failure of randomization. Randomization is only a mechanism to achieve an unbiased assignment to one of the two groups. The mechanism will, in the long run, produce equivalent groups, but at any particular sample size some differences can occur.

Having applied the statistical tools of *t* tests for continuous variables, an evaluator could ask whether the results were not significant because of violations in the assumptions, such as normality, independence between the two groups, or a representative random sample. A second series of questions, however, could be addressed. The initial one is whether there is evidence of a significant program effect. The lack of evidence could be due to the small sample size yielding the expected large variability, which makes such a small sample insufficient to detect any changes in the compliance index. The intervention may not have worked, which is a question an evaluator must ask even if it goes against prior beliefs and vested interests. Finally, a series of questions must be asked about sources of bias as described in Chapter 6. For example, one source of unequal performance between the interventions could be interviewer effects. In a health education intervention involving two types of therapists (one administering a dietary protocol and the other a compliance protocol), the skills of the therapists might be substantially different. Such differences may cause differences in results, which are related to the performance of those administering the treatments and not the treatments themselves. This is not apparent from the statistics computed or the tests performed on them. Each of the 12 types of bias given in Chapter 6 and their variations should be considered.

A very special form of bias often occurs when investigators look at only the individuals who had positive results. This potential bias is known as *stratification by response*. In general, it is a very dangerous form of analysis and harbors many biases not obvious to the evaluator. If evaluators look at only the individuals who had favorable improvements as a result of a treatment and ignore the rest, they risk showing overly positive results. They also may find correlates of success that are the opposites of the true relationship. For example, in the most extreme case, suppose you are going to mount an intervention designed to reduce stress, based on evidence that all individuals interviewed after having a heart attack (hence all who survived) were individuals who had high stress. You conclude that high stress leads to heart attacks. You could be making a serious mistake, however. Suppose that high stress protects against fatal heart attacks and that individuals who did not have conditioning through high stress died of their heart attacks. You concluded that stress is associated with heart attacks because those individuals interviewed exhibited it. If all the individuals who died did not possess the characteristic, the very characteristic you are setting out to reduce may actually be what allowed the others to survive! Intervening could have the adverse effect of increasing mortality. This is an extreme example of a misinterpretation by evaluation after stratifying by response.

The second type of two-group design is frequently called a *nonequivalent comparison group design* (Case Study 1, Chapter 5). In a community-based program, a comparison ($\underline{C}$) group is selected with similar demographic characteristics, a comparable pattern of utilization (if it is a utilization study), and as many of the same characteristics as can reasonably be matched. Frequently, such studies are used where the ultimate unit of analysis is an aggregate, such as a county, school, or defined geographic area. The design is selected because the addition of the comparison group improves the chances of attributing observed impacts to program efforts applied on this larger scale. In the cervical cancer screening program example, a $\underline{C}$ county, Marengo, was shown in Table 8.9. This county was a nonequivalent comparison group. It was selected on the basis of demographic characteristics, a comparable pattern of service use at the baseline, and the presence of an ongoing community-based cancer screening and detection program over a comparable time period. Marengo County was also chosen as the best county to compare with Hale because of its geographic proximity. An increase in new users in Marengo County can be seen in the second quarters of 1978 and 1979 in Table 8.9. This parallel increase with the intervention county raises some questions about the demonstrated impact for Hale County. Investigation suggested that the increased utilization may have been due to National Cancer Screening Month, which occurs generally in April or May. Special efforts occur throughout Alabama during that month to promote community awareness of and interest in cancer detection. This probably provided an increase in the utilization in both counties.

In the nonequivalent comparison group design, although t tests are used to compare continuous results, often studies are evaluated merely in terms of frequency data. The simplest form of analysis is to compare the increases in the magnitude of new users. A 493% increase in new users is observed for Hale County, 89 versus 15, whereas the magnitude of increase in Marengo is 40%, 45 versus 32. A gross estimate of the impact of the community intervention can be obtained by subtracting the increase noted in the $\underline{C}$ county, 40%, from that noted in the treatment county, 493%. A program using this approach might conclude that the "effect size" was approximately 450% in the intervention county. *Although this rather extensive difference is*

Table 8.13 New Users of Cervical Cancer Screening Clinics, Hale and Marengo Counties, 1979

County	Total New Users	Number in Quarter 2	Percentage
Hale	135	89	65.93
Marengo	140	45	32.14
Total	275	134	

SOURCE: Windsor and Cutter (1982).

likely not to be the true measure, analysis of data from nonequivalent comparison groups studies allows only cautious interpretation of any statistical techniques. In general, the percentage increase could be estimated and tested. Assuming a binomial or Poisson distribution for some of these increases, the means and or variances could be tested for equivalence (Windsor and Cutter, 1982).

More complicated methods could be used, such as fitting response curves to both sets of data and testing the equivalence of the two sets of parameters. Although these methods are generally well known, they are oversophisticated and often do not improve the evaluator's perception of what has taken place. This does not mean that elaborate techniques can never be valuable; however, given available resources and personnel, it is unlikely that such tools will be available to most evaluators. What is useful, though, is not simply an estimate of the percentage increase but also computing a confidence interval for the percentage increase. An approximate method was published by Bross (1954), demonstrating how to assess a percentage increase due to the second-quarter intervention. Table 8.13 shows new users in Hale and Marengo counties for 1979. The table shows total new users and new users in the intervention quarter alone. The percentage of all new users in 1979 who came in during the second quarter in Hale County was 65.93% compared with 32.14% in Marengo. Using this formulation of the data, you can estimate the percentage increase in the second quarter for Hale County compared with Marengo County. The formula is

$$\hat{\theta} = \frac{100(p_2 - p_1)}{p_1}$$

where $\hat{\theta}$ = estimated percentage increase
p_1 = percentage in group 1, or base percentage
p_2 = percentage in group 2, or increased percentage

Applying the data,

$$\hat{\theta} = \frac{100(0.6593 - 0.3214)}{0.3214} = 105.10$$

The percentage increase in the second quarter in Hale County was 105.10%. This shows a substantial increase in the utilization during the second quarter for this single 1-year intervention comparison. *It indicates a substantive effect, and program evaluators can be very comfortable reporting such a percentage increase.* This analytic method takes into account the increase that occurred in Marengo County due to the Cancer Society efforts and shows the additional impact obtained from the educational intervention occurring in Hale County. However, simply a point estimate, such as this percentage increase, may not be sufficient. With small numbers, the estimates vary markedly. Using the methods proposed by Bross (1954), an interval estimate or confidence interval can be obtained, which gives limits for the percentage increase, using the following formula. First, we need two interim values:

$$LL = \text{approximate lower limit} = r - [2\sqrt{r(1 - r)/n}]$$

$$UL = \text{approximate upper limit} = r + [2\sqrt{r(1 - r)/n}]$$

where r is the ratio of the number of individuals in a specified class of the baseline group (group 1), to the total in the class n. Applying the data from Table 8.13, using new users from Marengo County as the baseline group,

$$r = 45/(45 + 89) = 45/134 = 0.336$$

$$LL = 0.336 - [2\sqrt{(0.336)(0.664)/134}] = 0.254$$

$$UL = 0.336 + [2\sqrt{(0.336)(0.664)/134}] = 0.418$$

Thus, to obtain an approximate 95% confidence interval, we find,

$$L = \text{lower estimate} = \frac{100[n_1 - (n_1 + n_2)UL]}{n_2(UL)}$$

$$U = \text{upper estimate} = \frac{100[n_1 - (n_1 + n_2)LL]}{n_2(LL)}$$

where n_1 and n_2 are the total number of individuals in each group, respectively. For the above example,

$$L = \frac{100[140 - (140 + 135)(0.418)]}{135(0.418)} = 44.39\%$$

$$U = \frac{100[140 - (140 + 135)(0.254)]}{135(0.254)} = 204.58\%$$

Although these formulas appear to be rather difficult, reference to Bross's original paper or simply plugging through the formulas can yield the appropriate confidence intervals. Substitution into these formulas shows that the confidence interval for the percentage increase obtained for Hale over Marengo leads to 95% confidence limits of 44.39%–204.58%, *a confidence interval that conveys a sense of strong conviction that there was an additional educational impact in Hale County* (i.e., it does not contain 0).

With the nonequivalent comparison group design (or, in fact, the equivalent control group design) simple time-series analysis is often suitable to assess program impact. Referring to Table 8.9 on new user data for 1978–1980 for Hale County, analysis of the multiple–time series data might be attempted. The literature identifies the multiple–time series (MTS) design as an excellent quasi-experimental method. The data indicate that the baseline year for Hale County, 1978, was stable for the first, third, and fourth quarters, and new users increased during the second quarter, as shown in the table. The baseline data from Marengo County fluctuated more than in Hale, but the observed increase in the second quarter is consistent across counties. The increase in the second quarter in the first intervention year, 1979, was greater for Hale County than for Marengo County. Both E and $\underline{C}$ counties then reverted back to the new user frequencies approximating those in the preintervention quarter. The three quarters between intervention periods of 1979 and 1980 were marked by a relatively stable pattern of use for both E and $\underline{C}$ counties.

The data for the second intervention period in 1980 show a marked increase in Hale County, where the intervention was applied, although of a lesser magnitude than the previous year, and do not show a marked increase in the control county. Following the intervention quarter the frequency of new users again reverted to its original level in Hale County. It is possible that the observed increase from 29 to 40 cases in Marengo County in the third quarter may be attributable in part to another factor—this was the last year this screening clinic was to be open in the county. The basic difference between the patterns is not clear. The average numbers of new users per quarter for 1978, 1979, and 1980 in Hale County were 5, 10.4, and 7.2, respectively. In Marengo County, the averages were 4.4, 6.4, and 6.0, respectively. These data suggest that the observed patterns of change in Hale are somewhat larger than in Marengo. They are not, however, as impressive as the data presented in the visual analyses of the intervention quarters.

Analyses of the MTS designs are merely an extension of the methods of simple time series. If coefficients are estimated, comparisons of these coefficients can be made. Each coefficient is approximately distributed as a t distribution when standardized by its standard error. A two-sample t test can be used to assess the equality of these slopes. A second method is to use analysis of variance with repeated measures or chi-square procedures over both groups. The chi-square test for the quarterly frequency data uses two rows, one for each county, and twelve columns, one for each quarter. *The test answers the question, Are new users per quarter independent of county?* The data shown in Table 8.9 yield a chi-square of 63.85 with 11 d.f. or a p-value less than .0001. This chi-square test for independence suggests that the quarterly frequency is not independent of county, although this does not in itself demonstrate the success of the intervention. To get some idea of whether the intervention has had the desired effect, an evaluator could eliminate the two intervention periods from the computations and recompute the chi-square test. This yields a chi-square of 7.84 with 9 d.f., a result consistent with the independence hypothesis. That is, it suggests there is independence between county and quarter when the two intervention quarters, the second quarter of 1979 and the second quarter of 1980, are eliminated. *In combination, these two results suggest an intervention effect* (Windsor and Cutter, 1982).

Multiple-Group Designs

We merely mention the analyses of multiple groups in this chapter. Generally, these analyses involve some form of regression analysis, analysis of variance, or chi-square procedures. Use of these methods is an extension of the analyses of two-group designs. The title of this chapter conveys the notion that complex designs are not the subject of this chapter. Multiple-group designs, by their very nature, tend to be complex. From this perspective, it is our belief that, when you use such designs, you need a complete understanding of the tools required to analyze the program data before you implement the design. There are many times when multiple groups can be used, such as in studies of layered treatment effects (e.g., a dietary program to reduce cholesterol coupled with an exercise program and possibly a control group). Intervention programs might be used alone and in combination with drug treatments, leading to multiple groups. However, analyses of multiple-group comparisons present problems that are not straightforward in the sense of many of the other tools. Explicit designs should be used when more than two groups are envisioned, and the necessity for more than two groups should be carefully weighed. All too often, program planners invest enormous resources in multiple-group studies with small sample sizes, leading to results that are virtually uninterpretable. Because of the high variability in small samples, the results lack power to show differences in treatment effects. From an analytic perspective, the simpler methods often answer the more important questions. It is better to have a reasonable answer to a simple question than no answer to many questions.

Analysis of variance in the simplest form is a mere extension of the t test. Although the statistics used involve the F distribution rather than the t distribution, the basic computations and concepts are the same. The result of an analysis of variance is displayed as an analysis of variance table. The single test of the hypothesis answers the question of whether there are significant differences among the means of the treatments being considered. This test answers only a single question; the means are equal to each other or they are unequal. The basic procedure followed for the analysis of variance is to ascertain whether the variability that occurs among the various treatment groups is greater than the residual or random error occurring within the treatment groups. An F test is used to compare the size of the variability among the groups to the variability within groups. If there are substantial treatment effects, then the variability among the groups will be significantly greater than the variability within groups.

A second problem, known as a *multiple-comparison problem*, arises when dealing with multiple-group studies. Once the overall significance is found on an F test, evaluators tend to want to know which treatments are better. To learn this, they tend to make a series of paired comparisons. This ultimately leads to a problem in the overall chance of falsely rejecting a hypothesis of no difference, called a *Type I error*. To compensate for this, various procedures are applied that can be found in basic statistics books on analysis of variance. Simply, these procedures require the p-values to be smaller before a result is considered significant.

The use of regression analysis in multiple-group studies is generally done in one of several ways, but it yields results equivalent to those found by analysis of variance. Such techniques are described in the texts on regression analyses and are beyond the scope of this book. The overall use of the chi-square statistic is a straightforward extension of what was presented above for two-group designs. Instead of looking at two rows across interventions for frequency data, the evaluator has multiple groups and goes through the same process of identifying independence between, for example, the intervention period of response and the treatment group. More complicated chi-square techniques are available in the literature on categorical data analyses, as well as more general tools such as the logistic regression model.

SUMMARY

In this chapter, we have discussed simple tools to use in the analysis of program data and community health education evaluations. Although inappropriate uses can and do occur, there are no hard and fast rules for exactly when to use each tool. Experience is an artful teacher. Reacting with careful and clearly articulated questions is as much a necessity in the analysis process as choosing the tools to use.

This chapter has dealt with concepts of basic statistics: types of data—nominal, ordinal, and numerical; accuracy and precision; their equivalence to validity and reliability; and the statistical definition of bias. Some basic rules of data presentation in tables, graphs, and charts were discussed, emphasizing the need for clarity, simplicity, and purpose. A major section was devoted to descriptive statistics. These included: summary counts, measures of central tendency (mean, median, mode), measures of spread or dispersion, range, variance, standard deviation, and standard error. The concept of a distribution was introduced, and the binomial, Poisson, normal, t, chi-square, and F distributions were discussed. The notions of z scores, probability, p-values, and computing formulas were presented.

Two basic types of designs, single-group and two-group, formed the context for the remainder of the chapter. The use of chi-square tests and correlation for identifying associations was presented. Examples of pretest, posttest data, time series, and linear regressions were provided. The computation and interpretation of regression coefficients was given, along with testing their significance. The concept of use and identification of outliers in evaluation studies was explored, illustrated with examples of their use. Several examples of two-group designs were provided, along with a method of generating an estimate of a percentage increase and its confidence interval. Finally, the chapter gave an extended example and some mention of multiple-group designs.

The simple tools of this chapter can be used to enhance the health promotion and education efforts. The results need not always be positive for a thorough analysis to be useful. These tools can uncover the areas of success, failure, and uncertainty to which future efforts can be directed.

9

Cost Analyses

"Our director said she wants to see a cost analysis in future plans of work. What should we include?"

"Everybody talks about cost effectiveness. What is it?"

"I need a good example of cost effectiveness to present to my staff. Are there any good examples in the literature?"

"What is the difference between cost-effective analysis and cost–benefit analysis?"

Professional Competencies Emphasized in This Chapter

• Defining the terms *cost-effective analysis* (CEA) and *cost–benefit analysis* (CBA)

• Describing the steps to estimate personnel and nonpersonnel costs

• Interpreting results of cost analyses: CEA and CBA

• Performing a sensitivity analysis

• Comprehending the role a cost analysis plays in making policy and program-planning decisions.

The *Report of the President's Committee on Health Education* (U.S. Department of Health, Education and Welfare, 1971) recommended that "cost analysis studies should be made to determine the long term effectiveness of health education programs in reducing personal health care costs for persons with specific types of health problems." This represented one of the first national consensus statements about the need for cost analyses of health promotion and education programs. In the 1970s, very few applications of the principles and methods of cost analyses were apparent in the health promotion and education literature (Green, 1974). Rogers et al. (1981) reported one of the first reviews of the cost-effective health promotion programs. The importance of conducting cost analyses for health promotion and education programs is now well established. Documentation of successful program implementation, impact, and associated costs (efficiency evaluations) are recognized as important information for decision making by contemporary program managers and policymakers.

Although a large number of opportunities to conduct cost analysis were missed in the past, a different picture emerged in the 1980s. Multiple reports in peer review journals such as the *American Journal of Public Health, Public Health Reports, American Journal of Health Promotion, Health Education Quarterly*, and *Health Education Research* confirmed cost analyses of health promotion and education interventions for diverse problems, settings, and populations, including the following:

Motorcycle laws (Muller, 1980)

Hypertensive patients (Betera and Betera, 1981)

Childhood asthma (McNabb et al., 1985)

Prevention of high serum cholesterol levels (Oster and Epstein, 1986)

Exercise programs (Hatziandreu et al., 1988)

Health advertising (Freimuth et al., 1988)

Smoking cessation and prenatal care (Windsor et al., 1988; Windsor et al., 1993)

Cost of AIDS (Begley et al., 1990)

Work-site health promotion (Betera, 1990)

These readily available references provide useful case studies from which to gain knowledge about the application of cost analysis methods.

The report from the Brookings Institute, *Evaluating Preventive Care* (Russell, 1987), deserves special attention in a discussion of cost analyses of health promotion programs. This report, proceedings of a workshop held in May 1986, represents a thorough review of the efficacy of selected health promotion/disease prevention programs to improve the health of older people. It includes a review of the related literature for the health effects, type of interventions, and a cost-effective analysis in six health promotion and education program areas: drug therapy for hypertension control, smoking, exercise, dietary calcium uses, obesity counseling, and alcohol use. "Guidelines for Cost Effectiveness Evaluations" and a brief, related bibliography are presented. This report, the literature cited, and many other sources have provided an excellent knowledge base for future study in this area.

The purpose of this chapter is to provide a basic discussion of principles, methods, and applications of cost analyses for planning, implementation, and evaluation of health promotion and education programs. It is beyond the scope of this chapter to present a comprehensive review of all types of cost analyses. Thorough discussions are readily available in health economics literature. An excellent first choice as a referent is *Standards for the Socioeconomic Evaluation of Health Care Services* (Luce and Elixhauser, 1990). Luce and Elixhauser have identified six types of cost evaluation, including (1) cost–benefit analysis (CBA), (2) cost-effective analysis (CEA), (3) cost–utility analysis (CUA), (4) cost-minimization analysis (CMA), (5) cost of illness (COI), and (6) quality-of-life (QOL) assessment. This chapter focuses only on CEA and CBA, because they are the most common methods used to conduct cost studies for health promotion–health education–disease prevention programs.

COST-EFFECTIVE ANALYSIS

Cost-effective analysis (CEA) is an evaluation method designed to assess program alternatives according to costs and effectiveness in the production of a measurable impact or outcomes. The objective of a health promotion and education program evaluation is to determine which intervention method has produced a change ($+$ or $-$) in an impact rate from a baseline pattern or rate: for example, increased participant knowledge, increased skill, increased compliance, increased utilization of health services, or decreased workdays lost. Typically, health promotion and education program evaluations apply different educational–behavioral–communications interventions to an experimental (E) group or a control (or minimal intervention) (C) group. In performing a CEA, two intervention alternatives—E and C—are compared using common measurement methods to confirm the level of achievement of program objectives (end points). Effectiveness data (increases in knowledge, skill, behavior or changes in utilization of health services), representing increases in impact (*output*), are examined in the context of personnel and nonpersonnel costs (*input*) allocated to accomplish the observed degree of effectiveness. This computation enables the evaluator to identify which alternative provided the maximum effectiveness in the context of its cost.

COST–BENEFIT ANALYSIS

Cost–benefit analysis (CBA) represents an evaluation method in which two or more alternatives (E group vs. C group) are compared according to monetary costs (*input*) and monetary benefits (*output*): Program costs and program benefits are measured in dollars and cents. Because CBA compares each alternative in monetary terms, the evaluator ascertains whether a specific method has a benefit that exceeds its costs and which method has the lowest cost-to-benefit ratio. The major issue raised about CBA is the difficulty (methodological and philosophical) with placing a dollar value on *all* program benefits (Rice and Hodgson, 1982; Vladeck, 1984).

PURPOSE OF CEA AND CBA

It is necessary to document expended fiscal resources to implement a health promotion and education program in order to conduct a cost analysis. Furthermore, data confirming successful program implementation (process evaluation), measurement validity and reliability, and internal validity of results (impact evaluation) must be available. Thus, before embarking on a cost analysis, multiple, critical issues identified in Chapters 1 to 8 must be addressed. The general purpose of CEA and CBA is to serve as an analytic evaluation tool to provide insight about program efficiency, thus favoring better decisions about resource allocation. The principles and basic steps to apply the principles of CEA and CBA are well described in the literature. The application of these methods and the assignment of monetary values to human experience or a social program may, however, be problematic. In using CEA and CBA, it is critical to appreciate the technical sophistication of these two evaluation methods and when appropriate to seek special expertise to perform the analyses.

In their original formulation, CEA and CBA had several distinct differences. More recent developments in the health economics literature have brought these two analytic, evaluation methods closer together. Warner and Luce (1982) present a comprehensive discussion of the development and application of CEA–CBA methods.

COST ANALYSIS METHODS

In applying CEA and CBA, there are five sequential steps: (1) defining the problem and objectives; (2) specifying the program—interventions; (3) computing program costs—input; (4) documenting effect size of impact or outcome—output; and, (5) performing sensitivity analyses.

Step 1: Defining the Problem and Objective

The first step in a cost analysis is to document the extent of the problem (numerator) among a defined population-at-risk (denominator). The incidence, or prevalence rate of the problem is specified numerically in behavioral, clinical, or epidemiological terms. If the problem is, for example, high blood pressure or injuries among a cohort of employees, the rates of control, associated morbidity, and utilization of employee health services attributable to the problem can be defined. Each rate, if improved, may have an associated economic benefit.

In defining the baseline incidence, or prevalence rate of a problem—be it a national prevention program or workers at XYZ Company —another essential step is to identify the population-attributable risk (PAR), or causes of the health problem. Concurrently, as part of this step, appropriate health promotion and education "treatment or new intervention alternatives" are identified by staff. Following specification of the extent of the health or behavioral problem, the next step is specification of measurable objectives derived from a valid baseline against which intervention methods are to be compared. It is assumed, at this stage, that technical and program capabilities exist to measure highly valid and reliable *outputs:* behavioral *impact* or health *outcomes.* In some cases, the measurement of an objective may be complicated (e.g., measurement of the quality-of-life years added due to an intervention), but most health promotion program morbidity outcomes (e.g., uncontrolled hypertension, high blood cholesterol levels) or a behavioral outcome (e.g., smoking status, weight loss) can be measured in very reliable and valid ways. Multiple measurable health-status and risk-reduction objectives in *Healthy People 2000* (U.S. Department of Health and Human Services, 1990b) are excellent examples of "measurable objectives."

Multiple objectives for each program are possible. Most major health promotion objectives are measurable, and instruments and methods exist to confirm status at different times for a defined population-at-risk. In some cases, however, some objectives are not easily measurable, such as reduction of suffering or emotional stress. Thus, it is more difficult to establish these types of objectives as endpoints for your health promotion and education program. Description and quantification of program objectives in measurable terms and documentation of a baseline are critical steps for an evaluation and cost analysis.

Step 2: Specifying The Program—Interventions

In Chapters 3–5, we placed considerable emphasis on the essentiality of specifying components and the need to empirically confirm that the set of program procedures (the intervention) was delivered to the target population as planned. From the perspective of cost analysis, you must thoroughly delineate the "program" used to intervene for the health or behavioral problem identified: frequency of contact and duration. It is presumed (the literature and formative evaluation) that the intervention used had an opportunity to modify the specific objectives prepared in step 1. In a health promotion and education program, there will always be one or possibly two intervention alternatives. One alternative is the usual education or information intervention (control group). One or two special interventions (experimental group) are always provided.

A critical dimension in the selection of alternatives at the onset is feasibility and costs. In most cases in the development and decision to deliver health promotion and education programs, interventions are created or selected because they have a good fit to a setting— specific health or behavioral problem—and the population-at-risk.

Step 3: Computing Program Costs (Input)

This step requires documentation of the costs associated with program delivery: staff time per group or individual contact, number of contacts, and the amount of materials distributed. Discussions in Chapter 3 provided some background to budgeting. In the specification of costs, the evaluator is responsible for documenting all budgetary resources expended to provide the program. In general, these costs can be segmented into direct costs, personnel and nonpersonnel, and indirect costs, facilities rent, maintenance, and so on. Whether to use indirect costs in a computation is an individual program judgment and depends on the extent to which the organization requires these costs to be used—who is paying for it?

Personnel Costs. The major costs associated with the delivery of all health promotion and education programs is personnel time: typically 70%–90% of a budget. A detailed description of the intervention would specify how much individual staff time is expended to provide the different components of the intervention. For example, in an employee physical fitness program, a bachelor's-trained exercise physiologist might use 10 hours to deliver once per week a 10-week aerobics class for a group of 20 employees. The instructor may have to spend an additional 10 hours in preparation: 1 hour per session. If you assume a $30,000 per year salary for this person, with a 20% fringe benefit rate (.20 × $30,000 = $6000), then the total salary costs would be $36,000 per year. The hourly rate for this staff member would be $17.30 ($36,000 ÷ 2080 hours). Thus, the total personnel costs to deliver this type of program to employees would be $346.00 ($17.30 × 20 hours).

Other costs to the company could be considered, depending on whether the program was delivered on company time or employee time. It might be zero, if on employee time, or the average hourly wage of the 20 employees, if on company time. Costs for staff to communicate to employees and/or to set up the facilities at all will also be incurred.

Equipment and Material Costs. In marketing and delivering the program, materials such as books, paper, handouts, leaflets, and posters are used. In addition, specialized equipment may be needed (e.g., for an exercise class). Equipment costs used for multiple programs and purposes can be estimated with the estimation of dollars equivalent to that proportion of the time in which the equipment is used solely for your intervention. Materials and equipment costs must be documented.

Another dimension of a cost analysis may be participant co-payment to defray costs.

Facilities Costs. Facilities costs reflect the monetary value of use of the physical space in which a program is provided. All property can be valued. An estimate of the cost per square feet for classroom or meeting space can be computed. The cost per square feet times the hours of use divided by the total number of possible hours of use give you a crude estimate of facilities costs. In situations in which facilities are rented, a lease contract would specify facilities costs. Unless space has to be rented, on-site facilities costs are often not used in cost analyses.

A simple worksheet (see Chapter 3) can be constructed to estimate the total personnel or nonpersonnel input costs allocated to deliver your health promotion and education program.

Step 4: Documenting Effect Size of Impact or Outcome (Output)

The next step in the performance of a cost analysis is to confirm the educational or behavioral impact and/or health outcome specified in your program objective (effect size). In examining these *output* data, you must address the methodological issues related to internal validity. You cannot perform cost analysis unless you have conducted a methodologically rigorous evaluation to provide convincing evidence about the validity of results. You must be able to present empirical evidence to confirm that the outcomes observed are attributable to the methods used.

Data documenting effect size defines the level of intervention impact. A health promotion and education program (e.g., fitness and weight control) may document that method 1 produced at a 6-month follow-up an effectiveness level of "5% less weight than at baseline observation," whereas method 2 produced an effectiveness level of "5% more weight than at baseline observation." Thus, effectiveness or effect size (ES) equals employee group 1 (-5%) or group 2 ($+5\%$).

When comparing method 1 against method 2, you would consider the relative cost to delivery method 1 and method 2 and compare the data in the context of effectiveness (weight loss). This computation produces a cost-effective ratio (CER). Looking at this example from a CBA perspective, you might be able to examine the costs of method 1 and method 2 and document the benefits (if any can be expected) in monetary terms of the method (e.g., was a reduction in workdays lost and cost savings observed?). Absenteeism rates (if attributable to the method)—producing a decrease in workdays lost—could translate into monetary savings. In the CBA evaluation of method 1 versus method 2, a cost-to-benefit ratio (CBR) would be computed and total economic benefit reported.

Step 5: Performing Sensitivity Analysis

If a favorable cost savings and CBR are documented, you may then decide to examine these results in the context of variations of costs for *input* and *output* at different sites or with different groups of program participants. Before you establish a new policy or new program and commit a large amount of money to a new activity, you want to have a clear picture of program efficiency. The purpose of sensitivity analysis (SA) is to estimate costs using different assumptions to determine how the cost savings and the CER or CBR would change. For example, personnel and material costs vary from site to site. You might decide in your SA to increase personnel costs 10% or 20% and to decrease the observed level of effectiveness 10% or 20%. By applying these SA assumptions, you can document, using estimates (low-medium-high), what changes would occur in your conclusions about each method. It is important to emphasize that, in choosing and applying SA, your assumptions must be reasonable. It is also not always necessary to apply SA; a clear rationale is needed. Case Studies 1 and 3 provide an application of SA.

Sensitivity analysis may produce four important results for the evaluator: (1) the dependence on a specific assumption of a conclusion of effectiveness, (2) an assumption that does not significantly affect conclusion, (3) a confirmation of the assumption of minimum or maximum value that a cost factor must have for a program to appear worthwhile, and (4) issues and uncertainties deserving future cost analyses evaluation.

VALUATION: DISCOUNTING

A discussion of costs must also include consideration of the value of monetary resources for purposes other than allocation to health promotion and education programs. Simply put, if a company budgets (invests) $100,000 annually in a health promotion and education program, it is taking resources away from other investment opportunities. It is also important to realize that all program costs and expenditures are not incurred at the present time. Costs are incurred over a period of years and the benefits (real or estimated savings) occur over a longer period of time. The issue is estimating the costs and benefits of a program throughout its effective lifetime. Therefore, future dollar costs and benefits are reduced, or "discounted," to reflect the fact that dollars spent or saved in the future should not weigh as much as dollars spent or saved today.

The term used to consider the value of current and future dollars in a cost analysis is *discounting*. The choice of the most appropriate discount rate (typically 3%–5%) depends to a large extent on how inflation rates are addressed. If all items in the costs of the program are expected to increase at the same rate and at the same rate as inflation, there are two choices in discounting. First, inflate all future costs and use a larger discount rate to allow for the effect of inflation. This is called the "inflation-adjusted discount rate." Second, do not inflate any future costs and use a smaller discount rate to not allow for inflation. Some financial calculators have discount functions. Numerous financial software packages for personal computers can easily perform these calculations.

The basic premise of discounting is that an organization has the option to invest an amount of money in units (e.g., $10,000) to an activity. If $10,000 is invested, it may yield $500 at a CD rate of 5%, for a total of $10,500 each year. Concurrently, during this year the economy experiences an inflation rate. If the inflation rate during the coming year is 10%, then the sum of $10,000 will have the investment buying power of only $9000 in the next year.

In the applications of CEA and CBA, there are a number of health problems areas for which cost analyses are complex and imprecise. The literature must be reviewed and specific expertise sought for your program area to ascertain how each issue—discounting, inflation, and sensitivity analysis—needs to be addressed.

CASE STUDIES

The following three case studies provide examples of the application of cost analysis methods. Case Study 1 describes methods used to conduct a CEA of two different health education methods for patients in maternity care. Case Study 2 describes the application of CEA to health education methods for adults with asthma in a pulmonary medicine clinic. Case Study 3 presents an application of CBA to an evaluation of the impact and estimated savings from health education methods for pregnant smokers in public health maternity clinics for an entire state.

Case Study 1 CEA: Self-Help Smoking-Cessation Methods for Pregnant Women

SOURCE: R. A. Windsor, K. Warner, and G. Cutter, "A Cost Effectiveness Analysis of Self-Help Smoking Cessation Methods for Pregnant Women," *Public Health Reports* 103(1) (1988):83–87. (*See publication for references.*)

Introduction

The 1985 Institute of Medicine's report, "Preventing Low Birthweight," identified smoking during pregnancy as a contributing factor in 20–40 percent of low birth weights among infants of women receiving public assistance in the United States. A major recommendation of the report was to consider the issues of relative costs and benefits in formulating public health policy about health education methods designed to increase birth weight. Lack of adequate data prevented the committee from estimating the additional public expenditure required to finance the recommended public health education program. The Institute of Medicine's report and a recent review of the intervention research literature concluded that estimates of the cost effectiveness and cost benefit of health promotion and education methods to increase birth weight are not available.

Our paper presents the results of a cost-effectiveness derived from a recently completed randomized trial to evaluate the effectiveness of self-help smoking-cessation methods for pregnant women in public health maternity clinics. The research methods, self-help interventions, and results have been discussed in detail elsewhere.

Cost-effectiveness analysis refers in this paper to the comparative evaluation of the costs and behavioral impact of three cessation methods for pregnant smokers used in the randomized trial. These analyses were performed to provide decision makers, such as directors of maternal and child health and public health education programs, with information to evaluate cessation methods; the goal was to maximize the effective use of available resources.

Methods

A randomized pretest–posttest design was used in the trial. At the time of their first clinic visit, pregnant smokers—a total of 309 women from three prenatal clinics—were assigned to one of three groups. Baseline comparability of the three groups was confirmed. Group 1, the standard information control group, received information in a nonfocused interaction on smoking and pregnancy, requiring about 5 minutes during the first prenatal visit. Group 2 received the standard clinic information on smoking plus a copy of "Freedom from Smoking in 20 Days," a manual published by the American Lung Association (ALA). Group 3 received the standard clinic information plus the pregnancy-specific self-help manual, "A Pregnant Woman's Self-Help Guide to Quit Smoking."

The Pregnant Woman's Guide went through extensive internal and external review before it was given to Group 3. All skills were pilot tested with pregnant smokers at each of the clinics. A prototype of the guide was produced representing a standardized smoking cessation method that professionals in prenatal care could use to educate their patients. Three pregnant women who participated in the pilot study of 50 pregnant smokers and who had used the guide to become ex-smokers served as editorial consultants.

Groups 2 and 3 also received an informational packet entitled "Because You Love Your Baby" on the risks of smoking and the benefits of quitting that is disseminated by the ALA. The patient education methods used to teach the use of the self-help manuals for Groups 2 and 3 were standardized and presented in approximately 10 minutes at the first prenatal visit by the same woman, a baccalaureate-trained health education specialist. No smoking cessation intervention methods were used with the 309 women after their first visits.

Smoking status was confirmed at midpregnancy and end of pregnancy, using patient self-reports and saliva thiocyanate tests with a cutoff value of 100 micrograms per milliliter or less. Women lost to followup were counted as smokers.

Cost Analysis. Intervention costs were estimated by identifying associated resources, determining their unit values (prices), multiplying the number of units of each by its price, and summing across all resource categories. The principal resources used were personnel and the self-help educational materials. No cost for the use of facilities were estimated. The cessation methods were applied during normal clinic hours in the three public health facilities and thus did not produce incremental or differential facilities costs. Because almost no supplies were used beyond those used during the normal visits to the clinics, supply costs were treated as zero. The one exception was the supplies needed for the saliva thiocyanate tests. These tests are unlikely to be used in an everyday clinic setting and hence were not considered to be a resource cost associated with self-help methods. From a social perspective, the client's time also was a resource, although it would not be relevant to an agency director dealing with program budgets. For purposes of this analysis, we adopted the perspective of the agency.

Estimating Personnel Costs. A health education specialist with a bachelor of science was used to teach groups 2 and 3. However, a nurse with a BSN is the most likely person to provide smoking cessation methods as part of prenatal care. Personnel costs vary from State to State, by type of personnel and by level of training. Based on interviews with personnel unit officials of health departments of six major cities, we estimated the average wage (1986) for clinic health department nurses at $20,000, with fringe benefits totaling an additional 20 percent, for a total personnel cost of $24,000 per nurse per year. Thus, the hourly labor cost per nurse was estimated at $12 (assuming 40 hours per week and 50 workweeks per year).

As noted previously, the time spent at first visit in Groups 2 and 3 to educate the women about how to use the self-help guides was on the average about 10 minutes each. Two brief followup nonintervention contacts were conducted to collect saliva samples and self-reports of smoking status. Each followup took an additional 2–3 minutes. Although not designed to be part of the patient education intervention, patients may have perceived the followup contacts to be part of it. Additionally, in practice, prenatal staff are likely to make inquiries about patient smoking status at subsequent clinic encounters. For women in Groups 2 and 3 who had quit, a verbal statement of encouragement such as "keep up the good work" was made.

Actual personnel time per client should be counted for a total of approximately 15 minutes for Groups 2 or 3. Group 1 required 5 minutes of staff time per client at first visit, with an additional combined 5 minutes for the midpoint and end-of-pregnancy followups. Total personnel time per client in group 1 was about 10 minutes. In all cases, personnel time was valued at the appropriate fraction of the hourly rate defined previously. The cost of each ALA cessation manual to the project in 1983 was $4, and the cost of each Pregnant Woman's Guide was also $4. Thus, the total costs and personnel time were the same for Groups 2 and 3.

Results

The end-of-pregnancy quit rates were 2 percent in Group 1, 6 percent in Group 2, and 14 percent in Group 3. A quitter was confirmed by combining patients self-reports of smoking status at followup with their saliva thiocyanate values.

Table 9.1 represents the cost per patient and cost-effectiveness ratios by study group. The ratios suggest that the pregnancy-specified, tailored self-help methods provided to Group 3 patients were more cost effective in encouraging smoking cessation than either the standard smoking cessation information provided to Group 1 or the self-help methods for Group 2. These estimates suggest that the Group 3 methods can achieve smoking cessation at less than half the cost of either of the two

Table 9.1 Cost Effectiveness of 3 Smoking-Cessation Methods

Group	Cost per Patient	Percent Who Quit	Cost-Effectiveness
1. Information	$2.08	2%	$104.00
2. ALA manual	$7.13	6%	$118.83
3. Guide	$7.13	14%	$ 50.93

NOTE: Cost effectiveness = cost per patient divided by who quit (effectiveness).
Group 1 = information in a nonfocused interaction on smoking and pregnancy.
Group 2 = information plus the "Freedom from Smoking" manual of the ALA.
Group 3 = information plus a self-help guide for pregnant women.

alternatives tested. Group 1 methods were the least costly on a per patient basis, but the increase in effectiveness associated with the Group 3 methods is sufficiently greater than the increase in the per patient cost of delivery to make this intervention more cost effective. Compared with the Group 1 method, Group 2's greater effectiveness is not sufficient to compensate for its greater cost.

Discussion

Sensitivity Analysis. The reported findings are based on several assumptions about costs and effectiveness. We performed several sensitivity analyses to assess whether the basic conclusions depended on the precise estimates employed in the analysis. Specifically, we addressed the following questions:

1. *Is the finding of the greater efficiency of the Group 3 (Pregnant Woman's Guide) approach dependent on the precision of its effectiveness?* The guide is more cost effective because it shares the highest cost with the ALA Manual but is more effective (14 percent versus 6 percent). There is, however, a substantial margin for the Guide to be less effective than observed without losing its cost effectiveness. The observed quit rate could be halved, and the guide would remain the most cost effective of the three methods. We conclude, therefore, that the superiority of the pregnancy-specific method is not likely to be dependent on the precision of the estimate of its effectiveness. The Guide will remain preferred to the ALA Manual as long as its effectiveness is greater, a function of the identical cost. The guide must be 3.4 times more effective to maintain superiority over the standard informational approach. The 1988 cost of the guide of $4 versus the cost of $7 for the "new" ALA Manual for pregnant smokers makes the guide even more cost effective because of its significantly lower cost.
2. *Is the cost effectiveness of the Group 3 methods dependent on the precise estimate of the cost of staff time, the dominant cost of intervention?* Allowing the hourly rate for labor costs to vary by 20 percent above our estimate, equivalent to base annual salaries of $24,000, we find that the pregnancy-specific self-help cessation method substantially dominates the two alternatives even when the high hourly rate is used for the guide and the low hourly rate is used for the two alternatives.
3. *Do the cost estimates of the materials significantly affect the findings?* No. The cost of the Group 3 methods could be nearly twice that observed, the third alternative would remain the most cost effective.

Social Cost Versus Accounting Cost. From a social perspective, the value of patient's time could be included as a resource cost. From an agency perspective—the perspective adopted in the analysis presented —clients' time is not a resource on which departmental funds must be expended. Hence, it is not a program budget component. It may be useful, however, to consider briefly how inclusion of the value of the patient's time might affect our analysis. As in the case of personnel, only the incremental time required by the interventions represents an intervention cost. Time expended by patients traveling to clinics and waiting to be seen by the health professionals is not a relevant cost, because patients already incur these costs for regular periodic clinic exams. In this context, incremental clinic time spent by patients is identical to that of the staff.

For patients in Groups 2 and 3, however, there is an additional incremental cost, namely, the time to read and use the self-help packages. If this extra time totals about 1 hour (7 days × 8–10 minutes), patients in Groups 2 and 3 will spend 75 minutes on the intervention. Patients in Group 1, by contrast, will devote only the additional 10 minutes also experienced by staff. If we value patients' time at $3.35 per hour (minimum hourly wage), the value of each patient's time required for Group 1 methods is about $56 (0.166 per hour × $3.35), while that required for Group 2 and 3 interventions is $419 (1.25 per hour × $3.35). This adds 27 percent ($.56 divided by $2.08) to the per patient cost for Group 1 and 59 percent ($4.19 divided by $7.13) to the cost of Groups 2 and 3 methods; cost-effectiveness ratios increase similarly. Under these circumstances, the Group 3 methods remain the most cost-effective and Group 2 the least cost effective.

Program and Policy Implications. A clear responsibility exists to provide efficient and effective methods to pregnant women to help them quit smoking. Increased attention is also needed to assist maternal and child health programs in the planning, management, and evaluation of smoking-cessation programs for pregnant smokers. A comprehensive review of the literature and this analysis indicate that simple verbal statements about risk are ineffective and inefficient. These data, and data from other studies, suggest that the typical informational content and methods of prenatal care education in the United States related to smoking need to be significantly revised. It should include specific smoking-cessation and maintenance methods to help the pregnant woman become and remain a nonsmoker. If a public health department expects to achieve a quit rate greater than 2–3 percent, increases in resources and time will have to be allocated.

Personnel costs associated with the provision of effective cessation methods can be absorbed by most ongoing prenatal education programs with small allocations of personnel time. Training requirements for nurses to use self-help methods are also modest. Initial inservice training and periodic training for new prenatal care nurses on how to teach the use of self-help methods as part of prenatal education would take approximately 2 hours, resulting in a training cost of $24 per nurse (at $12 per hour). This cost, however, would be spread out over a year for counseling all pregnant smokers. An additional cost of approximately $.24 per patient would be incurred if 100 pregnant smokers were counseled. Training time and costs, therefore, could double from 2 to 4 hours ($24 to $38) and only increase the cost for 100 patients counseled to about $.50 each. Although not tested in this study, it is also likely that the $.24 to $.48 cost per patient would be reduced, because almost all prenatal care education programs would provide this type of patient education as part of a small group. Additionally, in cases where there was little staff turnover, the cost would be further reduced in proportion to the number of pregnant smokers counseled. Total training costs would be very low.

Because the 2 percent control group quit rate observed in this study (3) is comparable to other reported quit rates (2–4 percent) for pregnant smokers after initiating prenatal care, perhaps only 20,000–40,000 of the annual cohort of approximately 1 million pregnant smokers are being motivated to quit by information approaches after initiating prenatal care. If the pregnancy-specific self-help methods and corresponding 14 percent quit-smoking rate observed in this trial could be applied to this cohort, there might be 140,000 quitters. This estimate is likely to be conservative, however, because more affluent and educated pregnant smokers who are provided cessation methods exhibit quit rates of approximately 25 percent.

The estimated cost of prenatal care, including delivery and postpartum care for a normal delivery, is approximately $2,000–$3,000, while the cost of neonatal delivery in Level II or Level III hospitals using low-to-medium estimates is approximately $14,000–$20,000. Although estimating clinical outcomes and cost–benefit ratios were not purposes of this trial, we note that if this type of self-help method were used, additional direct costs might be avoided due to reduced hospitalization and morbidity related to increased birth weight.

Applying the cost estimates from Table 9.1 to the 1 million pregnant smokers who deliver each year, the total cost for universal application of self-help methods would be approximately $7 million. The total investment across the 50 states, therefore, would be small, an insignificant proportion of the total private or public sector costs associated with low birth weight. Although additional rigorous behavioral impact and cost-effectiveness studies are needed, the self-help health education methods tested in this trial and other methods show promise as solutions to part of the problem of improving the health and well-being of the next generation of pregnant women and their infants and children in the United States.

Case Study 2 CEA: Health Education Methods to Increase Medication Adherence Among Adults with Asthma

SOURCE: R. Windsor, W. Bailey, J. Richards, B. Manzella, S-j. Soong, and M. Brooks, "The Efficacy and Cost Effectiveness of Health Education Methods to Increase Medication Adherence Among Adults with Asthma," *American Journal of Public Health* 80(12) (1990): 1519–1521. *(See publication for references.)*

Introduction

The prevalence of asthma among adults in the United States is 3–6 percent. There are over 500,000 hospitalizations and 3,500 deaths from asthma per year. Multiple studies of adults with asthma confirm adherence levels of only 30–40 percent. Educational intervention studies have reported methodological problems, used small sample sizes, lacked cost analyses, and presented inconclusive results. This evaluation study was designed to document *Efficacy*—the level of behavioral impact produced by a Health Education Program with optimal resources and *Costs* (personnel and materials) needed to routinely deliver the program.

Methods

The study was conducted at a University-based Comprehensive Pulmonary Medicine Clinic. Patients who had a primary diagnosis of asthma, used medications daily, and met the following diagnostic criteria were eligible: recurrent episodes of wheezing or dyspnea; objective evidence of significantly increased airway resistance during episodes; and improvement in the airway when symptom-free. Of the 280 adults ≥17 years meeting the criteria screened between April 1986 to March 1987, 267 (95 percent) participated.

Following informed consent and baseline assessment, 135 patients were randomized to a control group and 132 patients to an experimental group. Prior to randomization, patients were stratified by level of asthma severity within each of 11 physician practices. Using pilot study data, an estimated possible improvement in adherence of 20 percent or more for 12-months, and an anticipated 10 percent attrition rate, we defined a need for at least 120 patients in each study group.

Health Education Intervention

The Experimental Group received a peak flow meter and a standardized program from a health education specialist:

> A 30-minute one-to-one session with instruction on peak flow–meter use, inhaler use skills, and use of *A Self-Help Guide to Asthma Control,*

> A 60-minute asthma support group session of 4–6 patients and asthma control partners, and

> Two brief telephone reinforcement calls within one month of the group session.

One-to-one discussions and a review of all methods and materials were conducted with clinic nurses and all 11 participating pulmonary physicians. Four focus group sessions with patients were held to develop the intervention. All educational components and evaluation methods were pilot tested.

Measurement

All patients received a baseline and 12-month follow-up medical and behavioral assessment including four behavioral outcomes: (1) correct in-

Table 9.2   Baseline Patient Characteristics by Study Group

Characteristics		Control Group N = 135	Experimental Group N = 132
Sex: female		71%	61%
Race: black		28%	32%
Median age		49	50
Median years of education		13	13
Current smoker		13%	10%
Asthma severity	Mild	39%	37%
	Moderate	45%	48%
	Severe	17%	16%

haler use, (2) inhaler adherence, (3) medication adherence, and (4) total adherence rating. A 10-item observational checklist documented inhaler use and skill (IU). Medication adherence (MA) and inhaler adherence (IA) were assessed using instruments adapted from the literature. Psychometric analyses (Cronbach Alpha) confirmed adequate reliability: r (MA) = .69, r (IA) = .64, and r (IU) = .78. Items analyses confirmed minimum item-discrimination coefficients: r ≥ .20. A Total Adherence Score was derived by combining patient scores on the medication and inhaler adherence scales.

Over 85 percent of the patients used an inhaled bronchodilator and continuous theophylline. Theophylline levels were analyzed on the two follow-up assessment days to indirectly corroborate patient adherence reports. Patients were informed that their theophylline level would be analyzed to assess adherence. While theophylline level is an imperfect measure of adherence and does not reflect adherence to non-theophylline medications, behavioral studies of adults who know a method is available to validate self-reports document a significant reduction in deception rates (bogus pipeline or pipeline effect).

Behavioral Intervention Results

A comparison of the 13 patients who refused (5% refusal rate) versus the 267 who participated confirmed no baseline differences by gender, race, age, education, and asthma severity. Data in Table 9.2 confirm group equivalence at baseline. Thirty-four of the control group patients (25%) and 8 of the experimental group patients (6%) were lost to follow-up. Analyses of baseline data confirmed that the 42 dropouts were not significantly different from the 238 participants. Within the intervention group, use of the *Asthma Guide* was reported by 124 patients (94%), 110 (89%) participated in the group session and 124 patients (94%) received both reinforcement calls.

The behavioral impact of the intervention is presented in Figure 9.1.

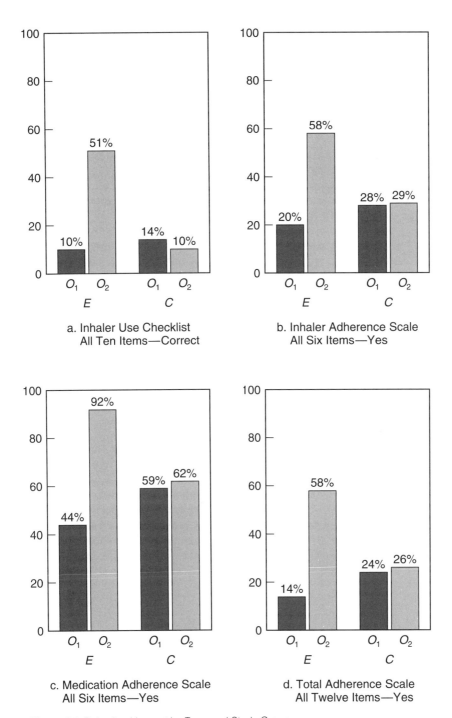

a. Inhaler Use Checklist
All Ten Items—Correct

b. Inhaler Adherence Scale
All Six Items—Yes

c. Medication Adherence Scale
All Six Items—Yes

d. Total Adherence Scale
All Twelve Items—Yes

Figure 9.1 Behavioral Impact by Type and Study Group

Table 9.3   Cost Effectiveness of the Health Education Program

Group	Cost per Patient	Adherence Score Improvement	Total Cost Effectiveness*
Control Group (N = 135)	$ 3.61	+ 2%	$243.68
Experimental Group (N = 132)	$32.03	+44%	$ 96.09

*Cost effectiveness = Total cost per group divided by Adherence Score Increase.

Using a 95% confidence interval (CI) to evaluate differences between rates of group improvement, a consistent pattern of adherence was confirmed for a 12-month period. Significant improvements for the intervention group in inhaler skills use (CI = .29, .61), inhaler adherence (CI = .24, .50), medication adherence (CI = .31, .57), and total adherence score 100 percent adherence (CI = .28, .56) were observed. Little behavior change was observed in the control group.

Cost Estimation and Analysis

Patient time and intervention development costs were not used to compute program costs. While an MPH-health education specialist provided the intervention, a nurse would be the typical provider. We used a salary of $25,000 plus a fringe benefit rate of 20% to estimate nursing cost: $30,000 per year/2080 hr. = $14.42/hr. Total personnel time costs for the experimental group were $24.30: Component #1 = $7.21, Component #2 = $14.42 and Component #3 = $2.40. The *Asthma Guide* cost $8.00 for a Total Intervention Cost = $32.03/patient. The total Control Group costs for a 10-minute general discussion about the importance of adherence and two brief follow-up contacts for a total of 15 minutes were $3.61/patient. Cost analyses presented in Table 9.3 confirmed the need to allocate resources to significantly increase patient adherence.

Discussion

The increase in adherence observed in our intervention group exceeded those of previous reports. While some proportion of patient self-reports of adherence may represent a "social desirability" response, psychometric analyses indicated good measurement of behavioral impact. Our high recruitment rate confirmed that adults with asthma are interested in taking an active role in their self-management and will participate in a health education program integrated into routine asthma care. Near unanimous positive anecdotal comments about the intervention by nurses, physicians, and patients were observed. Feasibility, patient and provider acceptance was very high. From an administrative and programmatic perspective, our experience indicated that this type of intervention has potential for adaptation by other asthma programs. However, in our attempt to maximize efficacy, an intervention was provided that may be too resource-intensive and costly for other asthma-care sites. Although the methods and results reported here and elsewhere were encouraging, future health education research needs to evaluate the impact of a streamlined health education program on health services utilization—for example, ambulatory care, emergency care, and hospitalization—and clinical outcomes.

Case Study 3 (CBA): Health Education Methods for Pregnant Smokers

SOURCE: R. A. Windsor, J. B. Lowe, L. L. Perkins, D. Smith-Yoder, L. Artz, M. Crawford, K. Amburgy, and N. R. Boyd, Jr., "Health Education Methods for Pregnant Smokers: Behavioral Impact and Cost Benefit," *American Journal of Public Health* 83(2) (1993):201–206.

Introduction

Maternal smoking causes infant morbidity and mortality. The elimination or reduction of active and passive maternal and fetal exposure to cigarette smoke represent a high priority for the decade. The need for effective smoking cessation methods among pregnant women, particularly high risk public health populations, is well defined.

Multiple randomized clinical trials and evaluation studies have reported estimates of the behavioral impact of cessation methods for pregnant smokers and assessed medical cost outcomes. Only one clinical trial has evaluated the behavioral impact and the cost effectiveness of cessation methods among pregnant smokers in a public health maternity setting. Cost benefit analyses of health education methods for that setting are not available.

This report presents the results of the Birmingham Trial II, an evaluation of the behavioral impact and cost benefit of a health education program for pregnant smokers in public health maternity clinics.

Methods

This study was conducted from 1986 to 1991 at the four highest census maternity clinics, representing 85% of the annual cohort, of the Jefferson County Health Department (JCHD) in Birmingham, Alabama. A fifth JCHD clinic with a small census did not participate.

A Formative Evaluation was conducted from July, 1986, to August, 1987: (1) to conduct a prospective, natural history study prior to pre-Trial II to document smoking prevalence and quit rates attributable to routine prenatal care and risk information; (2) to train the health counselors; and (3) to pilot-test the intervention, measurement, and data collection methods. Intervention, evaluation, and data collection methods were adapted from Trial I conducted at the JCHD from 1982 to 1985.

Screening interviews at the first prenatal visit from September 1, 1987, to November 30, 1989, identified 4,352 patients: 1,381 (31.7%) reported smoking at conception. Of the 1,381, 1,171 were current smokers (26.9%) and 210 patients were self-initiated quitters (4.8%) before their first visit. A current smoker was defined as: "a patient who self-reported during the first prenatal visit at least one puff of one cigarette in the last seven days." An assessment study using self-reports and salivary cotinine analyses confirmed that 74 (35%) of the 210 self-initiated quitters relapsed before delivery.

Of the 1,171 smokers screened, 110 (9.4%) were ineligible for one or more of the following reasons: (1) were not pregnant, (2) were ineligible for care, (3) were very late entry into care (≥ 32 weeks), (4) did not stay for the first visit, (5) did not return for care, (6) were Trial I participants, (7) were prisoners, and/or (8) had difficulty reading the baseline questionnaire. Of the 1,061 women eligible, only 67 patients (5.7%) refused to participate. Thus, 994 smokers were enrolled in Trial II.

Evaluation Design. A prospective randomized pre-test, post-test control group evaluation design with mid-pregnancy and end of pregnancy assessments of smoking status from self-reports and saliva cotinine tests was implemented. Random assignment of 994 patients was performed at the first prenatal visit after informed consent using a computer generated system: Experimental (E) Group = 493 patients and Control (C) Group = 501 patients. After randomization, 93 E Group and 87 C Group patients became ineligible due to withdrawal from the public health maternity system, a miscarriage, or an abortion. A total of 814 pregnant smokers were eligible for a follow-up: E Group = 400 and C Group = 414.

Formative and Process Evaluation. A Formative Evaluation was conducted at the four clinics with a sample of 269 patients (100 smokers and 169 non-smokers) recruited from 300 consecutive intakes. A 35% smoking prevalence rate (105/300) and a 10% refusal rate (31/300) was observed. The sample of 100 smokers served as a prospective, Historical Comparison Group (C/Group) to document pretrial baseline prevalence rates and "normal" quit rates from the first visit to the third trimester and childbirth. Data and saliva collection methods were reviewed by clinic nurses and administrators and field tested with the 269 patients.

Intervention time, barriers to routine use, and patient participation rates were documented for each clinic. Focus group discussions were held with five to eight patients at each clinic to field test the E Group intervention. As a part of the Formative Evaluation, the intervention was pilot tested, reestablishing the feasibility of routinely providing cessation methods and confirming patient and provider acceptance.

A Process Evaluation system was pilot tested with the sample of 269 patients. Monthly, quarterly, and annual clinic reports were prepared to document the level of implementation for the three intervention components and each measurement procedure.

Health Education Methods. The health education intervention had three components.

Component #1:   During the first visit, a standardized, health education cessation skills and risk-counseling session of approximately 15 minutes was provided from a trained female health counselor to E Group patients. Patients were taught how to use a seven day self-directed cessation guide (Windsor R, Amburgy K, and Artz L: Unpublished cessation Guide, 1987) with a sixth grade reading level. The guide and counseling session were modified methods from Trial I. Following completion of Trial II, the self-help *Guide* was revised for dissemination purposes.

During follow-up visits patients received components #2 and 3:

Component #2:   Clinic patient reinforcement methods were provided. A Chart Reminder Form was put in the medical record and a Medical Provider Letter was sent to patients within seven days.

Component #3:   Social support methods were provided in the form of: a buddy letter, a buddy contract and a buddy tip sheet. Each patient was also sent a one page quarterly "newsletter" with testimonial information on successful quitters, additional risk information, and cessation tips.

All 814 E and C Group patients were strongly urged to quit and were given two pamphlets: *Smoking and the Two of You* (an American Lung Association pamphlet) which provided risk and benefit information and *Where to Find Help if You Want to Stop Smoking* with a contact name, phone number and cost of local programs.

During a 30-minute group prenatal education class at the first visit as a part of the standard prenatal care process and content, the risks of smoking and the importance of quitting were presented to all patients in about 2 minutes by a nurse. No staff participated in continuing education on smoking cessation and no changes were observed in the staff counseling behavior during the study.

Measurement. Patients completed a one-page screening form, informed consent, and a self-administered questionnaire to document baseline smoking status, health beliefs, and commitment to quit. Saliva samples were tested using a standardized radioimmunoassay (RIA) protocol by the Clinical Biochemistry Laboratory of the American Health Foundation (AHF). Patients were informed that their saliva would be analyzed.

Smoking status was reassessed by self-reports and cotinine tests at approximately four to eight weeks after the first visit (mid-point observation) and as soon as possible after the 32nd week of gestation (end-point observation). Only one follow-up was performed for patients who started care during the 6th or 7th month of pregnancy. A cotinine value of ≤30 ng/ mL was used as the cut-off to validate self-reports of cessation.

Because a dose-response relationship exists between maternal smoking and intrauterine growth retardation, in addition to documenting quit rates, significant reduction rates were also documented for E and C Group patients. A patient was defined as a "significant reducer" if her follow-up cotinine value was 50% or less than her baseline value, e.g., 200 ng/mL to ≤100 ng/mL.

Compliance Assessment. Compliance needs to be documented to establish the feasibility of implementation and patient use of all health education methods or programs. E Group patients completed a self-administered questionnaire at the mid-point follow-up to document the number of days the *Guide* and cessation methods were used. They had to report use of the *Guide* four or more days and use of five or more cessation methods to be counted as "compliant."

Cost Estimation. Before health education programs are routinely used, a cost analysis should be performed. The cost to deliver the intervention was personnel time and educational materials. Because an agency perspective was used in our cost analyses, patient time, facilities cost, and intervention development costs were not used in our estimates. While a health counselor provided the intervention, a nurse would be the usual provider. A salary of $30,000 plus a fringe benefit rate of 20 percent was used to estimate staff cost ($36,000 per year/2,080 hours = $17.31 per hour). Personnel costs for routine use of the 15-minute intervention including brief reinforcement would be about $4.33/patient ($17.31 × 0.25). While the *Guide* costs were approximately $5.00/patient, large volume printing—5,000 copies—reduces the cost to about $1.25/patient. The cost of educational materials, reproduction, and labor costs is about $0.40. The total intervention cost is about $6.00/patient.

Two minutes were spent at the first visit to provide the C Group one-to-one risk information and materials. That, plus brief contacts at follow-up visits which may have served as reinforcement produced a total of five minutes, so total cost amounted to about $1.50/patient ($17.31 × 0.083).

Cost Benefit Analyses of Statewide Dissemination. Smoking population attributable risk (SPAR) for LBW has been documented at 20% to 35%. A low estimate of this risk was used to estimate the potential impact of statewide dissemination of the intervention on the LBW incidence in Alabama in 1990.

The benefit of dissemination, defined as the estimated number of LBW infants preventable by cessation, was based on the estimated net incremental health care costs of a LBW birth provided by the Office of Technology Assessment (OTA): $9,000 (low estimate) and $23,000 (high estimate). These estimates include three components: (1) hospitalization and physician costs at birth; (2) rehospitalization costs in the first year of life (hospital costs only); and (3) long-term health care costs of treating

Table 9.4   Comparability of Study Groups by Baseline Variables

Baseline Variable	C Group N = 100	E Group N = 400	C Group N = 414	Total N = 814	Refused N = 67
Mean age, years	23.8	24.1	24.7	24.6	27.5
Mean education, years	12.1	12.4	12.2	12.4	13.7
Mean EGA[a]	3.8	3.9	4.1	4.0	4.1
Race: % black	52	50	54	52	49
Cotinine (ng/ml)					
Mean	121	117	109	114	N/A
SD	103	100	91	96	N/A

[a]EGA = Estimated gestational age at entry into care (units = months).

an LBW infant. These estimates, including discounting by the OTA, were adjusted to 1990 dollars by the inflation rates of the consumer price index/ medical care component of the Bureau of Labor statistics: 5.8% (1987), 6.9% (1988), 8.5% (1989), and 9.6% (1990). The discounted, inflation-adjusted, OTA low estimate of $12,104 and the OTA high estimate of $30,935 were used in our cost benefit calculations.

Results

Data in Table 9.4 confirm the baseline equivalence of the E and C Groups. The C Group (Historical Comparison Group) of 100 pregnant smokers were comparable to the E and C Groups. The refusals were similar to the study participants. At baseline about 45% of the patients exhibited low (≤99 ng/mL) and 40 percent moderate (100 to 199 ng/mL) levels of cotinine exposure. No E versus C Group or Black versus White differences in mean baseline cotinine values were observed.

Process Evaluation. Process Evaluation data from monthly, quarterly, and annual clinic reports confirmed the following E Group exposure rates by health education component: Component #1 = 100%, Component #2 = 88%, and Component #3 = 100%. The intervention was successfully provided by nine different counselors to 400 patients at the four JCHD clinics over a 27 month period.

Patient Compliance Rates. Data confirmed that 63% of the E Group reported use of the *Guide* at least four days or more and use of five or more cessation methods. This rate was comparable to the E Group compliance rate of Trial I—65%. Eighty-two percent of the E Group and 60% of the C Group reported a quit attempt.

Behavioral Impact. The behavioral impact of the health education methods is reported in Table 9.5. Only patients who self-reported quitting at their first and second follow-up visit(s) and who had a cotinine value

Table 9.5 Quit Rates by Race and Study Group

Race	E Group Quit Rate %	N	C Group Quit Rate %	N	C̲ Group Quit Rate %	N	95% CI (E − C)	p = Value
Black	18.1[a]	210	10.7[b]	242	N/A		(0.8, 13.9)	0.03
White	10.0[a]	190	5.2[b]	172	N/A		(−0.6, 10.2)	0.08
Total	14.3	400	8.5	414	3.0	100	(1.4, 10.1)	0.01

[a]p = 0.03.
[b]p = 0.07.

Table 9.6 Quit Rates By Level of Baseline Cotinine Values

Baseline Cotinine (ng/ml)	E Group N = 57 %	C Group N = 35 %
Low ≤99	89	83
Moderate 100 to 199	9	14
High ≥200	2	3

≤30 ng/mL were counted as "quitters." Approximately 15 percent of the 814 patients were lost to follow-up: all were counted as failures. A comparison of the baseline characteristics of patients lost to follow-up and participants confirmed no significant differences.

As noted in Table 9.5, the E Group had significantly higher quit rates than the C and C̲ Groups. Among the E Group black patients the intervention increased quit rates by 7.4% and among E Group white patients the intervention increased quit rates by 4.9% (p = 0.03 for blacks, p = 0.08 for whites). Black patients in the E and C Group had substantially higher quit rates than white E and C Group patients.

Relapse was assessed from midpregnancy to delivery. The E Group had a significantly higher relapse rate (14%) than the C Group (8%) (p = 0.001).

Data in Table 9.6 confirmed that cessation occurred among both E and C Group with low to moderate cotinine levels.

Analyses of baseline variables—age, education, EGA, race, and cotinine value—to document cessation predictors revealed that E Group participation, baseline cotinine, and race were significant.

As noted in Table 9.7, although E and C Group White patients had lower quit rates than Black patients, E Group White patients had a significantly higher reduction rate than Black patients in the E Group (p = 0.05) or White patients in the C Group (p = 0.05). Although not statistically

Table 9.7 Significant Reduction Rates By Race and Study Group[a]

Race	E Group %	E Group N	C Group %	C Group N	95% CI	$p =$ Value
Black	12.9	210	11.6	242	(−4.8, 7.3)	.68
White	21.1	190	13.4	172	(0.0, 15.4)	.05
Total	16.8	400	12.3	414	(−0.4, 9.3)	.07

[a]Patients who quit were not counted as significant reducers.

significant (p = 0.07), overall, the E Group had a 27% higher reduction rate than the C Group. Including the quitters as significant reducers, the "behavior change rate" was 31.0% in the E Group versus 20.8% in the C Group (p = 0.001).

Sensitivity, specificity, and the positive predictive value of the cotinine test to validate end-of-pregnancy self-reports of smoking status were 86%, 74%, and 93% respectively. A comparison of self-reports to cotinine values of ≥31 ng/ml confirmed a total deception rate of 28%: E Group = 32% and C Group = 17%. No differences in deception rates, however, were observed between black and white patients in either the E or C Group.

Estimated Behavioral Impact of Statewide Dissemination. The E Group, C Group, and C̲ Group differences in quit rates were 6% (E − C) and 11% (E − C̲). However, the E Group and C̲ Group quit rates in Trial II (E = 14% versus C̲ = 3%) were comparable to Trial I (E = 14% versus C = 2%). Both trials were conducted at the same JCHD sites among patient cohorts equivalent at baseline by SES, age, education, EGA, cotinine values, and percent Black. However, only Component #1 was provided to the patients in Trial I. *The addition of five minutes of intervention time and Components #2 and #3 in Trial II did not produce a higher quit rate in the E Group.* Thus, a 10-minute time period, only intervention Component #1 and the average E − C quit rate difference of 12% (Trial I E − C = 12% and Trial II E − C̲ = 11%) was used to estimate the potential behavioral impact and cost benefit.

Although a 12% quit rate difference may be possible at many prenatal clinics, it may represent an estimate of the *efficacy* (best estimate) of the behavioral impact of the intervention. Accordingly, the 12% quit rate *difference* was attenuated to eight percent to reflect the *effectiveness* (typical estimate) of the intervention in routine use by prenatal nurses. If the intervention had been provided to the estimated 4,800 smokers (0.30 × 16,000 prenatal patients) in the 1990 Alabama public health cohort, an additional 384 quitters (0.08 × 4800) might have been produced.

Estimated Impact of Statewide Dissemination on LBW Rate. A low birthweight (LBW) rate of about 12% to 13% has been observed among the Alabama public health cohort for several years resulting in about

2,000 LBW infants each year (0.125 × 16,000). Using a LBW-SPAR = 0.20 (low estimate), about 400 smoking attributable LBW infants (0.20 × 2000) were born in the 1990 cohort. If the 8% difference to estimate the intervention's potential to reduce the incidence of smoking-attributable low birthweight had been used, an estimated 32 fewer LBW infants (0.08 × 400) might have been prevented by statewide dissemination and routine use of the intervention.

Estimated Cost Benefit of Statewide Dissemination. Based on the Office of Technology Assessment's discounted, inflation-adjusted estimates of excess health care costs (low estimate = $12,104 and high estimate = $30,935) 32 smoking attributable LBW infants cost an excess of between $387,328 and $989,920.

Because data from Trial I and Trial II confirmed that Component #1 delivered during a 10-minute session produced the behavioral impact, the total cost per patient can be reduced from $6.00 to $4.50 (staff time—15 to 10 minutes). Our cost benefit analysis was based on the prevention of LBW infants among the estimated Alabama public health maternity cohort of 4,800 smokers. Because the cost benefit of dissemination was expressed as a net cost difference (economic benefit minus cost) among all 4,800 women who might have received the intervention, not just quitters, our costs to disseminate the intervention to the estimated 4,800 pregnant smokers would be approximately $21,600/year (4,800 × $4.50).

The Cost Benefit Ratio for the low estimate is $1 : $17.9 and the high estimate is $1 : $45.8. The net difference between benefit and cost is $365,728 (low estimate) to $968,320 (high estimate) in favor of the intervention.

Sensitivity Analysis. Sensitivity analyses need to be performed in an assessment of the cost benefit of new prevention methods. We examined the sensitivity of our estimates in relation to changes in two parameters: intervention cost and estimated economic benefit. We varied the intervention cost from $4.50 (low estimate) to $9.00 (high estimate). We varied the health benefit by reducing the smoking population attributable risk from 0.20 to 0.15 thereby further reducing the estimated number of preventable low birthweights from 32 (low estimate) to 24 (very low estimate).

Data from evaluation studies confirmed that a quit rate difference (E minus C Group) of 6% to 12% is achievable. Because we used an effectiveness rate difference of 8% (low estimate), this parameter is likely to reflect the rate achievable in public health practice and is unlikely to vary substantially. However, costs for personnel and materials to routinely provide the intervention will vary. If we increase the total intervention costs by 50%—moderate increase—from $4.50 to $6.75 ($6.75 × 4800 = $32,400), the Cost to Benefit Ratio (CBR) is: low estimate = $1 : $12.0 and high estimate = $1 : $30.6. If costs were increased by 100%—high increase—($9.00 × 4,800 = $43,200) the CBR low estimate = $1 : $9.0 and high estimate = $1 : $22.9. The net difference between benefit and cost favors the intervention: $344,128 (low estimate) and $946,720 (high estimate).

If we increase the intervention cost by 100% (high increase) and decrease the estimated benefit (LBW-SPAR 0.20 to 0.15) by 25% (very low estimate), the CBR low estimate = $1 : $6.7 (24 × $12,104/$43,200) and high estimate = $1 : $17.2 (24 × $30,935/$43,200). Thus, for each $1 spent on smoking cessation, $7 to $17 in medical care costs might be saved. The net difference between the economic benefit and excess cost favors the intervention: the low estimate is $247,296 and the high estimate is $699,240.

Thus, variations in estimates of behavioral impact, smoking attributable risk, excess health care cost, or discount rates do not affect the conclusions about the cost benefit and potential net savings of the intervention. The estimated cost benefit ratios from this study and thus the net economic benefits are substantially higher than the Cost to Benefit Ratio of $1 : $3.4 for prenatal care reported by the Institute of Medicine.

Discussion

This evaluation recruited 94% of a cohort of pregnant smokers from multiple clinics over a 27 month period when considered along with evidence from Trial I, and results of other intervention studies, this study confirms that an additional 6% to 12% quit rate difference is achievable in public health clinics.

An evaluation study of WIC patients in Michigan, which adapted Trial I self-help methods and the ALA self-help cessation methods, reported quit rates of 11% (E_1 Group)—self-help methods, 7% (E_2 Group)—risk information methods, and 3% (C Group)—no intervention. Another evaluation study in Washington, D.C., undertaken among a predominately Black cohort of pregnant smokers who received the *Guide* plus one-to-one counseling and other intervention materials, reported a quit rate based on self-reports of "about one-third." If the 33% self-reported quit rate is adjusted by applying our 32% E Group deception rate, a 22% quit rate is derived. This quit rate is similar to the 18% quit rate of the E Group Black patients.

The 8% C Group quit rate in Trial II was much higher than the C Group quit rate in Trial I—2%, the observed quit rate among our Trial II C Group (Historical Comparison Group)—3%, and the C Group in the Mayer et al. WIC study—3%. The Mayer et al. study E_2—risk information group, however, exhibited a 7% quit rate which was comparable to the Trial II C Group rate of 8.5%. The E_2 Group in the Mayer et al. and the Trial II C Group both received brief, one-to-one verbal and written risk information, and strong encouragement to quit. These data suggest that as implemented the Trial II C Group may have become a "minimum intervention group." Strong, one-to-one advice to quit, reinforced with readable risk information and RN/MD reinforcement *may* increase the "normal" quit rate observed in public health settings from 2% to 4% to 6% to 8%.

No clear explanation was apparent for the large difference between C (8.5%) and C̱ (3.0%) Group quit rates. The difference may be attributable to a combination of reasons: (1) the presence, duration, and intensity of Trial II over a 27 month period, (2) the use of patient education reinforcement methods in Trial II but not used in Trial I or with the C̱ Group in our Formative Evaluation, and/or (3) greater societal, peer, and family pressure to quit placed on pregnant women during the Trial II intervention period (1987 to 1989) versus the Trial I intervention period (1984). Additionally, a meta-evaluation of smoking cessation and pregnancy intervention studies conducted after 1985 revealed a trend of small increases in C Group quit rates ranging from 5% to 8%. No evidence is available to indicate communication between E and C Group patients.

The compliance rate in Trial II, almost identical in both JCHD studies—Trial I = 65% and Trial II = 63%—and the compliance rate of 67% reported by Coates and Maxwell using the *Guide* plus one-to-one counseling, was encouraging. Qualitative data from the 102 E Group patients in Trial I also confirmed good patient ratings of the *Guide*. Patients in this setting, at HMOs, and at WIC clinics will use self-help methods. The qualitative and quantitative evidence from patients and providers is strong and consistent, supporting the internal and external validity of these methods for pregnant smokers. No adverse effects of the intervention were observed in the Trial I, Trial II or other evaluation studies.

This study also confirmed a large difference in quit rates between Black and White E and C Group patients. Although others have reported racial differences based on cotinine analyses, with Black female adults (18–30 years) serum cotinine levels consistently *higher* than white female adults (18–30 years), no baseline difference in mean saliva cotinine levels by race was observed in Trial II or in the mean saliva thiocyanate levels in Trial I. Additionally, our results, confirming a *higher* quit rate among Black smokers versus White smokers, were the opposite of other evaluation reports. White smokers are often *more* successful in quitting than Black smokers. *Although no explanation was apparent for the observed quit-rate differences by race, the substantially larger quit rate documented among Black pregnant smokers represents one of the most important findings of this study.* Smoking, active and passive, is a primary cause of LBW, and the Black LBW rate (13.2%) is twice the LBW rate observed for White infants (6.6%).

Our results and other efficacy and cost effectiveness analyses have also documented that dissemination of these methods may reduce the incidence of LBW and reduce associated, excess health care costs. Estimates of the impact of dissemination of "tested" health education methods to the 1990 U.S. Public Health Cohort of approximately 1 million pregnant women, 350,000 pregnant smokers and 120,000 LBW infants, indicate that approximately 1,920 fewer LBW infants (120,000 × PAR .20 × .08) might have been prevented. Assuming a cost per public health patient of $6.75, the total cost to deliver the intervention to the total 1990 U.S. cohort would have been approximately $2.4 million ($6.75 × 350,000 pregnant smokers). Thus, a net economic benefit of approximately $20 to $56 million might have been produced by dissemination. Annual dissemination to the U.S. maternity cohort of over 1 million pregnant smokers (4.0 + million × 0.25 smokers) may also help achieve approximately 31% to 78% of the *Healthy People 2000 Objectives* for pregnant smokers.

These estimates of impact, however, reflect only a small part of the economic, health and emotional benefit to women, infants, and their families. A national effort is needed in the 1990s to change prenatal-care policy and the health education process and content for pregnant smokers. Continuing education programs must be expanded to improve the cessation counseling methods and skills of health care practitioners. *The Handbook to Plan, Implement, and Evaluate Smoking Cessation Programs for Pregnant Women* will assist in these efforts, particularly in public health settings. As dissemination plans are prepared, evaluation research will also be needed to document the degree to which health education methods are adopted in public and private health maternity care settings and to measure their behavioral and clinical impact.

Summary

All evaluators should consider at the onset of planning the cost implications of their health promotion and intervention methods. The efficiency of intervention methods in producing either outcomes described in nonmonetary terms or outcomes described in dollars and cents should be documented. From a philosophical perspective, however, it is also important to emphasis that a singular preoccupation with cost analyses and solely judging a program's worth or value *only* on the basis of cost is not justifiable. The OTA of the U.S. Congress concluded in 1981 that health care decision making could be improved by the process of identifying and considering all the relevant costs and benefits of a decision. However, cost-effectiveness analysis/cost–benefit analysis (CEA-CBA) cannot serve as the sole or primary determinant of health care decision making. Program efficiency is only one part of the rationale to decide, for example, to provide drug education to children in elementary schools; or exercise, fitness, and diet classes to workers; or a mass-media program to influence use of prenatal care earlier in a pregnancy or high blood pressure medications. A broader range of issues reflecting concern for the welfare of a target population by an agency or organization and ethical and legal responsibilities must also guide decisions to allocate resources and provide programs.

APPENDIX A

The Evaluation Report

As discussed in Chapter 3, a good health education program most often results from the application of logical thinking to a public health problem and the behavior change expected to help alleviate or eliminate the problem. The evaluation report is the document that ties together a problem, program, analysis of program impact, and outcome. This synthesis is done by presentation of data to illustrate, if observed, cause-and-effect relationships. When a program fails to yield an expected impact, the report is a vehicle to explore explanations. The evaluation report is a medium of communication. Therefore, while you are preparing it, you must keep in mind the people to whom it is directed. If the audience is varied, you should prepare different forms of a report emphasizing in each the issues and ideas of greatest interest to a particular group of readers.

The evaluation report is not a massive historical document describing events and results for future generations, although such a document may be worth preparing. Rather, it is an immediate, dynamic, succinct communication to those with specific interest in the program. The report discusses program process and outcomes and serves to guide others in making future related health promotion and education decisions. It is not the length but the quality of the report that makes it acceptable. It may be used to decide if and how to revise the existing program, to expand the program to other sites or settings, or to increase, reduce, or rearrange staff or budget. The major evaluation concern covered in a report is the program's efficacy: Did it yield what was expected? If not, why not? In the following pages, we delineate the sections of a comprehensive report. The extent of each section depends on the specific audience to whom the report is directed.

THE AUDIENCE

To what audience must you communicate? In day-to-day practice, the unit administrator in the sponsoring organization will likely be the first person to see a draft of the report. Next the directors of the agency or organization may see it. If the program has been funded by outside grants, a report must communicate results of interest to the source of grant support. If the program results add to or clarify dimensions of health education practice, your colleagues will be interested. When a program complements medical or nursing practice, other providers may have an interest. If the program has brought about changes with strong implication for community health and health services, local residents and news media may be interested.

Reports that communicate to each of these audiences differ in range, length, complexity, and language. Each, however, draws from the same data set. Much of the material generated in developing the original program plan will be useful in writing each version. It is generally a mistake to try to write one report to address the interests of all the potential audiences. Although there may be some standard sections in all reports (the same material repeated in each), some sections must be specifically tailored toward target audiences and provide more complete material about their interests. The process of communicating to several audiences is made more efficient by preparing a document with interchangeable parts. The statistical analysis, for example, may be presented in great detail for some audiences and only briefly summarized for others. The administrative pattern for operating the program may be described elaborately for some readers and barely mentioned for others. The first question to ask yourself is, Who do I want to reach with this document? Then you ask, Which elements and aspects of the evaluation of the program are of greatest importance to that reader?

FORMAT

If you have followed the evaluation procedures discussed in this book and have collected data both at predetermined points in a program and at the end of the program period, then you will have much data in hand when report-writing time arrives. You will also have in hand a logically conceived program plan or blueprint to enumerate the ex-

Table A.1   Evaluation Report Outline

1. Title page
2. Executive summary (abstract)
3. Table of contents
4. Program purpose
   a. Aims and objectives
   b. Participant description
5. Program description
   a. Educational–behavioral methods
   b. Contents–process–time
   c. Staffing
6. Evaluation methods
   a. Process evaluation
   b. Impact–outcome evaluation
7. Results
   a. Quantitative analysis
   b. Qualitative analysis
   c. Cost analysis
8. Conclusions–Recommendations

pected impact and outcomes of the program. Preparing evaluation reports therefore should start with a review of the original plan, data, and analysis, and interpretation of the data. Organize this information into a clear, well-documented presentation. Table A.1 provides a suggested outline for the sections of this communication.

Executive Summary (Abstract)

The first section is the executive summary. Because most evaluators have been influenced by their academic training, some tend to prepare reports that assume the readers have a widespread academic interest and are willing to plod through voluminous material to find the important points. Few people have either the time or the patience to search through many pages to find the pearls. A good evaluation report presents its findings at the beginning. The readers know the results at the outset. One way to accomplish this is to prepare an executive summary and to make this the first page of the evaluation report. The summary should concisely describe the program's objectives, methods, processes, and results. Write the summary, like the report, without jargon and in the active voice. If you need to use scientific or technical words, define them for readers.

The summary should present essential evaluation material in language the intended readers will understand. The quality of the summary often dictates whether the full report will be read. It should be followed by a clearly numbered and accurately referenced table of contents. Some people refuse to read reports without a well-labeled table of contents. They may be justified because its absence demonstrates a significant deficiency in the report writers.

Program Purpose and Key Evaluation Questions

Readers of the report need to be told what the program intended to achieve. Readers also need to know why achieving the goal was important—the benefits. If the program expected, for example, to help overweight employees lose weight, why is this valuable? The reasons may be different for the reader who is the employee's spouse and for the reader who is the chief executive officer of the company.

It is important not to assume that the reader has background information about the program and its potential worth. Assume the reader does not. Prepare a clear, direct description of the program purpose and potential benefit—do not exaggerate. Describe the characteristics that make the program unique. Include a profile of the participants. Obviously, a program is valuable because of the particular people it aimed to assist. Why was it important to reach them?

The major evaluation questions should be spelled out in this section. They are the measuring sticks of whether the program achieved its purpose. This list of the questions that guided your evaluation, whether it is long or short, should be self-explanatory once the reader has gone through your description of purpose.

Program Description

Once readers have grasped the purpose of the program and reviewed the questions that guided evaluation of it, they will want to understand what the program "looked like." To say that the program was "self-management training" is not enough. What was the training? Where? When? How did it occur? You need to include five elements in this program description, more or less extensively depending on the audience for your report:

1. *The basic nature of the education.* What theoretical principles of education were used? For example, was the program based on social cognitive and social support theory? Was it a combination of organized peer group support and rehearsal of specific health skills? Was it counseling from professionals? Was it provision of information through various media? Was it based on group problem solving?

2. *The content of the program.* What material was presented? How was it presented at each learning session?

3. *The logistics and process of the program.* What was the location of the educational sessions, their frequency, and their duration? What number of hours, days, or weeks was assessed?

4. *The number of deployment of staff.* What kind of training did they receive before inception of the program? What was the average number of participants in the sessions?

5. *The administrative support provided.* What number and deployment of program managers, coordinators, secretaries, and other administrative personnel were used?

This description should enable readers to envision a learning session with the educators and participants doing what they would typically do. A complete narrative would include examples of the behavioral objectives set, how learners were enabled to reach the objectives, and how achieving the objectives was related to the overall purpose of the program.

Evaluation Methods

Describe for readers the methods of program assessment. The methods and design selected from the possibilities presented in Chapters 4 to 9 should be presented. Discuss two dimensions: the design (Chapter 5) that enabled you to ascertain the impact and outcomes of the program (e.g., whether employees changed their eating patterns and lost weight) and the process evaluation (Chapter 4) that enabled you to make judgments about the quality of the program (e.g., whether the staff performed as expected or the anticipated average level of participation in group discussions was reached). These two dimensions are best described separately. The quality assessment measures what actually occurred in the program. The evaluation design measures the results. In health education programs, both are exceedingly important and should be reported. Readers will have more or less interest in quality assessment, however. Your audience will be more interested in the design to determine the impact of the program. Once persuaded that this dimension was adequately addressed, many readers will want to know more about process. In this section, like the others, you must determine how much material is appropriate for the reader. When in doubt, mention the material in the body of the report. Include a narrative description in an appendix.

The description of your evaluation design should include use of control groups, sampling procedures, sample size, and the reliability and validity of the data. In describing these points, discuss not only what judgments each element allows you to make about the program but also what judgments cannot be made. Describe limitations of the study. As we discussed in previous chapters, using highly controlled evaluation techniques in natural settings is often difficult. Almost all quasi-experimental designs and all process assessment methods are flawed. It is your responsibility to recount the ways in which the evaluation procedures are deficient. This demonstrates to the readers that you have thought about and tried to account for evaluation weaknesses.

Next, present a description of the ways in which you collected data to answer each evaluation question. If you used several techniques, the limitations of each should be discussed. For example, if some data were collected in face-to-face interviews, how candid and forthcoming were respondents? How did you guard against interviewer bias? If you used hospital records as a source of data, how accurate and consistent were the records completed by health personnel? It is important for you to show that you anticipated, and wherever possible addressed, problems in data collection. Some readers like to see samples of questionnaires or other instruments for collecting data, but do not put questionnaires in the body of a report; put this in the appendix.

Results

Describe how you analyzed the data. If a large data set was collected and you used a computer, mention how the data were managed and what computer program you used. Few practitioners have the resources to write special statistical programs; most use standard packages. It is sufficient, in most cases, to name the program and mention why it was selected. Within each program, several statistical options are generally available. Report which statistical procedures were used for each kind of evaluation question. Describe any adjustments or corrections in the tests that were made. If your audience comprises measurement specialists and statisticians, however, you will have to give much more detail on why you selected these tests. You may also need to discuss more fully the limitations of the procedures in analyzing the given variables and the evaluation questions considered important.

If you collected primarily qualitative data or for some other reason did not use a computer and analyzed the data by hand, describe the methods used and the statistical tests applied. Some reports have only percentages computed by hand. However, as reported in Chapter 8, simple statistical procedures are easy to compute, especially with the pocket calculator. When you have made the effort to design an evaluation and collect quantitative data in the ways suggested in this text, you need to employ these simple tests. In reporting them, make clear the standards for accepting statistical significance. If statistically significant, was it important?

Some of your data will have been analyzed "qualitatively" (e.g., content analysis, rating by experts, tabulation of observations over time, or in other ways). Describe the methods used in enough detail so readers can judge how careful, comprehensive, and consistent the procedures were. If several raters have been used to review data, report interrater reliability. Similarly, discuss your view of the stability of the data. If there were major problems in analyzing the data, describe and clarify these problems in this part of the report.

The data analysis section should help readers see how the data were handled and in what ways they were interpreted by the evaluators. This section should illustrate that the results in the pages to follow are based on reliable data and a careful, generally conservative, analysis.

Program Costs

With increasing frequency, health promotion and education programs are being asked to comment in fiscal terms on the cost effectiveness and cost benefits of programs. Some administrators want a detailed cost analysis. As discussed in Chapters 3 and 9, there are several ways to ascertain the effectiveness and benefits of a program, given its costs. These formulas are rarely definitive, but where they can be applied they provide some indication of whether the goals attained were beneficial and whether the program was the most effective vehicle for reaching the goal. Often it is not possible to illustrate cost effectiveness or benefit because data needed from other sources are not available. Then, as discussed in Chapters 3 and 9, approximations are used and educated guesses made. Even when data are not available for a sophisticated analysis, you should be able to demonstrate what the program cost the sponsoring organization and estimate or give examples of the kinds of savings the education might yield. These figures, as described previously, are easy to compute.

Conclusions and Recommendations

Although this section is positioned fairly late in the report, it is frequently the one to which readers flip immediately after the executive summary. The focal point of the document, it answers the evaluation questions. There are at least two common errors report writers make here: (1) claiming more than the evidence suggests and (2) claiming things not suggested in the evidence at all. Both are lethal errors to be avoided at all costs.

In an evaluation report, you want to present not only positive findings (significantly more men in the program lost more weight than did men in the control group) but also negative ones (fewer men attended the second half of the program than the first half). The objective of this part of the report is both to present and interpret findings and to explore explanations for results. If fewer men attended as the program continued, what were some possible reasons? Did they tire of the program? Were the later sessions less relevant to their needs? Were there changes in their work schedules? Did every person reach his weight-loss goal early? The world rarely operates just as you expect, and an evaluation report that reads as if all went perfectly is at best inaccurate and at worst dishonest. The report gives you the opportunity to make guesses or present additional data to show why the intended results were not achieved and why your expectations were reached or exceeded.

It is important to present data for every evaluation question posed and to interpret the meaning of each finding in relation to the overall aims of the program. In other words, you need to say why a particular finding is more or less important, given the impact and outcomes expected. This lends a perspective of the programmatic significance of your results. The statistical significance of a finding is an indication that the changes observed from before to after the program did not occur randomly. Programmatic significance means that the changes had value to the participants and program planners, given all that the program tried to accomplish.

Tables and graphs are often useful to depict findings, but you should not overwhelm readers with them in the body of the report; append them. Only a few, very pertinent and revealing tables or graphs should be included in the findings section. Similarly, the narrative should not repeat what is shown in the tables. It should interpret, enhance, or expand on the data presented. You should describe all significant findings in the text in narrative form. Refer readers to tables in the appendix for further detail when data are extensive.

The section should end with a brief summary of the findings and some general conclusions about the program and its accomplishments. The more analytic the review of findings and conclusions, the better. This means thoughtful consideration of each result within the context of your program. It means not drawing conclusions about the program for which there are no empirical data (error 2 mentioned earlier) or making more of a finding than is really there (error 1). It seems only fair that you should explicitly caution readers about conclusions. The soundness of the program can be undermined by sloppy or grandiose "analysis" and presentation of its results. The findings and conclusion section is the most important part of the evaluation report and reflects your genuine understanding of the problem, what the program intended to accomplish, and the extent to which aims were met.

Many readers will expect you to make recommendations based on program outcomes. However, you must determine what kinds of recommendations are suitable based on the characteristics of the audience for the report. It is most appropriate for you to make programmatic rather than policy recommendations unless you were specifically asked to do the latter. A recommendation that a successful program be expanded to a larger audience is well within the prerogative of an evaluator. A recommendation that a hospital change its reimbursement pattern to accomplish this end is not. Recommendations, like conclusions, must be derived from the findings of the evaluation. Adding extraneous recommendations not supported by the data simply weakens the general effectiveness of the report. Some writers even refer to specific evidence in the body of the report when putting forward their suggestions.

Keep in mind—the most successful program can generally use fine-tuning. The recommendations section is an opportunity to call attention to ways a program may be made even stronger. Quality assessment data and findings that describe the processes of program implementation can be particularly useful in recommending change or adjustments in content and process. The questions usually addressed in a recommendations section are similar to those below:

1. Should the learning approach process or content of the program be revised? If so, in what way?
2. Should the program staffing patterns be changed in any way?
3. Should there be changes in the types of personnel implementing the program?
4. Should there be adjustments in the budget allocations to various elements of the program?
5. Is the program generalizable to other groups of learners? If so, in what way might it best be expanded? How might it best be replicated?

DISSEMINATION TO DECISION MAKERS

One of the biggest complaints of evaluators is the underutilization of data. Findings are rarely used as much as they could be. Getting the report read by the right people does not occur by magic. If you want your evaluation report to influence decisions, you must think through how best to reach the decision makers. One way to do this, as we have discussed, is to ensure that the material in your report is targeted to the interests of a specific audience. But there are other things you can do to generate interest.

According to Zweig and Marvin (1981), the education of any group (in this case, decision makers) by any other group (in this case, evaluators) cannot happen without a process that respects the institutions, culture, and practices of each. In other words, you must carefully consider the individuals or groups you hope will use your report. How can you present your case for using the report so that it respects their point of view? Zweig and Marvin also suggest that evaluators need a conception of evaluation that takes into account the secondary place of evaluative information in day-to-day decision making. The decision maker will use your data as only one input into the decision. Your report is primarily only to you. You must determine how your findings directly and indirectly relate to the priorities of the decision maker you want to reach. Spell out the uses of the data to that person's interests.

Sichel (1982) believes that it is critical to give key individuals previews of the report. We strongly agree. Relevant drafts of information should be shared with decision makers in advance of open discussion or submission of the report. By having them review the material, you accomplish two things. First, you increase the chances that your material will be accepted by the decision maker. When you speak with him or her on an individual basis, you can better address that person's individual concerns. You eliminate the element of surprise and can verify that you have been sensitive to the decision maker's position and perspective. Second, you can emphasize the policy implications and usefulness of the report to that particular decision maker. You also take the opportunity to sell the decision maker on using your findings.

A report that sits on the shelf is of little use. Develop a strategy for reaching key people and assisting them to make data-based decisions.

FINAL THOUGHTS

Anonymity

During the data-collection period, it is likely that you assured program participants that the actions and opinions they allowed you to document would be anonymous in all evaluation documents. It is crucial to honor this commitment. No section of the report should be written so that the identity of individuals is revealed or can be deduced. The institutions, organizations, and services that were part of your program may also wish to remain anonymous. Before writing the report, determine how specific you can be in your description of people, places, and events while not violating participants' anonymity.

Sensitivity

Few things can unnerve even people with the strongest egos more than the idea of being evaluated. Successful evaluators approach both their subjects and their task in a way that reassures people that they are not being judged or labeled in negative ways. The evaluation report must be written with sensitivity. Even in the rare case when only a few people will see the document, a large measure of sensitive wording and phrasing of ideas is the most professional approach. You also want to ensure that the report is not offensive to those who have participated. To accomplish this end, you might ask someone familiar with the program but outside the evaluation team to read a draft of the report before it is completed and distributed. The reviewer should be asked to judge its sensitivity to people, places, and events. This reader must, of course, be a trusted person who is pledged to keep confidential all that the document contains.

Confidentiality

Because evaluation reports—even glowingly positive ones—can be sensitive documents, you must accord them a certain confidentiality. Determine at the outset the readership of the report. With members of the program hierarchy, compile lists of those who are to receive the various forms of the document. Discuss with the administrators how the report is to be treated after its initial distribution. Will it be made freely available to all who express an interest in the program? Will it be given out only with the permission of someone within the sponsoring organization? Will it be marked "confidential"? Will it be piled at the doorway so that every visitor can pick it up? You need to know the ground rules for handling and distribution of the report.

Objectivity

The chapters of this text have stressed that the primary task of evaluators is to look objectively at a problem and the program designed to address it. Next, they must organize program descriptions and assessment data into clear communications for specific groups of readers. Objectivity must be reflected in every page of every evaluation report. In many ways, developing a health education program is the art of professional health education practice; evaluation is the science. To develop future programs to assist people to prevent and manage illness more fully, health educators must learn from the evaluations of current programs. In this sense, every health education program has the opportunity to contribute to the knowledge base of practice in addition to assisting individual learners. It is only by conducting careful, objective program evaluations and communicating the results to others in the most objective way that the art and science of health promotion and education can be enhanced.

APPENDIX **B**

Specification of the Role of the Entry-Level Health Educator

Area of Responsibility V:

The entry-level health educator, working with individuals, groups and organizations, is responsible for:

EVALUATING HEALTH EDUCATION (12%)

The entry-level health educator, working with individuals, groups and organizations, is responsible for:

Function: A. Participating in developing an evaluation design. (24%)

Skill: 1. The health educator must be able to assist in specifying indicators of program success.

Knowledge: The health educator must be able to:

   a. differentiate between what can and cannot be measured (e.g., knowledge gained, changes in morbidity rates due to health education).

   b. translate objectives into specific indicators (e.g., knowledge gained, values stated, behaviors mastered).

   c. describe range of methods and techniques

SOURCE: U.S. Department of Health and Human Services, Public Health Service, *Initial Role Delineation for Health Education. Final Report*, prepared for the National Center for Health Education, DHHS Publication no. (HRA) 80-44 (Washington, D.C.: Government Printing Office, 1980), pp. 78–82.

used for educational measurement (e.g., inventories, scales, competency tests).

d. list steps involved in evaluative activities (e.g., setting standards, specifying objectives, developing criteria for achievement of objectives).

Skill: 2. The health educator must be able to help to establish the scope for program evaluation.

Knowledge: The health educator must be able to:

a. define scope of evaluation efforts (e.g., match standards with goals, explain relationship between activities and outcomes).

b. describe feasibility of evaluative activities (e.g., time availability, resources, setting, nature of the program).

c. explain the beliefs and purposes behind health education activities (e.g., value to consumers, increased control over health matters, informed public).

Skill: 3. The health educator must be able to help develop methods for evaluating programs.

Knowledge: The health educator must be able to:

a. identify various measures for determining knowledge, attitudes and behavior (e.g., questionnaires, self-assessment inventories, knowledge tests).

b. describe data available for evaluation (e.g., program attendance, reports of behaviors, survey data, letters from consumers and others, test scores).

c. list strengths and weaknesses of various data collection methods (e.g., value of self-report, expense of observing behavior).

Skill: 4. The health educator must be able to participate in the specification of instruments for data collection.

Knowledge: The health educator must be able to:

a. describe advantages and disadvantages of "home made" and commercial instruments (e.g., utility, cost, timeliness).

b. identify sources of instruments (e.g., professional organizations, research organizations, consultants, textbook publishers).

Skill: 5. The health educator must be able to assist in the determination of samples needed for evaluation.

Knowledge: The health educator must be able to:
a. define sample concepts (e.g., stratified, random, convenience, universe).
b. identify strengths and weaknesses of sampling techniques (e.g., sampling error, skewed results, normal distributions, precision of estimates).

Skill: 6. The health educator must be able to assist in the selection of data useful for accountability analysis.

Knowledge: The health educator must be able to:
a. describe the uses of cost-benefit analysis (e.g., modify programs, select alternative(s) from competing choices).

The entry-level health educator, working with individuals, groups and organizations, is responsible for:

Function: B. Assembling resources required to carry out evaluation. (22%)

Skill: 1. The health educator must be able to acquire facilities, materials, personnel and equipment.

Knowledge: The health educator must be able to:
a. describe facilities, materials and equipment needed (e.g., telephones, typewriters, computers).
b. identify required expertise and sources for expertise (e.g., survey methodology from universities, physician for clinical study, experts in evaluation).
c. identify ways of obtaining necessary facilities, materials, expertise and equipment (e.g., personal visitations, formal requests, budgetary requisitions).

Skill: 2. The health educator must be able to train personnel for evaluation as needed.

Knowledge: The health educator must be able to:
a. describe the process for assessing training needs (e.g., listing skills needed, reviewing skills of available personnel, comparing skills with program requirements).
b. describe steps for implementing training programs (e.g., specifying learning objectives, selecting instructional methods, carrying out methods, evaluating).

Skill: 3.   The health educator must be able to secure the cooperation of those affecting and affected by the program.

Knowledge: The health educator must be able to:
a. describe how to involve relevant parties in the evaluation process (e.g., explaining importance, answering questions, asking for cooperation).
b. identify importance of safeguarding rights of individuals involved (e.g., explanation of purposes and procedures, confidential record-keeping).
c. explain methods to maintain interest in program evaluation (e.g., importance of the work, reinforcement of effort, communication techniques, presentation of evaluation results).

The entry-level health educator, working with individuals, groups and organizations, is responsible for:

Function: C.   Helping to implement the evaluation design. (30%)

Skill: 1.   The entry-level health educator must be able to collect data through appropriate techniques.

Knowledge: The health educator must be able to:
a. identify the applicability of various techniques to a given situation (e.g., observations, interviews, questionnaires, written tests).
b. describe how to acquire data from existing sources (e.g., scan newspapers, review journal articles, scan morbidity and mortality data, health records).

    c. distinguish between quantitative and quali-
tative data (e.g., counts vs. expressions of
satisfaction, changes in physical indices vs.
loss of interest).

Skill: 2. The health educator must be able to analyze collected data.

Knowledge: The health educator must be able to:

    a. identify basic statistical measures (e.g.,
counts, means, medians).

    b. describe processes of statistical analysis
(e.g., selected analysis based on stated
concern, collecting data, use of statistical
techniques).

    c. explain the results of statistical analysis
(e.g., report data, make inferences, draw
conclusions).

    d. identify steps in analyzing qualitative data
(e.g., developing categories, ascribing
meaning to data, making inferences).

    e. explain how data may be kept and used
as needed (e.g., record keeping system,
computer storage, filing systems, progress
reports).

Skill: 3. The health educator must be able to interpret results of program evaluation.

Knowledge: The health educator must be able to:

    a. identify relationships between analyzed
data and program objectives (e.g., objectives met, reasons for lack of achievement,
changes in program reflected in data).

    b. recognize importance of looking for unan-
ticipated results (e.g., appearance of seemingly unrelated results, significant deviations from what was expected).

    c. identify variables necessary for interpreta-
tion of data (e.g., SES, sex, age, medical
diagnosis).

    d. recognize risks of drawing conclusions not
fully justified by the data (e.g., program's
value to other fields, program successes,
program failures).

The entry-level health educator, working with individuals, groups and organizations, is responsible for:

Function: D.   Communicating results of evaluation. (25%)

Skill: 1.   The health educator must be able to report the processes and results of evaluation to those interested.

Knowledge: The health educator must be able to:
  a. describe how to organize, write and report findings (e.g., objectives, activities, results, interpretation, conclusions).
  b. translate evaluation findings into terms understandable by others (e.g., professionals, consumers, administrators).
  c. explain various ways to depict findings (e.g., graphs, slides, flipcharts).

Skill: 2.   The health educator must be able to recommend strategies for implementing results.

Knowledge: The health educator must be able to:
  a. list strategies that can be used for implementation (e.g., involve those affected, explain results to given audiences, propose new or modified programs).
  b. identify implications from findings for future programs or other actions (e.g., alert others beyond programs, publish reports on programs and their evaluation).

Skill: 3.   The health educator must be able to incorporate results into planning and implementation processes.

Knowledge: The health educator must be able to:
  a. describe how program operations can be modified based on evaluation results (e.g., discussions with personnel, proposed changes in objectives/methods/content).
  b. explain how evaluation results are part of the planning process (e.g., formative vs. summative evaluation, self-renewal of programs).

References

Aday, L. A. 1991. *Designing and conducting health surveys*. San Francisco: Jossey-Bass.

Alkin, M. C. 1980. A user focused approach. In *Conducting evaluations: Three perspectives*. New York: Foundation Center.

Alluisi, E. A. 1975. Optimum uses of psychobiological, sensorimotor, and performance measurement strategies. *Human Factors* 17(4):309–320.

Alvares, A. P.; Kappas, A.; Eiseman, J. L.; Anderson, K. E.; Pantuck, C. B.; Pantuck, E. J.; Hsiao, K. C.; Garland, W. A.; and Coriney, A. H. 1979. Intraindividual variation in drug disposition. *Clinical Pharmacology and Therapeutics* 26(4):407–419.

American College of Sports Medicine. 1980. The recommended quantity and quality of exercise for developing and maintaining fitness in healthy adults. *Journal of Physical Education and Recreation* 1:17–18.

American Lung Association (ALA). 1980a. *Freedom from smoking in 20 days*. New York: Author.

American Lung Association (ALA). 1980b. *A lifetime of freedom from smoking*. New York: Author.

American Public Health Association, Committee on Professional Education. 1957. Educational qualifications and functions of public health education. *American Journal of Public Health* 47:1.

American Public Health Association. 1987. Criteria for the development of health promotion programs. *American Journal of Public Health* 77(1): 89–92.

409

American Society for Healthcare Education and Training. 1990. American Hospital Association, 840 North Lake Shore Drive, Chicago, IL 60611.

Anderson, A. 1976. Policy experiments: Selected analytic issues. In *Validity issues in evaluative research*, ed. I. N. Bernstein, 17–34. Sage Contemporary Social Science Issues, vol. 23. Beverly Hills, Calif.: Sage.

Anderson, R.; Kasper, J.; Frankel, M. R.; et al. 1979. *Total survey error: Applications to improve health surveys.* San Francisco: Jossey-Bass.

Andrasik, F., and McNamara, J. R. 1977. Optimizing staff performance in an institutional behavior change system: A pilot study. *Behavior Modification* 1(2):235–248.

Andrasik, F.; McNamara, J. R.; and Abbott, D. M. 1978. Policy control: A low resource intervention for improving staff behavior. *Journal of Organizational Behavior Management* 1:125–133.

Aneshencel, C. S.; Frerichs, R. R.; Clark, V. A.; and Yokopenic, P. A. 1982. Telephone versus in-person surveys of community health status. *American Journal of Public Health* 72(9):1017–1021.

Argyris, C. 1970. *Intervention theory and method: A behavioral science view.* Reading, Mass.: Addison-Wesley.

Axelrod, M. 1975. Ten essentials for good qualitative research. *Marketing News* 10 (Mar. 14):10–11.

Babbie, E. R. 1979. *Practice of social research.* Belmont, Calif.: Wadsworth.

Baggaley, J. 1982. Electronic analysis of communication technique. *Media in Education and Development* 15(2):70–73.

Baggaley, J., and Smith, K. 1982. *Formative research in rural education.* Institute for Research in Human Abilities Research Bulletin no. 82-003. St. John's: Memorial University of Newfoundland.

Bailar, B. A.; and Lanphier, C. M. 1978. *Development of survey methods to assess survey practices.* Washington, D.C.: American Statistical Association.

Baker, F., and McPhee, C. 1979. Approaches to evaluating quality of health care. In *Program Evaluation in the Health Fields*, vol. 2, ed. H. C. Schulberg and F. Baker, 187–204. New York: Human Sciences Press.

Bales, R. 1951. Interaction process analysis. Reading, Mass.: Addison-Wesley.

Bandura, A. 1977. *Social learning theory.* Englewood Cliffs, N.J.: Prentice Hall.

Bandura, A. *Social foundations of thought and action: A social cognitive theory.* 1986. Englewood Cliffs, N.J.: Prentice Hall.

Baranowski, T. 1978a. Defining a strategy for statewide health education needs assessment. Paper presented to the Second National Conference on Need Assessment in Health and Human Services, Louisville, Ky.

Baranowski, T. 1978b. Implications of the concepts of need for health education needs assessment strategy. Paper presented to the Second National Conference on Need Assessment in Health and Human Services, Louisville, Ky.

Baranowski, T. 1989–1990. Reciprocal determinism at the stages of behavior change: An integration of community, personal, and behavioral perspectives. *International Quarterly of Community Health Education* 10(4):297–327.

Baranowski, T. 1992–1993. Beliefs as motivational influences at stages in behavior change. *International Quarterly of Community Health Education* 13(1):3–29.

Baranowski, T.; Bee, D.; Rassin, D.; Richardson, J. D.; Brown, J.; Guenther, N.; and Nader, P. R. 1982. Social support, social influence, ethnicity and the breastfeeding decision. *Social Science and Medicine* 17(21):1599–1611.

Baranowski, T.; Bee, D.; Rassin, D.; Richardson, J.; and Palmer, J. 1990. Expectancies toward infant-feeding methods among mothers in three ethnic groups. *Psychology and Health* 5:59–75.

Baranowski, T.; Domel, S.; Gould, R.; Baranowski, J.; Leonard, S.; Treiber, F.; and Mullis, R. 1993. Increasing fruit and vegetable consumption among 4th and 5th grade students: Results from focus groups using reciprocal determinism. *Journal of Nutrition Education* 25(3):114–120.

Baranowski, T.; Evans, M.; Chapin, J.; Wagner, G.; and Warren S. 1980. Utilization and medication compliance for high blood pressure: An experiment with family involvement and self-blood pressure monitoring in a rural population. *American Journal of Rural Health* 6(1–6):51–67.

Baranowski, T.; and Fuller, C. 1981. Third party reimbursement for health education services in rural primary care clinics. *American Journal of Rural Health* 7(2):13–25.

Baranowski, T.; Henske, J.; Dworkin, R.; Clearman, D.; Dunn, J. K.; Nader, P. R.; and Hooks, P. 1986. The accuracy of children's self reports of diet: The Family Health Project. *Journal of the American Dietetic Association* 86(10):1381–1385.

Baranowski, T.; Henske, J.; Simons-Morton, B.; Palmer, J.; Hooks, P.; Tiernan, K.; and Dunn, J. K. 1990. Dietary change for CVD prevention among Black-American families. *Health Education Research* 5(4):433–443.

Baranowski, T., and Simons-Morton, B. 1991. Children's physical activity and dietary assessment: Measurement issues. *Journal of School Health* 61(5):195–197.

Baranowski, T.; Sprague, D.; Henske, J.; Seale, D.; and Harrison, J. 1991. Accuracy of maternal dietary recall for preschool children: Socioeconomic status and day care factors. *Journal of the American Dietetic Association* 91(6):669–674.

Baranowski, T.; Tsong, Y.; and Brodwick, M. 1990. Scaling of response scale adverbs among Black-American adults. *Perceptual and Motor Skills* 71:547–559.

Baric, L. 1980. Evaluation: Obstacles and potentialities. *International Journal of Health Education* 23(3):142–149.

Barker, R. F., and Blankenship, A. B. 1975. The manager's guide to survey questionnaire evaluation. *Journal of the Market Research Society* 17(4):233–241.

Bartko, J. J., and Carpenter, W. T. 1976. On the methods and theory of reliability. *Journal of Nervous and Mental Disease* 163(5):307–317.

Basch, C. E. 1987. Focus group interview: An underutilized research technique for improving theory and practice in health education. *Health Education Quarterly* 14(4):411–448.

Basch, C.; Sliepcevich, E.; Gold, R.; et al. 1985. Avoiding type III errors in health education program evaluation: A case study. *Health Education Quarterly* 12(3):315–331.

Becker, M. H. 1976. Sociobehavioral determinants of compliance. In *Compliance with therapeutic regimens*, ed. D. C. Sackett and R. B. Haynes, 40–50. Baltimore: Johns Hopkins University Press.

Becker, M. H., and Green, L. W. 1975. A family approach to compliance with clinical treatment. *International Journal of Health Education* 18:1–11.

Becker, M., and Maiman, L. 1975. Sociobehavioral determinants of compliance. *Medical Care* 13:10–24.

Begley, C. E., et al. 1990. Estimating the mortality cost of AIDS: Do estimates of earnings differ? *American Journal of Public Health* 80(10):1268–1271.

Beland, F.; Maheux, B.; and Lambert, J. 1991. Measurement of attitudes and behaviors in public health surveys. *American Journal of Public Health* 81(6): 103–105.

Berdie, D. F., and Anderson, J. F. 1974. *Questionnaires: Design and use.* Metuchen, N.J.: Scarecrow Press.

Bernstein, I. N., ed. 1976. *Validity issues in evaluative research.* Sage Contemporary Social Science Issues, vol. 23. Beverly Hills, Calif.: Sage.

Bernstine, R. L., and Baranowski, T. 1976. *Development, testing and evaluation of a Washington State prehospital emergency medical care reporting form.* Report to the Washington State Department of Social and Health Services. Seattle: Battelle Memorial Institute.

Bertera, E. M., and Bertera, R. L. 1981. The Cost-effectiveness of telephone vs. clinic counseling for hypertensive patients: A pilot study. *American Journal of Public Health* 71(6):626–629.

Bertera, R. L. 1990. The effects of workplace health promotion on absenteeism and employment costs in a large industrial population. *American Journal of Public Health* 80(9):1101–1105.

Bertrand, J. 1978. *Communications pretesting.* Chicago: University of Chicago, Community and Family Study Center.

Biron, P. 1975. Dosage, compliance and bioavailability in perspective. *Canadian Medical Association Journal,* 115:102–113.

Boatman, R.; Levin, L.; Roberts, B.; and Rugen, M., ed. 1966. Professional preparation in health education in schools of public health: A report prepared for the 1965 annual meeting, Association of Schools of Public Health, Ad Hoc Committee on Health Education. *Health Education Monographs* 21:1–35.

Bonham, G. S., and Corder, L. S. 1981. *NMCES household interview instru-*

ments: Instruments and procedures 1. DHHS Publication no. (PHS) 81-3280. Washington, D.C.: National Center for Health Services Research.

Bonjean, C.; Maclemore, D.; and Hill, R. 1967. *Sociological measurement.* San Francisco: Chandler.

Boruch, R. 1976. Coupling randomized experiments and approximations to experiments in social program evaluation. In *Validity issues in evaluative research,* ed. I. N. Bernstein, 35–57. Sage Contemporary Social Science Issues, vol. 23. Beverly Hills, Calif.: Sage.

Bosanac, E. M.; Petersen, V. E.; Forren, G. L.; and Baranowski, T. 1982. A resource inventory approach to needs assessment: Examples from a statewide hypertension control program. *Social Science and Medicine* 16: 1301–1307.

Boyd, N. F.; Pater, J. L.; Ginsburg, A. D.; and Myers, R. E. 1979. Observer variation in the classification of information from medical records. *Journal of Chronic Diseases* 32:327–332.

Boyd, R., and Windsor, R. Fall 1993. A meta-evaluation of nutrition education research among pregnant women. *Health Education Quarterly* 20(3): 327–345.

Boyer, J. F., and Langbein, L. I. 1991. Factors influencing the use of health evaluation research in Congress. *Evaluation Review* 15(5):507–532.

Bradburn, N. M., and Sudman, S. 1979. *Improving interview method and questionnaire design.* San Francisco: Jossey-Bass.

Bravo, G., and Potvin, L. 1991. Estimating the reliability of continuous measures with Cronbach's alpha or the intraclass correlation coefficient: Toward the integration of two traditions. *Journal of Clinical Epidemiology* 44:381–390.

Brehony, K. A.; Frederiksen, L. W.; and Solomon, L. J. 1984. Marketing principles and behavioral medicine: An overview. In *Marketing health behavior: Principles, techniques, and applications,* ed. L. W. Frederiksen, L. J. Solomon, and K. A. Brehony. New York: Plenum.

Broskowski, A. 1979. Management information systems for planning and evaluation in human services. In *Program evaluation in the health fields,* vol. 2, ed. H. C. Schulberg and F. Baker, 147–171. New York: Human Sciences Press.

Bross, I. 1954. A confidence interval for a percentage increase. *Biometrics* 13(2):245–250.

Brownell, K., and Stinkard, A. J. 1978. Behavioral treatment of obesity in children. *American Journal of Diseases of Children* 132:403–412.

Brownell, K. D., et al. 1978. The effect of couples training and partner cooperativeness in the behavioral treatment of obesity. *Behavior Research and Therapy* 16:323–333.

Bruner, J. S. 1973. *Beyond the information given.* New York: Norton.

Bruvold, W. 1993. A meta-analysis of adolescent smoking prevention programs. *American Journal of Public Health* 83(6):872–880.

Buros, O. K. 1972. *Mental measurements yearbook*. 7th ed. Highland Park, N.J.: Gryphon Press.

Cambre, M. 1978. The development of formative evaluation procedures for instructional film and television: The past fifty years. PhD diss., Indiana University, Bloomington.

Cambre, M. 1981. Historical overview of formative evaluation of instructional media products. *Education Communications and Technology Journal* 29(1): 3–25.

Campbell, D. 1969. Reforms as experiments. *American Psychology* 24(4):409–429.

Campbell, D. 1975. Assessing the impact of planned social change. In *Social research and public policies*, ed. G. M. Lyons. Hanover, N.H.: Dartmouth College, Public Affairs Center.

Campbell, D., and Stanley, J. 1966. *Experimental and quasi-experimental designs for research*. Chicago: Rand McNally.

Cannell, C. F.; Lawson, S. A.; and Hausser, D. L. 1975. *A technique for evaluating interviewer performance*. Ann Arbor, Mich.: Institute for Social Research.

Cannell, C. F.; Marquis, K. H.; and Laurent, A. 1977. *A summary of studies of interviewing methodology*. Vital and health statistics: Data Evaluation and Methods Research, series 2, no. 69. DHEW Publication no. (HRA) 77-1343. Rockville, Md.: National Center for Health Statistics.

Cannell, C. F.; Oksenberg, L.; and Converse, J. M., eds. 1977. *Experiments in interviewing techniques: Field experiments in health reporting, 1971–1977*. DHEW Publication no. (HRA) 78-3204. Washington, D.C.: National Center for Health Services Research.

Carey, L. C. 1972. The quality form. *Journal of Systems Management* 6(June): 28–30.

Cartwright, D., and Zander, A. 1968. *Group dynamics, research and theory*. 3rd ed. New York: Harper & Row.

Clark, N. M. 1978. Spanning the boundary between agency and community. *American Journal of Health Planning* 3(4):40–46.

Clark, N. M. 1981. Should adult education be competency based? In *Examining controversies in adult education*, ed. B. W. Kreitlow, 126–142. San Francisco: Jossey-Bass.

Clark, N. M.; Feldman, C.; Evans, D.; Duzey, O.; Levison, M. J.; Wasilewski, Y.; and Mellins, R. B. 1986. Managing better: Children, parents, and asthma. *Patient Education and Counseling* 8:27–38.

Clark, N. M.; Feldman, C. H.; Evans, D.; Millman, E. J.; Wasilewski, Y.; and Valle, I. 1981. The effectiveness of education for family management of pediatric asthma: A preliminary report. *Health Education Quarterly* 8(2): 166–174.

Clark, N. M.; Feldman, C. H.; Freudenberg, N.; Millman, E. J.; Wasilewski, Y.; and Valle, I. 1980. Developing education for children with asthma through study of self-management behavior. *Health Education Quarterly* 7(4):278–297.

Clark, N., and Gakuru, O. N. 1982. The effects on health and self-confidence of collaborative learning projects. *International Journal of Health Education* 1(2):47–56.

Clark, N. M., and Pinkett-Heller, M. 1977. Developing HSA leadership: An innovation in board education. *American Journal of Health Planning* 2(1): 9–13.

Clark, N. M., and Pinkett-Heller, M. 1979. The institution of administrative change in the home health service agency. *Home Health Services Quarterly* 1(1):7–17.

Clark, N. M., and Wolderufael, A. 1977. Community development through integration of services and education. *International Journal of Health Education* 20(3):189–199.

Cohen, J. 1960. A coefficient of agreement for nominal scales. *Educational and Psychological Measurement* 20:37–46.

Cohen, J., and Cohen, P. 1975. *Applied multiple regression/correlation for the behavioral sciences.* Hillsdale, N.J.: Erlbaum.

Conner, R. F. 1979. The evaluator–manager relationship: An examination of the sources of conflict and a model for a successful union. In *The evaluator and management,* ed. H. C. Schulberg and J. H. Jerrel. Sage Research Progress Series in Evaluation, vol. 4. Beverly Hills, Calif.: Sage.

Connolly, T., and Porter, A. L. 1980. A user focused model for the utilization of evaluation. *Evaluation and Program Planning* 3:131–140.

Cook, T. D., and Campbell, D. T. 1979. *Quasi-experimentation: Design and analysis for field settings.* Boston: Houghton Mifflin.

Cook, T. D., and Campbell, D. T. 1983. The design and conduct of quasi-experiments and true experiments in field settings. In *Handbook of industrial and organizational psychology,* ed. M. D. Dunnette. New York: Wiley.

Cook, T. D., and Reichardt, C. S., eds. 1979. *Qualitative and quantitative methods in evaluation research.* Beverly Hills, Calif.: Sage.

Corroll, V. 1980. Employee fitness programs: An expanding concept. *International Journal of Health Education* 23(1):35–41.

Cox, D. R., and Snell, E. J. 1979. The choice of variables in observational studies. *Journal of the Royal Statistical Society,* series C, 23(2):51–59.

Cox, G. B. 1977. Managerial style: Implications for the utilization of program evaluation information. *Evaluation Quarterly* 1(3):499–508.

Coyle, S.; Boruch, R.; and Turner, C. (eds.). 1991. *Evaluating AIDS prevention programs* (expanded edition). Prepared by the Panel on the Evaluation of AIDS Interventions, National Research Council. Washington, D.C.: National Academy Press.

Creer, T.; Renne, C.; and Christian, W. 1976. Behavioral contributions to rehabilitation and childhood asthma. *Rehabilitation Literature* 37:226–232.

Cronbach, L. J. 1951. Coefficient alpha and the internal structure of a test. *Psychometrika* 16:297–334.

Cummings, A. R. 1992. Quality control principles: Applications in dietetics practice. *Journal of the American Dietetic Association* 92:427–428.

Dale, E., and Chall, J. 1948. A formula for predicting readability. *Educational Research Bulletin* 27(Jan. 2):11–20, (Feb. 17):37–54.

Daltroy, L., and Goeppinger, J. 1993. Arthritis health education [Special issue]. *Health Education Quarterly* 20(1).

Deeds, S.; Chwalow, A.; Green, L.; and Levine, D. 1975. Operational constraints on the design and implementation of health education research in a teaching hospital setting. Paper presented at the annual meeting of the American Public Health Association, Chicago.

Deeds, S.; Hebert, B.; and Wolle, J., eds. 1979. *A model for patient education programming*. Special Project Report. Washington, D.C.: American Public Health Association, Public Health Education Section.

Deeds, S., and Mullen, P., eds. 1981. Managing health education in health maintenance organizations: Part 1. *Health Education Quarterly* 8(4):279–375.

Deeds, S., and Mullen, P., eds. 1982. Managing health education in health maintenance organizations: Part 2. *Health Education Quarterly* 9(1):3–95.

Delbecq, A. L. 1974. Contextual variables affecting decision making in program planning. *Decision Sciences* 5(4):726–742.

Delbecq, A. L. 1978. Relating need assessment to implementation strategies: An organizational perspective. Paper presented to the Second National Conference on Need Assessment in Health and Human Services, University of Louisville, Ky.

Delbecq, A. L.; Van de Ven, A. H.; and Gustafson, D. 1975. *Group techniques for program planning: A guide to Nominal Group and Delphi processes*. Glenview, Ill.: Scott, Foresman.

Deniston, O., and Rosenstock, I. 1968a. Evaluation of program effectiveness. *Public Health Reports* 83(4):323–335.

Deniston, O., and Rosenstock, I. 1968b. Evaluation of program efficiency. *Public Health Reports* 83(7):603–610.

Deniston, O., and Rosenstock, I. 1973. The validity of nonexperimental designs for evaluating health services. *Health Service Reports* 88(2):153–164.

Dial, C., and Windsor, R. A. 1985. A formative evaluation of a health education-water exercise program for class II and class III adult rheumatoid arthritics. *Patient Education Counseling* vol. 7(1).

Dickey, B., and Hampton, E. 1981. Effective problem-solving for evaluation utilization. *Knowledge: Creation, Diffusion, Utilization* 2(3):361–374.

Dillman, D. A. 1978. *Mail and telephone surveys: The total design method*. New York: Wiley.

Dinkel, N.; Zinober, J.; and Flaherty, E. 1981. Citizen participation in CMHC program evaluation: A neglected potential. *Community Mental Health Journal* 17(1):54–65.

Doak, C. C.; Leonard, G.; and Root, J. H. 1985. *Teaching patients with low literacy skills.* Philadelphia: Lippincott.

Domel, S.; Baranowski, T.; Davis, H. C.; et al. 1993 (in press). Measuring fruit and vegetable preferences among 4th and 5th grade students. *Preventive Medicine.*

Domel, S.; Baranowski, T.; Davis, H. C.; et al. 1993 (in press). Accuracy of 4th and 5th grade student diaries compared to school lunch observation. *American Journal of Clinical Nutrition.*

Donabedian, A. 1966. Evaluating the quality of medical care, Part 2. *Milbank Memorial Fund Quarterly* 44:166–206.

Donabedian, A. 1968. Promoting quality through evaluating the process of patient care. *Medical Care* 6:191–202.

Dunn, W. 1980. The two communities metaphor and models of knowledge use. *Knowledge: Creation, Diffusion, Utilization* 1(4):515–536.

DuRant, R. H.; Baranowski, T.; Davis, H.; Thompson, W. O.; Puhl, J.; Greaves, K.; and Rhodes, T. 1992. Reliability of heart rate monitoring in three, four, and five year old Anglo-, Black-, and Mexican-American children. *Medicine and Science in Sports and Exercise* 24:265–271.

Dwyer, F., and Hammel, R. 1978. An experimental study: Patient package inserts and their effects on hypertensive patients. *Urban Health* 7(June):46.

Easton, E.; Easton, M.; and Levy, M. 1977. Medical and educational malpractice issues in patient education. *Journal of Family Practice* 4(2):276.

Ehrenberg, A. C. S. 1982. Writing technical papers and reports. *American Statistician* 36(4):326–329.

Emerson, R. M. 1981. Observational field work. *Annual Review of Sociology* 7:351–378.

Employee Health Fitness editors. 1980. Absenteeism drop linked to hospital health promotion. *Employee Health Fitness* 2(11):135.

Evans, D.; Clark, N. M.; Feldman, C. H.; Rips, J.; Kaplan, D.; Levison, M. J.; Wasilewski, Y.; Levin, B.; and Mellins, R. B. 1987. A school health education program for children with asthma aged 8–11 years. *Health Education Quarterly* 14(3):267–279.

Farquahar, J.; Maccoby, N.; et al. 1977. Community education for cardiovascular health. *Lancet* 1(June 4):1192–1195.

Feinstein, A. R. 1970. Quality of data in the medical record. *Computers and Biomedical Research* 3:426–435.

Feinstein, A. R. 1977. Clinical biostatistics XLI: Hard science, soft data, and the challenges of choosing clinical variables in research. *Clinical Pharmacology and Therapeutics* 22(4):485–498.

Ferber, B. 1968. Problems in abstracting and using data from hospital medical records. *Inquiry* 5(1):68–73.

Fink, A., and Kosecoff, J., eds. 1979. How to write an evaluation report. *How to Evaluate Health Programs.* Washington, D.C.: Capitol Publications.

Finnegan, J., et al. 1989. Measuring and tracking education program implementation: The Minnesota Heart Health Program experience. *Health Education Quarterly* 16:77–90.

Fitz-Gibbon, C., and Morris, L. 1978. *How to design a program evaluation.* Beverly Hills, Calif.: Sage.

Flanders, N. 1960. Interaction analysis: A technique for quantifying teacher influence. Paper distributed by Far West Laboratory for Educational Research and Development, San Francisco.

Flay, B. R. 1987. Evaluation of the development, dissemination and effectiveness of mass media health programming. *Health Education Research* 2(2): 123–129.

Fleiss, J. 1981. *Statistical methods for rates and proportions.* New York: Wiley.

Flesch, R. 1948. A new readability yardstick. *Journal of Applied Psychology* 32:221–233.

Freimuth, V. S., et al. 1988. Health advertising: Prevention for profit. *American Journal of Public Health* 78(5):557–561.

French, J. L., and Becker, S. W. 1975. Organizational intervention. In *The diffusion of medical technology,* ed. G. Gordon and G. L. Fisher. Cambridge, Mass.: Ballinger.

Freudenberg, N. 1989. *Preventing AIDS: A guide to effective education for the prevention of HIV infection.* Washington, D.C.: American Public Health Association.

Freudenberg, N.; Feldman, C. H.; Clark, N. M.; Millman, E. J.; Valle, I.; and Wasilewski, Y. 1980. The impact of bronchial asthma on school attendance and performance. *Journal of School Health* 50(9):522–526.

Fry, E. 1968. A readability formula that saves time. *Journal of Reading* 11: 513–516, 575–578.

Garber, A. M., et al. 1989. *Costs and effectiveness of cholesterol screening in the elderly.* Paper 3 of Preventive Health Services under Medicare.

Glanz, K. 1980. Compliance with dietary regimens: Its magnitude, measurement, and determinants. *Preventive Medicine* 9:787–804.

Glanz, K.; Lewis, F. M.; and Rimer, B. K. 1990. *Health behavior and health education: Theory, research, and practice.* San Francisco: Jossey-Bass.

Glanz, K., and Rudd, J. 1990. Readability and content analysis of print cholesterol education materials. *Patient Education and Counseling* 16:109–118.

Glaser, E. M., and Taylor, S. H. 1973. Factors influencing the success of applied research. *American Psychologist* 28:140–146.

Glass, G. V.; McGaw, B.; and Smith, M. L. 1981. *Meta-analysis in social research.* Beverly Hills, Calif.: Sage.

Glass, G.; Willson, V.; and Gottman, J. 1975. *Design and analysis of time series experiments.* Boulder: University of Colorado, Laboratory of Educational Research.

Gorry, G. A., and Goodrich, T. J. 1978. On the role of values in program evaluation. *Evaluation Quarterly* 2(4):561-572.

Gottlieb, B. H. 1987. Using social support to protect and promote health. *Journal of Primary Prevention* 8:49-70.

Green, L. 1974. Toward cost-benefit evaluations of health education: Some concepts, methods, and examples. *Health Education Monographs* 2(1): 34-64.

Green, L. 1977. Evaluation and measurement: Some dilemmas for health education. *American Journal of Public Health* 67(2):155-161.

Green, L., and Kreuter, M. 1991. *Health promotion planning: A diagnostic approach.* Mountain View, Calif.: Mayfield.

Green, L., and Brooks-Bertram, P. 1978. Peer review and quality control in health education. *Health Values: Achieving High Level Wellness* 2(4):191-197.

Green, L., and Figa-Talamanca, I. 1974. Suggested designs for evaluation of patient education programs. *Health Education Monographs* 2(1):54-71.

Green, L.; Levine, D.; and Deeds, S. 1975. Clinical trials of health education for hypertensive outpatients: Design and baseline data. *Preventive Medicine* 4:417-425.

Green, L. W., and Lewis, F. M. 1986. *Evaluation and measurement in health education.* Mountain View, Calif.: Mayfield.

Green, L.; Werlin, S.; and Schauffler, H. 1976. *Research demonstration issues in self care.* Cambridge, Mass.: Little.

Green, S. B. 1981. A comparison of three indexes of agreement between observers: Proportion of agreement, G-index, and kappa. *Educational and Psychological Measurement* 41:1069-1072.

Greene, R. 1976. *Assuring quality in medical care.* Cambridge, Mass.: Ballinger.

Greer, A. L. 1977. Advances in the study of diffusion of innovation in health care organizations. *Milbank Memorial Fund Quarterly, Health and Society* 19:505-532.

Groves, R. M. 1979. A researcher's view of the SRC computer-based interviewing system: Measurement of some sources of error in telephone survey data. In *Health survey research methods, third biennial conference,* ed. S. Sudman. DHHS Publication no. (PHS) 81-3268. Washington, D.C.: National Center for Health Services Research.

Groves, R. M., and Kahn, R. L. 1979. *Surveys by telephone: A national comparison with personal interviews.* New York: Academic Press.

Grubbs, F. E. 1969. Procedures for detecting outlying observations in samples. *Technometrics* 11:1-21.

Guba, E., and Lincoln, Y. 1989. *Fourth generation evaluation.* Newbury Park, Calif.: Sage.

Gurel, L. 1975. The human side of evaluating human services programs: Problems and prospects. In *Handbook of evaluation research*, vol. 2, ed. M. Guttentag and E. L. Struening. Beverly Hills, Calif.: Sage.

Guydatt, G.; Walter, S. W.; Norman, G. R. 1987. Measuring change over time: Assessing the usefulness of evaluative instruments. *Journal of Chronic Disease* 40:171–178.

Guyer, B. 1989. *Injury prevention: Meeting the challenge* [Special issue]. *American Journal of Preventive Medicine* 28 (suppl.)

Haggerty, R. 1977. Changing life styles to improve health. *Preventive Medicine* 6:276–289.

Handbook for certification of health education specialists. 1990. New York: National Commission of Health Education Credentialing.

Hatziandreu, E. I., et al. 1988. A cost-effectiveness analysis of exercise as a health promotion activity. *American Journal of Public Health* 78(11):1417–1421.

Hawkins, J.; Rorfman, R.; and Osborne, P. 1978. Decision makers' judgments: The influence of role, evaluative criteria, and information access. *Evaluation Quarterly* 2(3):435–454.

Health Education Monographs editors. 1977. Guidelines for health education preparation and practice. *Health Education Monographs* 5(1):1–18.

Hecht, R. 1978. Guide to media program development. Stanford, Calif.: Stanford University, School of Medicine, Division of Instructional Media.

Herbert, J., and Attridge, C. 1975. A guide for developers and users of observation systems and manuals. *American Educational Research Journal* 12(1):1–20.

Hill, R. A.; Standen, P. J.; and Tattersfield, A. E. 1989. Asthma, wheezing, and school absence in primary schools. *Archives of Disease in Childhood* 64:246–251.

Hladik, W., and White, S. 1976. Evaluation of written reinforcement used in counseling cardiovascular patients. *American Journal of Hospital Pharmacy* 33:155–159.

Hochbaum, G. 1962. *Evaluation: A diagnostic procedure.* Studies and Research in Health Education, vol. 5. Geneva: World Health Organization, International Union for Health Education, International Conference on Health and Health Education.

Hochbaum, G. 1965. Research to improve health education. *International Journal of Health Education* 8(1):141–148.

Holzbach, R. L.; Piserchia, P. V.; McFadden, D. W.; Hartwell, T. D.; Herrmann, A.; and Fielding, J. E. 1990. Effect of a comprehensive health promotion program on employee attitudes. *Journal of Occupational Medicine* 32(10):973–978.

House, A. E.; House, B. J.; and Campbell, M. B. 1981. Measures of interobserver agreement: Calculation formulas and distribution effects. *Journal of Behavioral Assessment* 3(1):37–57.

Hughes, G.; Hymowitz, N.; Ockene, J.; Simon, N.; and Vogt, T. 1981. The multiple risk factor intervention trial (MRFIT), V: Intervention on smoking. *Preventive Medicine* 10(4):476–500.

Hunter, J. E., and Schmidt, F. L. 1990. *Methods of meta-analysis.* Newbury Park, Calif.: Sage.

Inui, T. 1978. A common bond: Exploring the interface between health education and quality assurance. *Journal of Quality Assurance* 10(Oct.):6–7.

Isaac, S., and Michael, W. 1971. *Handbook in research and evaluation.* San Diego: Knapp.

Israel, B. A., and Rounds, K. A. 1987. Social networks and social support: A synthesis for health educators. In *Advances in health education and promotion: A research annual,* ed. W. B. Ward, S. K. Simonds, P. D. Mullen, and M. Becker. Greenwich, Conn.: Jai Press.

Iverson, D., guest ed. 1981. Promoting health through the schools: A challenge for the eighties. *Health Education Quarterly* 8(1):1–117.

Iverson, D., and Kolbe, L. 1983. Evaluation of the national disease prevention and health promotion strategy: Establishing a role for schools. *Journal of School Health* 53:294–302.

Janis, I., and Mann, L. 1977. *Decision making.* New York: Free Press.

Janz, N. K., and Becker, M. H. 1984. The health belief model: A decade later. *Health Education Quarterly* 11(1):1–47.

Jenkins, C. D.; Rosenman, R. H.; and Zyzanski, S. J. 1974. Prediction of clinical coronary heart disease by a test for the coronary-prone behavior pattern. *New England Journal of Medicine* 290(23):1271–1275.

Jobe, J. B., and Mingay, D. J. 1990. Cognitive laboratory approach to designing questionnaires for surveys of the elderly. *Public Health Reports* 105:518–524.

Johnson, S. M., and Bolstad, O. D. 1973. Methodological issues in naturalistic observation: Some problems and solutions for field research. In *Behavior change: Methodology, concepts, and practice,* ed. L. A. Hamerlynck, L. C. Handy, and E. J. Mash. Champaign, Ill.: Research Press.

Joint Committee on Standards for Education Evaluation. 1981. *Standards for evaluations of educational programs, projects, and materials.* New York: McGraw-Hill.

Jordan, L. A.; Marcus, A. C.; and Reeder, L. G. 1979. Response styles in telephone and household interviewing: A field experiment from the Los Angeles health survey. In *Health survey research methods, third biennial conference,* ed. S. Sudman. DHHS Publication no. (PHS) 81-3268. Washington, D.C.: National Center for Health Services Research.

Kalton, G.; Collins, M.; and Brook, L. 1978. Experiments in wording opinion questions. *Applied Statistics* 27(2):149–161.

Kaplun-le Meitour, A., ed. 1973. Twenty years of health education: Evaluation and forecast. *Proceedings of the 8th International Conference on Health Education.* Paris: International Union on Health Education.

Kelly, K. 1979. Evaluation of a group nutrition education approach to effective weight loss and control. *American Journal of Public Health* 69(8): 813–814.

Kenny, D. 1975. A quasi-experimental approach to assessing treatment effects in the nonequivalent control group design. *Psychology Bulletin* 82:345–362.

Kerlinger, F. 1973. *Foundations of behavioral research.* 2d ed. New York: Holt, Rinehart & Winston.

Kish, L. 1965. *Survey sampling.* New York: Wiley.

Kish, L. 1987. *Statistical design for research.* New York: Wiley.

Klare, G. 1974–1975. Assessing readability. *Reading Research Quarterly* 1: 62–102.

Klesges, R. C.; Cigrang, J.; and Glasgow, R. E. 1989. Worksite smoking modification programs: A state-of-the-art review and directions for future research. In *Applications in health psychology,* ed. M. Johnston and T. Marteau. New Brunswick, N.J.: Transaction Publishers.

Knutson, A. 1952. Application of pretesting in health education. *Public Health Monographs* 42(6):1–10.

Knutson, A. 1959. The influence of values on education. *Health Education Monographs* 3:32–40.

Koskela, K.; Puska, P.; and Tuomilehto, J. 1976. The North Karelia project: A first evaluation. *International Journal of Health Education* 19(1):59–66.

Kouzes, J. M., and Mico, P. R. 1979. Domain theory: An introduction to organizational behavior in human service organizations. *Journal of Applied Behavioral Science* 15:449–469.

Kouzes, J. M., and Mico, P. R. 1980. How can we manage divided houses? *New Directions for Mental Health Services* 8:43–57.

Kreuter, M. 1985. Results of the school health education evaluation. *Journal of School Health* 8.

Krueger, R. A. 1988. *Focus groups: A practical guide for applied research.* Newbury Park, Calif.: Sage.

Kurtz, D. L., and Boone, L. E. 1981. *Marketing.* New York: Dryden Press.

Laboratory Standardization Panel of the National Cholesterol Education Program. 1990. *Recommendation for improving cholesterol measurement.* NIH Publication no. 90-2964. Bethesda, Md.: National Heart, Lung, and Blood Institute.

Larry, R., chair. 1973. *Report of the president's committee on health education.* New York: Public Affairs Institute.

Lau, R. R., and Ware, J. F., Jr. 1981. Refinements in the measurement of health-specific locus-of-control beliefs. *Medical Care* 19(12):1147–1158.

Laurent, A.; Cannell, C. F.; and Marquis, K. F. 1972. *Reporting health events in household interviews: Effects of an extensive questionnaire and a diary procedure.* National Center for Health Statistics, Data Evaluation and Methods Research, series 2, no. 49. DHEW Publication no. (HSM) 72-1049. Rockville, Md.: Health Services and Mental Health Administration.

LeVee, W. ed. 1989. *New perspectives on HIV-related illnesses: Progress in Health Services Research*. National Center for Health Services Research, Public Health Service, U.S. Department of Health and Human Services. Washington, D.C.: Government Printing Office.

Leventhal, H.; Nerenz, D. R.; and Steele, D. J. 1984. Illness representation and coping with health threats. In *Handbook of psychology and health*, ed. A. Baum, S. E. Taylor, and J. E. Singer, 219–252. Hillsdale, N.J.: Erlbaum.

Levin, L.; Katz, A.; and Holst, E. 1976. *Self-care: Lay initiatives in health*. New York: Prodist.

Levine, A., and Levine, M. 1977. The social context of evaluation research: A case study. *Evaluation Quarterly* 1(4):515–542.

Ligouri, S. 1978. A quantitative assessment of the readability of PPIs. *Drug Intelligence and Clinical Pharmacy* 12:712–716.

Little, A. 1976. *A survey of consumer health education programs*. Final Report submitted to the Office of the Assistant Secretary for Planning and Evaluation/Health on Contract no. HEW 100-75-0082. Washington, D.C.: Department of Health, Education and Welfare.

Liu, K.; Cooper, R.; McKeever, J.; Byington, R.; Soltero, I.; Stamler, R.; Gosch, F.; Stevens, E.; and Stamler, J. 1979. Assessment of the association between habitual salt intake and high blood pressure: Methodological problems. *American Journal of Epidemiology* 110(2):219–226.

Lofland, J. 1971. *Analyzing social settings*. Belmont, Calif.: Wadsworth.

Loftus, E.; Klinger, M. R.; Smith, D. K.; and Fiedler, J. 1990. A tale of two questions: Benefits of asking more than one question. *Public Opinion Quarterly* 54(3):330–345.

Lowe, J. B.; Windsor, R. A.; Adams, B.; Morris, J.; and Reese, Y. 1986. Use of a bogus pipeline method to increase accuracy of self-reported alcohol consumption among pregnant women. *Journal of Studies on Alcohol* 47: 173–175.

Lowe, J.; Windsor, R.; and Valois, R. 1989. Quality assurance methods for managing employee health promotion programs: A case study in smoking cessation. *Health Values* 13(2):12–23.

Luce, B., and Elixhauser, A. 1990. *Standards for the socioeconomic evaluation of health care services* (A. Culyer, ed.) (pp. 1–160). New York: Springer-Verlag.

Luck, D. J.; Wales, A. G.; Taylor, D. A.; and Rubin, R. S. 1978. *Marketing research*. New York: Prentice Hall.

Manning, D. 1981. Writing readable health messages. *Public Health Reports* 96(5):464–466.

Manzella, B. A.; Brodes, C. M.; Richards, J. M., Jr.; Windsor, R. A.; Soong, S-j.; and Bailey, W. C. 1989. Assessing the use of metered dose inhalers by adults with asthma. *Journal of Asthma* 26:223–230.

McKnight, J. L. 1978. Community health in a Chicago slum. *Development Dialogue* 1:62–68.

McLaughlin, G. 1969. SMOG grading—a new readability formula. *Journal of Reading* 12(May):639–646.

McLeroy, K.; Bibeau, D.; Steckler, A.; and Glanz, K. 1988. An ecological perspective on health promotion programs. *Health Education Quarterly* 15(3): 351–378.

McLeroy, K. R.; Steckler, A.; and Glanz, K. 1984. Assessing the effects of health promotion in worksites: A review of the stress program evaluations. *Health Education Quarterly* 11(4):379–401.

McNabb, W. L., et al. Self-management education of children with asthma: Air wise. *American Journal of Public Health* 75(10):1219–1220.

McNagny, S. E., and Parker, R. M. 1992. High prevalence of recent cocaine use and the unreliability of patient self-report in an inner-city walk-in clinic. *Journal of the American Medical Association* 267:1106–1108.

McNutt, K. 1980. Dietary advice to the public: 1957–1980. *Nutrition Reviews* 38(10):353–360.

McShane, L. M.; Clark, L. C.; Combs, G. F., Jr.; and Turnbull, B. W. 1991. Reporting the accuracy of biochemical measurement for epidemiologic and nutrition studies. *American Journal of Clinical Nutrition* 53:1354–1360.

Meals for Millions Foundation. 1981. *Healthy lifestyle for seniors.* Santa Monica, Calif.: Meals for Millions Foundation.

Mezirow, J.; Darkenwald, G.; and Knox, A. 1975. *Last gamble on education.* Washington, D.C.: Adult Education Association.

Michnich, M.; Shortell, S.; and Richardson, W. 1981. Program evaluation: Resource for decision making. *Health Care Management Review* 6:25–35.

Miller, J., and Lewis, F. 1982. Closing the gap in quality assurance: A tool for evaluating group leaders. *Health Education Quarterly* 9(1):55–66.

Mojonnier, M. L.; Hall, Y.; Berkson, D. M.; et al. 1980. Experience in changing food habits of hyperlipidemic men and women. *Journal of the American Dietetic Association* 77:140–148.

Morley, J., and Levine, A. 1982. The role of the endogenous opiates as regulators of appetite. *American Journal of Clinical Nutrition* 35:757–761.

Morris, J. 1980. Vigorous exercise in leisure: Protection against coronary heart disease. *Lancet* 8206:1207–10.

Morris, J., and Windsor, R. A. 1985. Personal health practices of urban adults in Alabama: Davis Avenue Community Study. *Public Health Reports* 100: 531–539.

Morris, L. L., and Fitz-Gibbon, C. T. 1978. *Evaluator's handbook.* Beverly Hills, Calif.: Sage.

Moss, A. J., and Adams, F. A. 1963. Index of indirect estimation of diastolic blood pressure. *American Journal of Diseases of Children* 106:364–367.

Mullen, P.; McCuan, R.; and Iverson, D. 1986. Evaluation of health education and promotion programs: A review of qualitative methods. *Advances in Health Education and Promotion* 1:467–498.

Mullen, P., and Zapka, J. 1982a. *Guidelines for health education and promotion services: Completing an HMO program.* Washington, D.C.: Department of Health and Human Services, Office of Health Information, Health Promotion, Physical Fitness and Sports Medicine.

Mullen, P., and Zapka, J. 1982b. *Guidelines for health promotion and education services in HMOs.* Washington, D.C.: U.S. Department of Health and Human Services, Public Health Service.

Muller, A. 1980. Evaluation of the costs and benefits of motorcycle helmet laws. *American Journal of Public Health* 70(6):586–592.

Multiple Risk Factor Intervention Trial (MRFIT). V: Intervention on smoking. 1981. *Preventive Medicine* 10(4):476–500.

Mumford, E.; Schlesinger, H. J.; and Glass, G. V. 1982. The effects of psychological intervention on recovery from surgery and heart attacks: An analysis of the literature. *American Journal of Public Health* 72(2):141–151.

Nader, P. R.; Gilman, S.; and Bee, D. E. 1980. Factors influencing access to primary health care via school health services. *Pediatrics* 65(3):585–591.

National Center for Health Education. 1980. Health education and credentialing: The role delineation project. *Focal Points* 3(July):1–31.

National Center for Health Statistics. 1990. *Health United States, 1989.* U.S. Department of Health and Human Services Publication no. (PHS) 90-1232. Hyattsville, Md.: Public Health Service.

Neaton, J.; Broste, S.; Cohen, L.; Fishman, E.; Kjelsberg, M.; and Schoenberger, M. 1981. The Multiple Risk Factor Intervention Trial (MRFIT), VII: A comparison of risk factor changes between the two study groups. *Preventive Medicine* 10(4):519–543.

Nickerson, R. 1979a. The formative evaluation of instructional television programming using the program evaluating analysis computer. In *Experimental research in TV instruction,* vol. 2, ed. J. Baggaley. St. John's: Memorial University of Newfoundland.

Nickerson, R. 1979b. Program evaluation using the program evaluation analysis computer (PEAC). Paper presented at the 1979 convention of the Association for Educational Communications and Technology, New Orleans.

Noelle-Neumann, E. 1970. Wanted: Rules for wording structured questionnaires. *Public Opinion Quarterly* 34:191–201.

Nunnally, J. C. 1978. *Psychometric theory.* 2d ed. New York: McGraw-Hill.

Ogden, H. 1978. Recent developments in health education policy. *Health Education Monographs* 6(suppl. 1):67–73.

Ogden, H. 1980. Health education as an element of U.S. policy. *International Journal of Health Education* 23(3):150–155.

Oster, G., and Epstein, A. M. 1986. Primary prevention and coronary health disease: The economic benefits of lowering serum cholesterol. *American Journal of Public Health* 76(6):647–656.

Ostrom, D. 1978. *Time series analysis: Regression techniques.* Series: Quantitative Applications in the Social Sciences. Beverly Hills, Calif.: Sage.

Parcel, G., and Baranowski, T. 1981. Social learning theory and health education. *Health Education* 12(3):14–18.

Parkinson, R.; Green, L.; Beck, R.; Pearson, C.; McGill, A.; Collings, G., Jr.; Eriksen, M.; Merwin, D.; and Ware, B. 1982. *Managing health promotion in the workplace: Guidelines for implementation and evaluation.* Palo Alto, Calif.: Mayfield.

Patton, M. 1980. *Qualitative evaluation methods.* Beverly Hills, Calif.: Sage.

Patton, M. 1990. *Qualitative evaluation and research methods.* Newbury Park, Calif.: Sage.

Patton, M.; Grimes, P.; Guthrie, K.; Brennan, N.; French, B.; and Blythe, D. 1977. In search of impact: An analysis of the utilization of federal health evaluation research. In *Using social research in public policy making,* ed. C. H. Weiss, 59–81. Lexington, Mass.: Heath.

Perry, C.; Kelder, S.; Murray, D.; and Klepp, K. 1992. Communitywide smoking prevention: Long-term outcomes of the Minnesota Heart Health Program and the Class of 1989 Study. *American Journal of Public Health* 82(9): 1210–1216.

Perry, C.; Killen, J.; Telch, M.; Slinkard, L. A.; and Danaher, B. G. 1980. Modifying smoking behavior of teenagers: A school-based intervention. *American Journal of Public Health* 70(7):722–725.

Pilisuk, M., and Minkler, M. 1980. Supportive networks: Life ties for the elderly. *Journal of Social Issues* 36(2):95–116.

Pless, I., and Pinkerton, P. 1975. *Chronic childhood disorder promoting patterns of adjustment.* London: Kempton.

Polivka, L., and Steg, E. 1978. Program evaluation and policy development: Bridging the gap. *Evaluation Quarterly* 2(4):696–707.

Porras, J. I., and Silvers, R. C. 1991. Organizational development and transformation. *Annual Review of Psychology* 42:51–78.

Porter, A., and Chibocos, T. 1975. Common problems of design and analysis in evaluative research. *Sociological Methods and Research* 3:235–257.

Pratt, H. J. 1976. *The gray lobby.* Chicago: University of Chicago Press.

Public Health Reports editors. 1980. Special section: Health promotion at the worksite. *Public Health Reports* 95(2):99–200.

Puhl, J.; Greaves, K.; Baranowski, T.; Gruben, D.; and Seale, D. 1990. Description and calibration of a Children's Activity Rating Scale (CARS). *Research Quarterly for Exercise and Sport* 61(2):26–36.

Puska, P.; Koskela, K.; and McAlister, A. 1979. A comprehensive television smoking cessation programme in Finland. *International Journal of Health Education* 22(4, suppl.):1–28.

Reeder, L. G., ed. 1978. *Health survey research methods, second biennial confer-*

ence. DHEW Publication no. (PHS) 79-3207. Washington, D.C.: National Center for Health Services Research.

Reeder, L. G.; Ramacher, L.; and Gorelnik, S. 1976. *Handbook of scales and indices of health behavior.* Pacific Palisades, Calif.: Goodyear.

Reppucci, N. D. 1973. Social psychology of institutional change: General principles for intervention. *American Journal of Community Psychology* 1(4): 330–341.

Rice, D. P., and Hodgson, T. A. 1982. The value of human life revisited. *American Journal of Public Health* 72(6):536–537.

Richards, J. M., Jr.; Dolce, J. J.; Windsor, R. A.; Bailey, W. C.; Brooks, C. M.; and Soong, S-j. 1989. Patient characteristics relevant to effective self-management: Scales for assessing attitudes of adults toward asthma. *Journal of Asthma* 26:99–108.

Rimer, B. 1986. Research and evaluation programs related to health education for older persons. *Health Education Quarterly* 13(4).

Robinson, J. P., and Shaver, P. R. 1973. *Measures of social psychological attitudes.* Ann Arbor: University of Michigan, Institute for Social Research.

Rocella, E. J., and Ward, G. W. 1984. The National High Blood Pressure Education Program: A description of its utility as a generic program model. *Health Education Quarterly* 11(3):225–242.

Rogers, P.; Eaton, E.; and Brown, J. 1981. Is health promotion cost-effective? *Preventive Medicine* 10:324–339.

Roghmann, K. J., and Haggerty, R. J. 1972. The diary as a research instrument in the study of health and illness behavior: Experiences with a random sample of young families. *Medical Care* 10(2):143–163.

Roos, N. P. 1974. Influencing the health care system: Policy alternatives. *Public Policy* 22(2):139–167.

Rosenstock, I. 1960. Gaps and potentials in health education research. *Health Education Monographs* 8:21–27.

Rosenstock, I. 1975. General criteria for evaluating health education programs. In *Proceedings of the NHLI working conference on health behavior, May 12–15,* ed. S. M. Weiss. DHEW Publication no. (NIH) 76-868. Washington, D.C.: Government Printing Office.

Rosenstock, I. M.; Strecher, V. J.; and Becker, M. H. 1988. Social learning theory and the health belief model. *Health Education Quarterly* 15(2): 175–183.

Rosenthal, B. S.; Allen, G. S.; and Winter, C. 1980. Husband involvement in the behavioral treatment of overweight women: Initial effects and long-term follow-up. *International Journal of Obesity* 4:165–173.

Ross, H., and Mico, P. 1980. *Theory and practice in health education.* Palo Alto, Calif.: Mayfield.

Rossi, P. H., and Freeman, H. E. 1993. *Evaluation: A systematic approach.* 5th ed. Newbury Park, Calif.: Sage.

Rossi, P.; Freeman, H.; and Wright, S. 1979. *Evaluation: A systematic approach.* Beverly Hills, Calif.: Sage.

Rossi, P., and Williams, W., eds. 1972. *Evaluating social programs: Theory, practice and politics.* New York: Seminar Press.

Roter, D. 1977. Patient participation in the patient-provider interaction: The effects of patient question asking on the quality of interaction, satisfaction, and compliance. *Health Education Monographs* 5(4):281–315.

Rubin, D. 1974. Estimating causal effects of treatments in randomized and nonrandomized studies. *Journal of Educational Psychology* 56(5):688–701.

Rundall, T. G., and Bruvold, W. H. 1988. A meta-analysis of school-based smoking and alcohol use prevention programs. *Health Education Quarterly* 15:317–334.

Russell, L. B. 1987. *Evaluating preventive care: Report on a workshop.* Washington, D.C.: Brookings Institute.

Saccone, A. J., and Israel, A. C. 1978. Effects of experimental vs. significant other controlled reinforcement and choice of target behavior on weight loss. *Behavior Therapy* 9:271–278.

Sallis, J. F.; Howell, M. F.; Hofstetter, C. R.; Elder, J. P.; Caspersen, C. J.; Hackley, M.; et al. 1990. Distance between homes and exercise facilities related to the frequency of exercise among San Diego residents. *Public Health Reports* 105:179–185.

Schafer, R. B. 1978. Factors affecting food behavior and the quality of husbands' and wives' diets. *Journal of the American Dietetic Association* 72:138–143.

Schlundt, D. G. 1988. Accuracy and reliability of nutrient intake estimates. *Journal of Nutrition* 118:1432–1435.

Schulberg, H. C., and Jerrel, J. H., eds. 1979. *The evaluator and management.* Sage Research Progress Series in Evaluation, vol. 4. Beverly Hills, Calif.: Sage.

Schuman, H., and Presser, S. 1977. Question wording as an independent variable in survey analysis. *Sociological Methods and Research* 6(2):151–170.

Schwarz, N.; Knauper, B.; Hippler, H-J.; Noelle-Neumann, E.; and Clark, L. 1991. Rating scales, numeric values may change the meaning of scale labels. *Public Opinion Quarterly* 55:570–582.

Sechrest, L.; Perrin, E.; and Bunker, J., eds. 1990. *Research methodology: Strengthening causal interpretations of non-experimental data.* Rockville, Md.: AHCPR.

Sechrest, L.; Freeman, H.; and Mulley, A., eds. 1989. Health Services Research methodology: A focus on AIDS, conference proceedings. National Center for Health Services Research, Public Health Service, U.S. Department of Health and Human Services. Washington, D.C.: Government Printing Office.

Sepulveda, J.; Fineberg, H.; and Mann, J., eds. 1982. *AIDS prevention through education: A world view*. New York: Oxford University Press.

Shadish, W.; Cook, T.; and Leviton, L. 1991. *Foundations of program evaluation*. Newbury Park, Calif.: Sage.

Shaw, M. E., and Wright, J. M. 1967. *Scales for the measurement of attitudes*. New York: McGraw-Hill.

Sherwin, R.; Kaelber, D.; Kezdi, R.; Kjelsberg, M.; and Thomas, H., Jr. 1981. The multiple risk factor intervention trial (MRFIT), II: The development of the protocol. *Preventive Medicine* 10(4):402–425.

Shinn, M.; Lehmann, S.; and Wong, N. W. 1984. Social interaction and social support. *Journal of Social Issues* 40(4):55–76.

Shortell, S., and Richardson, W. 1978. *Health program evaluation*. St. Louis: Mosby.

Sichel, J. 1982. *Program evaluation guidelines*. New York: Human Sciences Press.

Siemiatycki, J. 1979. A comparison of mail, telephone and home interview strategies for household health surveys. *American Journal of Public Health* 69:238–244.

Simmons, J., ed. 1975. Making health education work. *American Journal of Public Health* 65(Oct., suppl.):1–49.

Simmons, J. J.; Salisbury, Z. T.; Kane-Williams, E.; Kauffman, C. K.; and Quaintance, B. 1989. Interorganizational collaboration and dissemination of health promotion for older Americans. *Health Education Quarterly* 16(4): 529–550.

Simon, S.; Howe, L.; and Kirschinbaum, H. 1972. *Values clarification*. New York: Hart.

Simons-Morton, B., and Baranowski, T. 1991. Observation methods in the assessment of children's dietary practices. *Journal of School Health* 61(5): 204–207.

Society for Public Health Education, Ad Hoc Committee. 1968. *Statement of functions of community health educators and minimum requirements for their professional preparation with recommendations for implementation*. Professional Preparation of Community Health Educators, National Commission on Accrediting. Washington, D.C.: Department of Health, Education and Welfare, Public Health Service, Center for Disease Control.

Society for Public Health Education, Ad Hoc Task Force on Professional Preparation and Practice of Health Education. 1977a. Guidelines for the preparation and practice of professional health educators. *Health Education Monographs* 5(1):75–89.

Society for Public Health Education, Committee on Professional Preparation and Practice of Community Health Educators at the Baccalaureate Level. 1977b. Criteria and guidelines for baccalaureate programs in community health education. *Health Education Monographs* 5(1):90–98.

Somers, A., ed. 1976. *Promoting health: Consumer education and national policy.* Germantown, Md.: Aspen Systems.

Sonstroem, R. J. 1984. Exercise and sport sciences reviews. In *Exercise and self-esteem*, ed. R. L. Teying, 123–155. Lexington, Mass.: Collamore Press.

Spector, P. 1981. *Research designs.* Quantitative Applications in the Social Sciences Series, no. 023, ed. J. L. Sullivan. Beverly Hills, Calif.: Sage.

Spiegel, C., and Lindaman, F. 1977. Children can't fly. *American Journal of Public Health* 67(12):1143–1147.

Squyres, W. 1979. Using media in hospitals. In *Handbook of health education*, ed. P. Lazes, 133–162. Germantown, Md.: Aspen Systems.

Staggs, E. W. 1972. Maybe it's your forms. *Journal of Systems Management* 23(Mar.):8–12.

Starfield, B. 1974. Measurement of outcome: A proposed scheme. *Milbank Memorial Fund Quarterly* 5(1):39–50.

Steckler, A. 1989. The use of qualitative evaluation methods to test internal validity. *Evaluation and the Health Professions* 12:115–133.

Steckler, A.; McLeroy, K. R.; Goodman, R. M.; Bird, S. T.; and McCormick, L. 1992. Toward integrating qualitative and quantitative methods: An introduction. *Health Education Quarterly* 19(1):1–135.

Stevens, R.; Feucht, T.; and Roman, S. 1991. Effects of an intervention program on AIDS related drug and needle behavior among intravenous drug users. *American Journal of Public Health* 81(5):727–729.

Stone, E.; Perry, C.; and Luepker, R. 1989. Synthesis of cardiovascular behavioral research for youth health promotion. *Health Education Quarterly* 16(1):155–169.

Stoner, S., and Fioullo, M. 1976. A program for self-concept improvement and weight reduction for overweight adolescent females. *Psychology* 13: 30–35.

Strauss, M. A., and Brown, B. W. 1978. *Family measurement techniques: Abstracts of published instruments, 1935–1974.* Rev. ed. Minneapolis: University of Minnesota Press.

Suchman, E. 1962. *What people know and do about health—more scientific rigor is needed.* Studies and Research in Health Education, vol. 5. Geneva: World Health Organization, International Union for Health Education, International Conference on Health and Health Education.

Suchman, E. 1967. *Evaluative research: Principles and practice in public service and social action programs.* New York: Russell Sage Foundation.

Sudman, S. 1976. *Applied sampling.* New York: Academic Press.

Sudman, S., ed. 1979. *Health survey research methods, third biennial conference.* DHHS Publication no. (PHS) 81-3268. Washington, D.C.: National Center for Health Services Research.

Sudman, S., and Lannom, L. B. 1980. *Health care surveys using diaries.* DHHS

Publication no. (PHS) 80-3279. Washington, D.C.: National Center for Health Services Research.

Sukhatme, P., and Margen, S. 1982. Autoregulatory homeostatic nature of energy balance. *American Journal of Clinical Nutrition* 35:355–365.

Sullivan, D., ed. 1977. *Educating the public about health: A planning guide.* Health Planning Methods and Technology Series. DHEW Publication no. (HRA) 78-14004. Washington, D.C.: Department of Health, Education and Welfare, Public Health Service.

Survey Research Center. 1976. *Interviewer's manual.* Rev. ed. Ann Arbor: University of Michigan, Institute for Social Research.

Sussman, S.; Burton, D.; Dent, C. W.; Stacy, A. W.; and Flay, B. R. 1991. Use of focus groups in developing an adolescent tobacco use cessation program: Collective norm effects. *Journal of Applied Social Psychology* 21:1772–1782.

Taylor, W.; Baranowski, T.; and Sallis, J. 1992. Family determinants of childhood physical activity: A social cognitive model. In *Exercise adherence: Its impact on public health,* 2nd ed., ed. R. K. Dishman. Champaign, Ill.: Human Kinetics Publishers.

Thomas, S. D.; Hathaway, D. K.; and Arheart, K. L. 1992. Face validity. *Western Journal of Nursing* 14:109–112.

Thornberry, O. J., Jr., and Massey, J. T. 1978. Correcting for undercoverage bias in random digit dialed national health surveys. In *Proceedings, Survey Research Methods Section, American Statistical Association,* 224–229. Washington, D.C.: American Statistical Association.

Tinsley, H. E. A., and Weiss, D. J. 1975. Interrater reliability and agreement of subjective judgments. *Journal of Counseling Psychology* 22(4):358–376.

Tripi, S. J. 1984. Clients' control in organizational settings. *Journal of Applied Behavioral Science* 20(1):39–47.

United Nations Fund for Population Activities. 1984. *Indepth evaluations of programs.* New York: United Nations.

U.S. Congress, House. 1975. National Health Planning and Resources Act of 1974, Public Law 93-641, 93rd Congress.

U.S. Congress, House. 1976. National Consumer Health Information and Health Promotion Act of 1976, Public Law 94-317, 94th Congress.

U.S. Congress. 1988. *How effective is AIDS education?* Office of Technology Assessment. Washington, D.C.: Government Printing Office.

U.S. Department of Health, Education and Welfare. 1971. *Findings and recommendations: National activities in support of health education.* Report of the President's Committee on Health Education. Washington, D.C.: Government Printing Office.

U.S. Department of Health, Education and Welfare. 1977. *Handbook for improving high blood pressure control in the community.* National Institutes of Health, National Heart, Lung, and Blood Institute. Washington, D.C.: Government Printing Office.

U.S. Department of Health, Education and Welfare. 1978a. *Preparation and practice of community, patient, and school health educators.* DHEW Publication no. (HRA) 78-71. Washington, D.C.: Government Printing Office.

U.S. Department of Health, Education and Welfare. 1978b. *Pretesting in cancer communications.* National Institutes of Health. DHEW Publication no. (NIH) 78-1493. Washington, D.C.: Government Printing Office.

U.S. Department of Health, Education and Welfare. 1979a. *Asthma and other allergic diseases.* National Institutes of Health, National Institute of Allergy and Infectious Disease Task Force. NIH Publication no. 79-397. Washington, D.C.: Government Printing Office.

U.S. Department of Health, Education and Welfare. 1979b. *Healthy people: The surgeon general's report of health promotion and disease prevention.* Washington, D.C.: Government Printing Office.

U.S. Department of Health, Education and Welfare. 1980a. *Health message testing service.* National Institutes of Health. NIH Publication no. 80-2042. Washington, D.C.: Government Printing Office.

U.S. Department of Health, Education and Welfare. 1980b. *Smoking and health: Report of the surgeon general.* Public Health Service. DHEW Publication no. (PHS) 79-50066. Washington, D.C.: Government Printing Office.

U.S. Department of Health, Education and Welfare. 1981. *Printed aids for high blood pressure education: A guide to evaluated publications.* National Institutes of Health, National Heart, Lung, and Blood Institute. DHEW Publication no. 81-3268. Washington, D.C.: Government Printing Office.

U.S. Department of Health and Human Services. 1979a. *Biennial conference.* Public Health Service, National Center for Health Services Research. DHHS Publication no. (PHS) 81-3268. Washington, D.C.: Government Printing Office.

U.S. Department of Health and Human Services. 1979b. *Reliability testing in cancer communications.* National Institutes of Health, National Cancer Institute, Office of Cancer Communications. NIH Publication no. 79-1689. Washington, D.C.: Government Printing Office.

U.S. Department of Health and Human Services. 1980a. *Initial role delineation for health education: Final report,* prepared for the National Center for Health Education. Public Health Service. DHHS Publication no. (HRA) 80-44. Washington, D.C.: Government Printing Office.

U.S. Department of Health and Human Services. 1980b. *Pretesting in health communications: Methods, examples, and resources for improving health messages and materials.* National Institutes of Health, National Cancer Institute. NIH Publication 81-1493, rev. Nov. Washington, D.C.: Government Printing Office.

U.S. Department of Health and Human Services. 1980c. *Promoting health/preventing disease: Objectives for the nation.* Public Health Service. Washington, D.C.: Government Printing Office.

U.S. Department of Health and Human Services. 1984. *Report on the standards and criteria for the development and evaluation of a comprehensive employee assistance program.* Public Health Service. Washington, D.C.: Government Printing Office.

U.S. Department of Health and Human Services. 1986. *A mid-course review.* Office of Disease Prevention and Health Promotion. Washington, D.C.: Government Printing Office.

U.S. Department of Health and Human Services. 1989a. *Guide to clinical preventive services.* Preventive Services Task Force. Washington, D.C.: Government Printing Office.

U.S. Department of Health and Human Services. 1989b. Making health communication programs work: A planner's guide. National Institutes of Health. NIH Publication no. 89-1493. Washington, D.C.: Government Printing Office.

U.S. Department of Health and Human Services. 1990a. *Development and evaluation of comprehensive federal physical fitness programs.* Washington, D.C.: Government Printing Office.

U.S. Department of Health and Human Services. 1990b. *Healthy people 2000: National health promotion and disease prevention objectives.* Washington, D.C.: Government Printing Office.

U.S. Department of Health and Human Services. 1992a. *Cultural competence for evaluators,* ed., M. Orlandi, R. Weston, and L. Epstein. OSAP Cultural Competence Series. DHHS Publication (SAMHA) no. 92-1884. Washington, D.C.: Government Printing Office.

U.S. Department of Health and Human Services. 1992b. *Health behavior research in minority populations,* ed., D. Becker, R. Hill, J. Jackson, et al. NIH Publication (NHLBI) no. 92-2965. Washington, D.C.: Government Printing Office.

Uzzel, D. 1978. Four roles for the community researcher. *Journal of Voluntary Action Research* 8(pts. 1, 2):62–75.

Van de Ven, A. H. 1980a. Problem solving, planning and innovation, part I: Test of the program planning model. *Human Relations* 33(10):711–740.

Van de Ven, A. H. 1980b. Problem solving, planning and innovation, part II: Speculations for theory and practice. *Human Relations* 33(11):775–779.

Van de Ven, A. H., and Koenig, R., Jr. 1976. A process model for program planning and evaluation. *Journal of Economics and Business* 28(3):161–170.

Verbrugge, L. M. 1980. Health diaries. *Medical Care* 18(1):73–95.

Vladeck, B. C. 1984. The limits of cost-effectiveness. *American Journal of Public Health* 74(7):652–653.

Wang, V. L.; Ephross, P.; and Green, L. 1975. The point of diminishing returns in nutrition education through home visits by aides: An evaluation of EFNEP. *Health Education Monographs* 3(1):70–88.

Warner, K. E., and Luce, B. R. 1982. *Cost benefit and cost effectiveness analysis in health care.* Ann Arbor, Mich.: Health Administration Press.

Webb, E. J.; Campbell, D. T.; Schwartz, R. D.; and Sechrest, L. 1966. *Unobtru-*

sive measures: Nonreactive research in the social sciences. Chicago: Rand McNally.

Weeks, E. 1979. The material use of evaluation findings. In *The evaluator and management,* ed. H. C. Schulberg and J. H. Jerrel. Sage Research Progress Series in Evaluation, vol. 4. Beverly Hills, Calif.: Sage.

Weick, K. E. 1968. Systematic observational measures. In *Handbook of social psychology,* ed. G. Lindzey, and E. Aronson. Reading, Mass.: Addison-Wesley.

Weingarten, V.; Goodfriend, S.; and Harris, C. 1976. *Health education demonstration at Roosevelt Hospital.* New York: Institute of Public Affairs.

Weiss, C. 1972. *Evaluation research: Methods for assessing program effectiveness.* Englewood Cliffs, N.J.: Prentice Hall.

Weiss, C. 1973a. Between the cup and the lip. *Evaluation* 1(2):49–55.

Weiss, C. 1973b. Where politics and evaluation research meet. *Evaluation* 1(3):37–45.

Weller, L.; Arad, T.; and Levit, R. 1977. Self concept, delayed gratification and field dependence of successful and unsuccessful dieters. *Israel Annals of Psychiatry and Related Disciplines* 15:41–46.

Wholey, J.; Scanlon, J.; Duffy, H.; Fukumoto, J.; and Vogt, L. 1970. *Federal evaluation policy: Analyzing the effects of public programs.* Washington, D.C.: Urban Institute.

Wilkie, W. 1974. Analysis of effects of information load. *Journal of Marketing Research* 11:462–466.

Windle, C. 1979. The citizen as part of the management process. In *The evaluator and management,* ed. H. C. Schulberg and J. H. Jerrel. Sage Research Progress Series in Evaluation, vol. 4. Beverly Hills, Calif.: Sage.

Windle, C., and Cibulka, J. G. 1981. A framework for understanding participation in community mental health services. *Community Mental Health Journal* 17(1):4–18.

Windle, C., and Paschall, N. C. 1981. Client participation in CMHC program evaluation: Increasing incidence, inadequate involvement. *Community Mental Health Journal* 17(1):66–76.

Windsor, R. A. 1973. Mood modifying substances usage among 4H and non-4H youth in Illinois. *Journal of Drug Education* 3(3):261–273.

Windsor, R. A. 1981. Improving patient education assessment skills of hospital staff: A case study in diabetes. *Patient Counseling and Health Education* 3(1):26–29.

Windsor, R. A. 1984. Planning and evaluating community health education programs in rural areas: Theory into practice. In *Case studies in health education practice,* ed. H. Cleary, J. Kichen, and P. Ensor. Palo Alto, Calif.: Mayfield.

Windsor, R. A. 1986. The utility of time series analysis in evaluating health promotion and education programs. *Advances in Health Education and Promotion* 1:435–465.

Windsor, R. A., and Cutter, G. 1981. Methodological issues in using time series designs and analysis: Evaluating the behavioral impact of health communication programs. In *Progress in clinical and biological research*, vol. 83: *Issues in screening and communications*, ed. C. Mettlin and G. Murphy, 517–535. New York: Liss.

Windsor, R. A., and Cutter, G. 1982. Quasi-experimental designs for evaluating cancer control programs in rural settings. In *Advances in cancer control research and development*, Proceedings of the Third Conference on Cancer Control, ed. C. Mettlin and G. Murphy, 517–555. New York: Liss.

Windsor, R. A.; Cutter, G.; and Kronenfeld, J. 1981. Communication methods and evaluation design for a rural cancer screening program. *American Journal of Rural Health* 7(3):37–45.

Windsor, R. A.; Bailey, W.; Richards, J.; Manzella, B.; Soong, S-j.; and Brooks, M. 1990. The efficacy and cost effectiveness of health education methods to increase medication adherence among adults with asthma. *American Journal of Public Health* 80(12):1519–1521.

Windsor, R. A.; Baranowski, T.; Clark, N.; and Cutter, G. 1984. *Evaluation of health promotion and education programs*. Mountain View, Calif.: Mayfield.

Windsor, R. A.; Boyd, N. R.; and Orleans, T. A meta-evaluation and meta-analysis of smoking cessation intervention research among pregnant women: Improving the Science and Art. *Health Education Quarterly*, in press 1994.

Windsor, R.; Cutter, G.; Morris, J.; et al. 1985. Effectiveness of self-help smoking cessation interventions for pregnant women: A randomized trial. *American Journal of Public Health* 76(12):1389–1392.

Windsor, R.; Dalmat, M.; Orleans, T.; and Gritz, E. 1990. *The handbook to plan, implement, and evaluate smoking cessation programs for pregnant women.* White Plains, N.Y.: March of Dimes Foundation.

Windsor, R. A.; Kronenfeld, J.; Cain, M.; Cutter, G.; Goodson, L.; and Edwards, E. 1981. Increasing utilization of a rural cervical cancer detection program. *American Journal of Public Health* 71(6):641–643.

Windsor, R. A.; Kronenfeld, J.; Crawford, M.; Graves, L.; and Gams, R. 1983. *Using concepts of social marketing to plan a new statewide cancer information service*, vol. 76, ed. P. Hobbs. Public Education About Cancer, UICC Technical Report Series. Geneva: International Union for Cancer Control.

Windsor, R. A.; Kronenfeld, J.; Ory, M.; and Kilgo, J. 1980. Method and design issues in evaluation of community health education programs: A case study in breast and cervical cancer. *Health Education Quarterly* 7(3): 203–218.

Windsor, R. A.; Lowe, J. B.; and Bartlett, E. E. 1988. The effectiveness of a worksite self-help smoking cessation program: A randomized trial. *Journal of Behavioral Medicine* 11(4).

Windsor, R. A.; Lowe, J. B.; Perkins, L. L.; Smith-Yoder, D.; Artz, L.; Crawford, M.; Amburgy, K.; and Boyd, N. B., Jr. 1993. Health education for pregnant smokers: Behavioral impact and cost benefit. *American Journal of Public Health* 83(2):201–206.

Windsor, R. A., and Orleans, C. T. 1986. Guidelines and methodological standards for smoking cessation intervention research among pregnant women: Improving the science and art. *Health Education Quarterly* 13(2): 131–161.

Windsor, R. A.; Roseman, J.; Gartseff, G.; and Kirk, K. A. 1981. Qualitative issues in developing educational diagnostic instruments and assessment procedures for diabetic patients. *Diabetes Care* 4(4):468–475.

Windsor, R. A.; Warner, K.; and Cutter, G. 1988. A Cost-effectiveness analysis of self-health smoking cessation methods for pregnant women. *Public Health Reports* 103(1):83–87.

Winkler, J.; Kanouse, D.; Berry, S.; Hayes-Roth, B.; Rogers, W.; and Garfinkle, J. 1981. *Informing patients about drugs, V: Analysis of alternative designs for erythromycin leaflets.* Santa Monica, Calif.: Rand Corp.

Witschi, J. C.; Singer, M.; Wu-Lee, M.; and Stare, F. J. 1978. Family cooperation and effectiveness in a cholesterol lowering diet. *Journal of the American Dietetic Association* 72:384–388.

World Health Organization, Expert Committee on Health Education of the Public. 1954. *First report.* WHO Technical Report Series, no. 89. Geneva: World Health Organization.

World Health Organization, Expert Committee. 1969. *Planning and evaluation of health education services.* WHO Technical Report Series, no. 409. Geneva: World Health Organization.

World Health Organization. 1980. *Health program evaluation: Guiding principles for application of the managerial process for national health development.* Geneva: World Health Organization.

World Health Organization. 1981. *Development of indicators for monitoring progress toward health for all by the year 2000.* Geneva: World Health Organization.

Yalom, I. 1970. *Theory and practice of group psychotherapy.* New York: Basic Books.

Yammarino, F. J.; Skinner, S. J.; and Childers, T. L. 1991. Understanding mail survey response behavior. *Public Opinion Quarterly* 55(4):613–639.

Yen, L. T.; Edington, D. W.; and Witting, P. 1992. Prediction of prospective medical claims and absenteeism costs for 1284 hourly workers from a manufacturing company. *Journal of Occupational Medicine* 34:428–435.

Zapka, J., ed. 1982. *Research and evaluation in health education.* SOPHE Heritage Collection of Health Education Monographs, vol. 3. Oakland, Calif.: Third Party Publishing.

Ziegenfuss, J. T., Jr., and Lasky, D. I. 1975a. *Manual of topics for evaluation: A working document.* Harrisburg, Pa.: Dauphin County Executive Commission on Drugs and Alcohol.

Ziegenfuss, J. T., Jr., and Lasky, D. I. 1975b. A rationale for evaluating the quality of services in drug and alcohol programs: Purpose, process, outcome. *Drug Forum* 5(2):171–184.

Ziegenfuss, J. T., Jr., and Lasky, D. I. 1980. Evaluation and organizational development: A management-consulting approach. *Evaluation Review* 4(5):665–676.

Zinober, J. W.; Dinkel, N. R.; Landsberg, G.; and Windle, C. 1980. Another role for citizens: Three variations of citizen evaluation review. *Community Mental Health Journal* 16(4):317–330.

Zweig, F., and Marvin, K., eds. 1981. *Educating policymakers for evaluation.* Sage Research Progress Series in Evaluation, vol. 9. Beverly Hills, Calif.: Sage.

Index

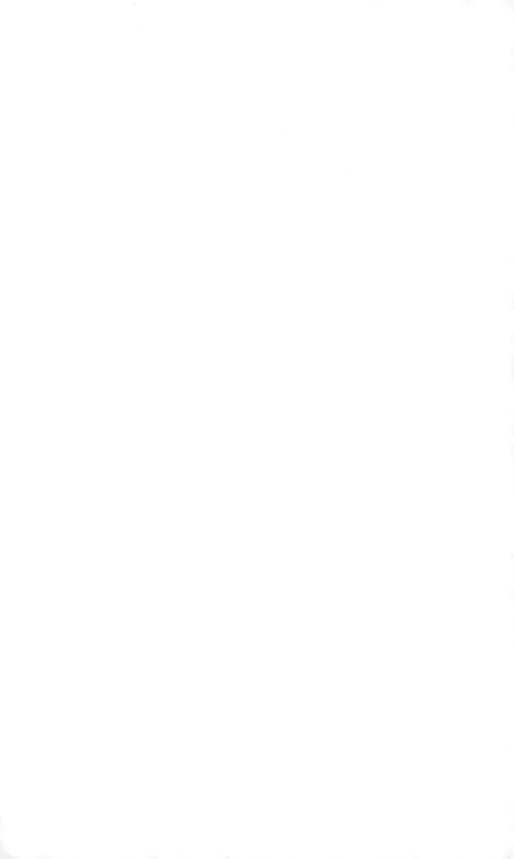